T0401962

Ryoichi Oyasu, Ximing J. Yang, Osamu Yoshida

Questions in Daily Urologic Practice
Updates for Urologists and Diagnostic Pathologists

Ryoichi Oyasu, Ximing J. Yang,
Osamu Yoshida

Questions in Daily Urologic Practice

Updates for Urologists and Diagnostic Pathologists

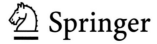 Springer

Ryoichi Oyasu, M.D.
Joseph L. Mayberry Sr. Professor of
Pathology and Toxicology Emeritus;
Professor of Urology Emeritus,
Northwestern University Feinberg School
of Medicine
303 East Chicago Ave. Chicago, IL 60611,
USA

Osamu Yoshida, M.D., Ph.D.
President, Nara Medical University;
Professor of Urology Emeritus, Kyoto
University Postgraduate School of Medicine
Shijo Machi 840, Kashihara, Nara 634-8521,
Japan

Ximing J. Yang, M.D., Ph.D.
Professor of Pathology, Surgical Pathology,
Northwestern Memorial Hospital,
Northwestern University
251 E Huron, Feinberg 7-338, Chicago,
IL 60611, USA

ISBN 978-4-431-72818-4   e-ISBN 978-4-431-72819-1

Library of Congress Control Number: 2007940951

Printed on acid-free paper

Springer is a part of Springer Science+Business Media
springer.com

Typesetting: SNP Best-set Typesetter Ltd., Hong Kong
Printing and binding: Kato Bunmeisha Co., Ltd., Japan

Contents

Part 2. Kidney

Part 3. Urinary Bladder

Part 4. Testis

Part 5. Adrenals

Preface

The principal role of the diagnostic surgical pathologist is to serve a patient by assisting the clinician in charge of the patient's care. In that capacity, the pathologist provides the vital information that should be directly and indirectly useful in guiding the clinician toward the most appropriate therapy. The material pathologists receive most commonly is a biopsy or a part of an organ removed after a definitive procedure. To extract useful information, pathological evaluation proceeds according to a set of guidelines. Simply reporting a diagnosis of cancer is inadequate. Detailed additional information is needed so that the clinician can go on to establish a therapeutic plan as needed. To best serve the patient, close interaction between the clinician and the pathologist is vital.

In the field of urological pathology, there are problems specific to this system. Typically, in the prostate, because of its location, there is little room for a surgeon to work to obtain adequate resection margins, unlike with many other organs. As a result, questions arise such as "What constitutes an adequate surgical margin?" "What is the significance of extraprostatic extension of neoplasm that is still inside the resection margin?" and "What is the significance of neoplastic glands found on the resection margin marked with the ink?" It has been shown that a prostate needle core biopsy can generate much information that is immediately useful in predicting the extent of cancer in the prostate and, consequently, the outcome for the patient. For example, the number of biopsy cores involved with cancer, the maximum percent of the core involved with cancer, and the location of the core positive for cancer have all been shown to have predictive value in anticipating the stage of cancer in the prostate. Is the pathologist providing these specific findings? If so, does the urologist understand and utilize the reported information to his or her full advantage?

In an attempt to improve the communication between urologists and pathologists, three of us, two pathologists and one urologist, solicited urologists for questions they may have raised in their daily practice. Based on their practice, the pathologists also contributed to the pool of questions. Thus, the book is unique; it is not a standard textbook. Using a question-and-answer format followed by comments, we discuss the communication of information that is vital between urologists and pathologists.

In this endeavor, we have attempted to extract "correct" data reported in the world literature and to provide as in-depth an answer as possible to every question. More often than not, conflicting results are reported. In such cases, we have tried to draw a conclusion based on the best of our knowledge and judgment. If that was not feasible, we have introduced both views with our comments.

We believe that this series of questions and answers will be useful not only for urologists but also for diagnostic surgical pathologists. We welcome and encourage critical comments and questions from readers, which can only serve to improve the quality of the book and achieve the goal that we have envisioned.

Ryoichi Oyasu, Ximing J. Yang, and Osamu Yoshida

Acknowledgment

The authors express their sincere gratitude to Mr. Masayuki Shakudo and his staff of Inter Medica, Tokyo, for providing the material used for the figures and tables found in this book.

Part 1. Prostate

Question 1

Does a prostatic capsule exist? Pathologists and urologists use the word "capsule" when evaluating the extent of prostatic cancer in prostatectomy specimens

Answer

In a very strict sense, the prostate lacks an intact capsule. For practical reasons, however, the prostate has a capsule along its dorsolateral aspect extending from the base down close to the apical margin. The ventral (anterior) middle third does not have a capsule but, instead, is invested by a thick smooth muscle layer that extends dorsally (posteriorly) in the midline and invests the urethra as a preprostatic sphincter. We now prefer the term "extraprostatic extension" (EPE) when prostate cancer extends outside the prostate. This is to avoid the argument of the presence or absence of a prostatic capsule.

Comments

Despite the use of an expression such as capsular penetration or perforation, the prostate lacks a well-defined capsule as an anatomic structure that encloses an organ or body part [1]. In some areas, a fibromuscular layer does exist between the most peripheral portion of nonneoplastic prostate parenchyma and the edge of the prostate, giving the appearance of a capsule (Fig. 1-1-1). Because this condensed fibromuscular layer is regarded as condensed prostate stroma, it cannot be considered a true capsule. External to the dorsal aspect of the prostate is Denonvilliers' fascia, which is an inverted triangle of fibromuscular tissue that covers the posterior aspect

of the prostate and surrounds the seminal vesicles. This structure consists of multiple layers that are fused not only together but also to the stroma of the prostate and the seminal vesicles [2]. During radical prostatectomy, Denonvilliers' fascia is separated from the rectal wall and is submitted with the prostate. Medially, this fascia is fused with the prostate "capsule" into a single sheath and contains a thick smooth muscle bundle in continuity with the prostate stroma.

The question, then, is how much of the "capsular" structure covers the outer surface of the prostate. In an attempt to answer this question, after initial microscopic examination the paraffin block of the apical cone was deparaffinized, cut into several thin sections in the sagittal plane, and processed for microscopic examination. Lateral views of each piece were photographed at low power to assess the extent of the capsule, and prints were combined to compose a panoramic view (Fig. 1-1-2). As is clear, in a prostate

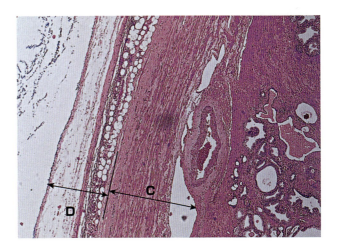

FIG. 1-1-1. This is a section of the left lateral aspect of the prostate. Denonvilliers' fascia (*D*) is made up of a loose fibrous layer, a thin smooth muscle layer, and a layer of adipose tissue. Inside this layer is a broad band of smooth muscle stroma of the prostate designated the "capsule" (*C*)

Panoramic lateral view of the apex of the prostate (View from right side)

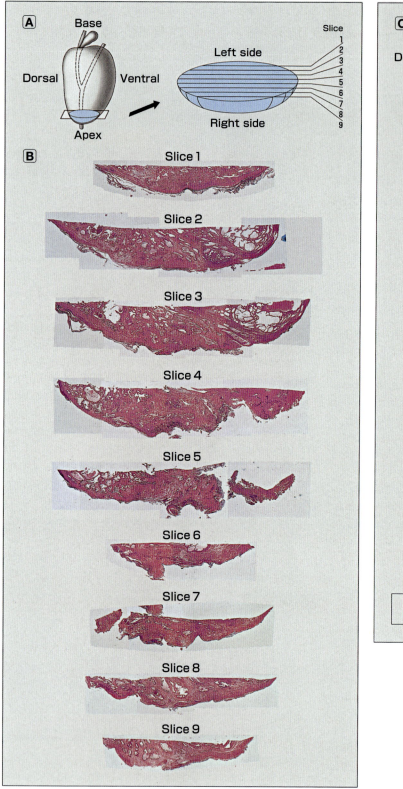

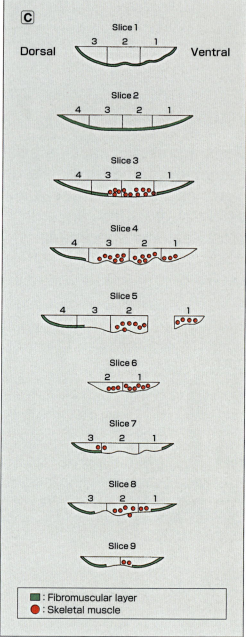

Fig. 1-1-2. **A** Right lateral view of the prostate. The apical cone was amputated, sliced sagittally into multiple pieces, and laid down from the left to right. **B** Low-power photographs of each piece were combined to create a panoramic view. **C** The pieces of slices shown in **B**

Structures which make up the external aspect of the prostate

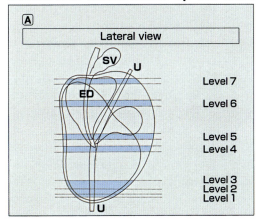

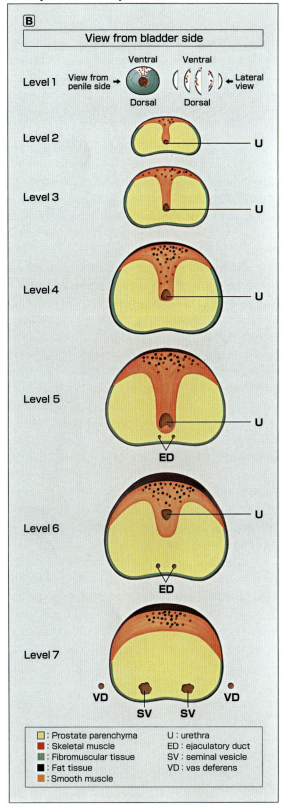

FIG. 1-1-3. **A** Right lateral view of the prostate. After fixation the prostate was step-sectioned from the apex to the base. Seven representative levels are depicted. **B** Each slice was laid down from the apex to the base. At level 1, a three-dimensional view from the penile side is shown. On the right side of the level 1 drawing are lateral views of the sliced apical cone. Structures represented by different colors: *green*, fibromuscular tissue ("capsule"); *red*, skeletal muscle; *orange*, smooth muscle; *black*, adipose tissue; *yellow*, prostate parenchyma. *U*, urethra; *ED*, ejaculatory duct; *SV*, seminal vesicle; *VD*, vas deferens

removed by an experienced surgeon, a "capsule" invests almost three-quarters of the circumference of the apex. The anterior third, however, lacks a "capsule" and consists of a mixture of smooth muscle and skeletal muscle enmeshed in loose fibrous tissue that surrounds the urethra as a distal striated sphincter. The skeletal muscle is the remnant of the urethral sphincter that invested the urethra before puberty [3].

Although the apex reportedly lacks a "capsule" [1, 4], we are able to trace a layered fibromuscular structure ("capsule") all the way down to the apex in the lateral and posterior walls (Fig. 1-1-2).

We also made a detailed study on the remaining portion of the prostate, and the structures are depicted in different colors in Fig. 1-1-3. Toward the base, the capsular structure diminishes, and the anterior third is covered by a thick smooth muscle layer originating from the prostate parenchyma, which in the midline extends posteriorly, encompassing the proximal urethra to become the preprostatic sphincter. Furthermore, the anterior muscle layer merges in the midline with the smooth muscle that extends downward from the bladder neck [4]. If one defines a capsule as a layered fibromuscular structure, this smooth muscle layer, of varying thickness in the anterior third, cannot be regarded as a capsule, but it does constitute a barrier against cancer invasion.

External to the capsule, one observes a layer of adipose tissue of varying thickness. It is abundant in the proximal half along the midline. The amount of fat tissue attached to radical prostatectomy specimens varies from case to case.

In conclusion, the prostate does not have a true capsule but is limited by a definable fibromuscular layer along the posterolateral aspect from the base to the apex. The semantics involved in whether one prefers to call this fibromuscular band a capsule is not as important as its true histologic configuration [1].

Well then, what are messages to the urologist and the pathologist? The histologic information is important for the urologist when evaluating the extent of carcinoma. A tumor that reaches or invades this band (capsule) but is still confined to the prostate does not have prognostic significance. However, transgression of the tumor through the fibromuscular band (perforation/penetration) does constitute an extension of the tumor outside the prostate and has clinical significance. To this end, the pathologist must evaluate the surgical margins, including the apical margin, carefully. Special attention should be paid to the apex. Removed by a skilled surgeon, the apical cone of the prostate should have a "capsule" extended close to the urethral stump. Thus, the concept of extraprostatic extension (EPE) or extracapsular extension (ECE) of the carcinoma should also apply to most of the apex. Furthermore, from well-oriented microscopic sections, the pathologist should be able to make more detailed comments, such as if a tumor is confined within the "capsule" or whether and where the margin is positive because an iatrogenic incision was made. EPE and ECE are the terms preferred for describing the pathologic diagnosis, rather than "capsular perforation" and "capsular penetration."

References

1. Ayala G, Ro JY, Babaian R, Troncoso P, Grignon DJ (1989) The prostate capsule: does it exist? Its importance in the staging and treatment of prostate carcinoma. Am J Surg Pathol 13:21–27.
2. Villers A, McNeal JE, Freiha FS, Boccon-Gibod L, Stamey TA (1993) Invarion of Denonvilliers' fascia in radical prostatectomy specimens. J Urol 149:793–798.
3. Oelrich T (1980) The urethral sphincter muscle. Am J Anat 158:229–246.
4. McNeal JE (1988) Normal histology of the prostate. Am J Surg Pathol 12:619–633.

Question 2

What is the anatomic structure of the prostate? Where is the transition zone? Where does carcinoma develop? Where does benign prostatic hyperplasia occur?

Answer

The prostate consists of four zones: anterior fibromuscular stroma, central zone, peripheral zone, and transition zone. The transition zone is a balloon-shaped component of the prostate that is located in the periurethral region. Most prostatic adenocarcinomas develop in the peripheral zone, although some arise in the transition zone. The transition zone is the exclusive site of benign prostatic hyperplasia (BPH). Both adenocarcinomas and BPH affecting the transition zone may cause urinary obstruction. Carcinomas that develop in the transition zone are generally of the well to moderately differentiated type (Gleason grades 1, 2, 3). Additionally, tumor cells characteristically have pale to clear cytoplasm.

Comments

According to the detailed study by McNeal [1], the human prostate is made up of several glandular and nonglandular components that are tightly fused together to form four zones: anterior fibromuscular stroma, central zone, peripheral zone, and transition zone [1] (Fig. 1-2-1). The nonglandular component makes up much of the anterior medial part and is composed of fibromuscular tissue that extends downward from the bladder neck over the anteromedial surface of the prostate (Fig. 1-2-2). The urethra is the anatomic landmark that runs through the midline of the prostate and is divided into proximal and distal halves of equal length. The proximal half is tilted forward and is connected to the vertically oriented distal half at a 35° angle. The proximal urethra is surrounded by a sleeve of smooth muscle fibers called

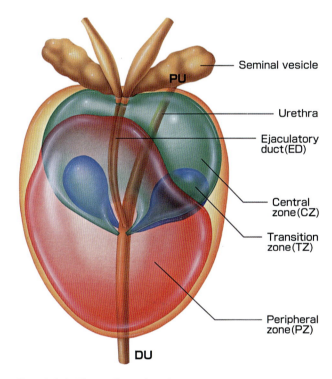

FIG. 1-2-1. Three-dimensional structure of the prostate viewed from the right posterolateral angle and drawn based on the model by McNeal [1]. The urethra, which runs through the midline, is divided into proximal (*PU*) and distal (*DU*) halves of equal length. The *PU* is tilted ventrally and is surrounded by a sleeve of smooth muscle fibers called the preprostatic sphincter. The distal end of the *PU* receives ducts derived from the transition zone (*TZ*) just proximal to the angulation. The central zone (*CZ*) ducts drain into the *DU* immediately surrounding the ejaculatory duct (*ED*) orifices. The ducts of the peripheral zone (*PZ*) open into the *DU* from the base of the verumontanum to the prostate apex

7

Schematic view of zonal distribution (Reconstructed based on McNeal's prostate drawing)

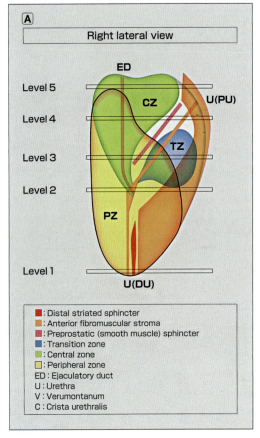

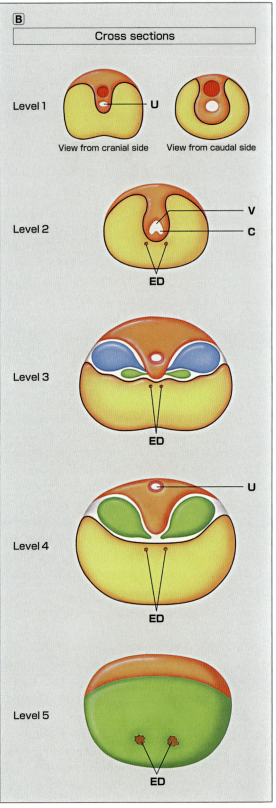

F_{IG}. 1-2-2. **A, B** Structure of the prostate and approximate location of the central, transition, and peripheral zones. Restructured based on the model of McNeal [1]

the preprostatic sphincter (Fig. 1-2-2). Crista urethralis is a longitudinally extending triangular ridge located on the posterior wall just distal to the angulation; it dilates into an oval enlargement called the verumontanum (Fig. 1-2-2). The distal urethral segment receives the ejaculatory ducts and the ducts of about 95% of the glandular prostate. The ejaculatory ducts extend cranially from the verumontanum to the base of the prostate, running for a short distance parallel to the distal segment of the urethra. The proximal urethra moves ventrally and continues to ascend.

The peripheral zone makes up about 70% of the mass of the glandular prostate. It is a concave structure, with the superior portion occupying the dorsal aspect of the base of the prostate and the basal portion taking up the entire glandular prostate below the level of the urethral angle. Thus, cancer developing in the apex is of peripheral zone origin. Its ducts open into the distal urethra as a double row extending from the base of the verumontanum to the prostate apex. The ducts divide as they extend into the parenchyma and give rise to numerous acini, the secretory unit of the prostate. The acini consist of a layer of luminal secretory cells that are prostate-specific antigen (PSA)-positive by immunohistochemistry and a layer of basal cells that are PSA-negative but positive for high-molecular-weight keratin (34β12E) surrounded by a basement membrane. Basal cells are not myoepithelial cells analogous to those of the breast or the salivary glands; they do not contain myofilaments. They are a distinctive component of the prostatic epithelium. The peripheral zone is the most susceptible to cancer and inflammation.

The central zone comprises about 25% of the prostate mass. Its ducts arise in a small focus on the convexity of the verumontanum and immediately surrounding the ejaculatory duct orifices [1]. The central zone extends cranially and posteriorly to form a conical structure and makes up almost the entire base of the prostate (Fig. 1-2-1). Glandular lobules in the central zone are separated by bands of compact smooth muscle fibers, and there is an abrupt contrast in the stromal structure that delineates the boundary between the central zone and the peripheral zone [1] (Fig. 1-2-3). Microscopically, central zone acini and ducts are similar to those in the peripheral zone and consist of an inner secretory cell layer and a surrounding basal cell layer. Unlike those in the periph-

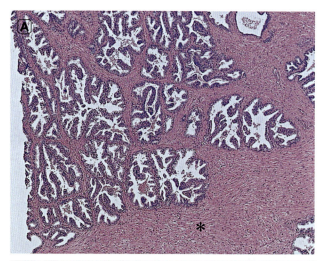

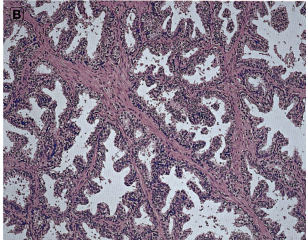

FIG. 1-2-3. Microscopic appearance of the CZ. The lobules are separated from the PZ by a broad band of smooth muscle fibers (*) (**A**). Unlike the cells of PZ, the secretory cells have basophilic cytoplasm and project to the lumen supported by stroma (**B**). Their nuclei are irregular in the cytoplasmic location unlike those of the PZ cells. Note that the basal cells form a prominent line because of dark-staining nuclei and scanty cytoplasm

eral zone, however, the lining cells project into the lumen supported by the stroma to form complex large glandular structures (Fig. 1-2-3). Furthermore, the secretory cells have granular, variably dark cytoplasm (unlike the pale cytoplasm of the peripheral zone); and unlike those in the peripheral zone, their nuclei are irregular regarding their cytoplasmic location. The central zone is relatively resistant to both carcinoma and inflammation [1].

The transition zone consists of two small balloon-shaped lobes and normally makes up 5%–10% of the glandular mass. The ducts leave the posterolateral recesses of the urethral wall just proximal to the point of the urethral angulation and extend laterally and anteriorly along the lower border of the preprostatic sphincter. The transition zone stroma is composed of compact, interlacing, smooth muscle bundles that blend with the anterior fibromuscular stroma. The transition zone and the periurethral region are the exclusive sites of benign nodular (prostate) hyperplasia (BPH). BPH in the periurethral region may protrude as a midline nodule (median bar/midline lobe) at the bladder neck into the bladder lumen.

A transurethral resection specimen consists of nodules of varying size and usually represents portions of the transition zone tissue and periurethral tissue; occasionally, portions of the ejaculatory ducts are removed. Cancer may arise in the transition zone; most tumors found incidentally at a transurethral resection are derived from this zone. Carcinoma arising in the transition zone is of low Gleason grades (grades 1, 2, 3) and consists typically of cells with pale to clear cytoplasm (Fig. 1-2-4).

Patients typically experience erectile dysfunction following non-nerve-sparing radical prostatectomy. It was Patrick Walsh and his colleagues who conducted elegant studies elucidating the cause of impotence. They concluded that impotence results from injury to the pelvic nerve plexus, which sends off branches to innervate the corpora cavernosa. Readers who are interested in their work are referred to the landmark papers published in 1983 [2] and 1987 [3]. Their findings can be highlighted as follows: The autonomic innervation of the pelvic organs and external genitalia arises from the pelvic plexus, which is formed by parasympathetic visceral efferent preganglionic fibers that arise from the sacral center (S2–S4) and sympathetic fibers from the thoracolumbar center (T11–L2). The pelvic plexus is located retroperitoneally beside the rectum and supplies fibers to the bladder, ureters, seminal vesicles, prostate, rectum, urethra, and corpora cavernosa. The branches to the prostate travel outside the "capsule" of the prostate and the Denonvilliers' fascia until they perforate the "capsule" and enter the prostate. The branches to the urethra and the corpora cavernosa also travel outside the prostate "capsule". The studies by Walsh demonstrated that the branches that innervate the corpora cavernosa are located dorsolaterally between the prostate and rectum.

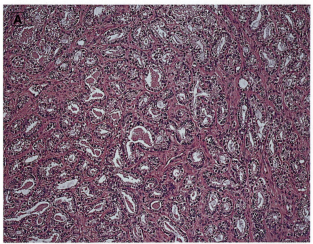

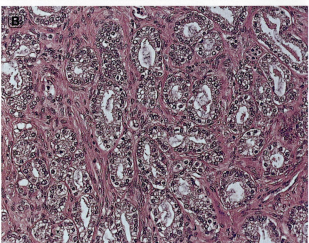

Fig. 1-2-4. **A, B** Typical transition zone carcinoma. It consists of small acini of equal size separated by a small amount of prostate stroma. Tumor cells have pale cytoplasm, and nuclei are regularly placed at the basal part of the cytoplasm, are round, and show an occasional prominent nucleolus. Note the total lack of desmoplastic reaction created by cancer cells, a characteristic feature of prostate carcinoma. Gleason score: 2 + 2

The prostate receives its blood supply mainly from the prostatovesicular artery, which is a branch of the hypogastric artery. The prostatovesicular artery terminates in two large groups: the urethral branches, which enter the prostate at the posterolateral vesicolateral junction and supply the vesical neck and periurethral portion of the prostate; and the capsular branches, which supply mainly the periphery of the parenchyma. These vessels run along the posterolateral surface of the gland and are closely accompanied by an extensive network of nerves and hence are referred to as a *neurovascular bundle* (Fig. 1-2-5). To

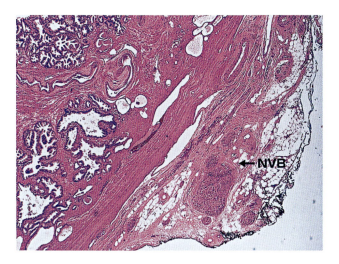

Fɪɢ. 1-2-5. Neurovascular bundle (*NVB*). This is a transverse section of the prostate vertical to the DU. In this prostatectomy specimen the neurovascular bundle was not saved. It is located at the posterolateral border of the prostate and consists of several nerve fibers, the largest of which contains ganglion cells. Adjacent to nerves are several veins and small arteries. The *black ink* denotes the surgical margins

preserve potency, this neurovascular bundle is saved by making an incision in the lateral pelvic fascia anterior to the neurovascular bundle, but the line of dissection should be extended outside Denonvilliers' fascia along the posterior surface of the resected prostate. According to Walsh, unilateral preservation of one functional neurovascular bundle may be sufficient to maintain sexual potency with some age dependence [3].

References

1. McNeal JE (1992) Normal histology of the prostate. Am J Surg Pathol 12:619–633.
2. Walsh PC, Lepor H, Eggleston JC (1983) Radical prostatectomy with preservation of sexual function: anatomical and pathological consideration. Prostate 4:473–485.
3. Walsh PC, Epstein JI, Lowe FC (1987) Potency following radical prostatectomy with wide unilateral excision of the neurovascular bundle. J Urol 138:823–827.

Question 3

What is the clinical significance of perineural invasion reported on prostate needle core biopsy?

Answer

Although the clinical significance of perineural invasion is a controversial issue, it does not appear to be an independent predictor of extraprostatic extension of cancer. Perineural invasion observed in a prostate needle core biopsy specimen is significantly associated with an increased risk of extraprostatic extension (by univariate logistic analysis), but it is not possible to quantify the magnitude of the risk.

Comments

Radical prostatectomy is considered one of the most appropriate treatments for men with organ-confined prostate cancer. Thus, it is highly desirable to know the extent of disease preoperatively. The probability of extraprostatic extension (EPE) is correlated with the clinical stage. However, the current clinical staging system for localized cancer is notoriously inaccurate for assessing its pathologic stage. Men with a high clinical tumor stage, large tumor volume, multiple positive biopsies, high preoperative prostate-specific antigen (PSA), and high Gleason score are more likely to have EPE [1].

Cancer in general spreads by direct invasion of the surrounding tissue matrix by actions of various proteases that are released from the cancer cells themselves or stromal cells. A second mechanism for spreading is via the perineural space. The perineural space is a route of spread favored by carcinomas of certain organs. Prostate carcinoma is one of them. In the past, it was accepted that tumors grow in the perineural space because it is the tissue space of least resistance [2]. However, this model of perineural invasion (PNI) failed to explain the fact that only certain tumors display neurotropism. Recently, Li et al. [3] demonstrated that neural cell adhesion molecule (N-CAM) expression was upregulated in the nerves with perineural cancer cell spread compared with nerves without carcinoma. They postulated that prostate carcinoma cells, through a yet-to-be-established paracrine loop, signal the nerve to increase N-CAM production and increase adhesion. The upregulation of N-CAM in nerves may reciprocally facilitate cancer cells to migrate toward nerves and enhance the process of perineural adhesion and spread. Many cancers use both mechanisms of spreading described above. With prostatic adenocarcinoma, PNI appears to be the predominant mechanism of spreading, at least during the initial stage, and the Stanford group has clearly demonstrated that this is indeed the case [4]. Cancer cells eventually penetrate lymphatics or vessels and reach regional lymph nodes or distant organs.

In the prostate, nerves within the neurovascular bundle supply branches at two sites: the large superior pedicle near the base and the small inferior pedicle at the apex. According to Villers et al., nerve bundles derived from the superior pedicle take a fairly long course of 0.5–1.5 cm before penetrating the parenchyma over the posterolateral surface. The inferior pedicle, which is small and located at the apex, sends off branches that extend for only 0.2–0.5 cm along the prostate capsule in Denonvilliers' fascia and behind the membranous urethra at the superior aspect of the rectourethral muscle. Thus, prostate cancer favors these two sites for EPE. Of the 78 stage B carcinomas with EPE [4], the penetration in 39 (50%) consisted exclusively of PNI immediately outside the "capsule." Most often PNI followed the oblique vertical course of nerve branches that extended cranially to the superior pedicle near the prostate base. Among the remaining 39 of 78 carcinomas, direct invasion through the "capsule" unassociated with PNI was observed at varying frequency in combination with perineural routes. In only 4 cases was direct spread judged to be the mode of EPE. Areas of direct "capsular" extension occurred at random and were common only in large-volume cancers. Extraprostatic extension by PNI occurred more commonly in the middle and superior thirds, but in 18 cases EPE occurred at the inferior pedicle and in 16 it resulted in positive surgical margins.

Thus, the suggestion that PNI seen in prostate needle core biopsy (PNB) specimens is a predictor of EPE is understandable. Therefore, based on the suggestion that PNI in PNB specimens could be used to direct surgical or radiation therapies, it is advised that PNI be routinely reported for biopsy specimens.

Several studies have investigated the significance of PNI for predicting EPE. We have tabulated some of their data in Table 1-3-1. To make the data comparable, we have calculated and added additional statistical numbers based on data presented in the articles. In all studies, PNI was defined as carcinoma cells tracking along or around a nerve in the perineural space (Figs. 1-3-1, 1-3-2, 1-3-3). Focal attachment to a nerve should not automatically be considered invasion, as this phenomenon, called benign perineural indentation, can be observed with benign glands (Fig. 1-3-4).

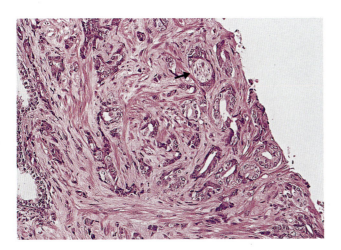

FIG. 1-3-1. Perineural invasion (*arrow*) detected in a prostate needle core biopsy showing a carcinomatous gland that completely encircles a nerve, a characteristic feature of perineural space invasion

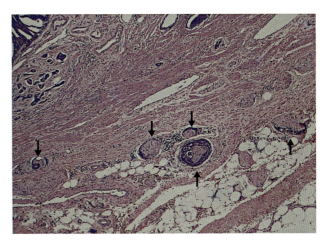

FIG. 1-3-3. Extraprostatic extension of carcinoma by extensive perineural space invasions (*arrows*)

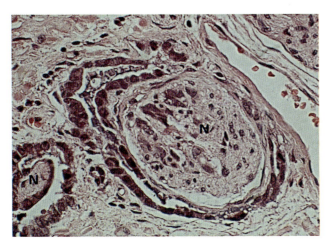

FIG. 1-3-2. Another example of perineural invasion. Two nerve fibers (*N*) are completely surrounded by cancerous cells

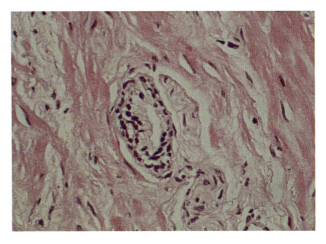

FIG. 1-3-4. Benign gland attached to a nerve (benign perineural indentation)

TABLE 1-3-1. Presence of perineural invasion vs. extraprostatic extension of cancer

Study	PNB No.	PNI	Extra prostatic extension	Sensitivity (%)	Specificity (%)	Radical prostatectomy PPV (%)	NPV (%)	Significance by Univ. analysis	Multiv. analysis	Other factors significant on multivariate analysis
Vargas [7]	340 (1995–1997)	Present 57 (17%) Absent 283 (83%) Total	22 (38%) 50 (18%) 72 (21%)	31[a]	88[a]	39[a]	82[b]	Yes	Yes[c]	PSA, no. of positive cores in biopsy
Egan [6]	349 (1991–1995)	Present 132 (38%) Absent 217 (62%) Total	65 (49%) 62 (29%) 127 (36%)	51	70	49	71	Yes	No	Gleason score, PSA, proportion of Ca in PNB
Bastacky [5]	302 (1986–1989)	Present 61 (20%) Absent 241 (80%) Total	57 (93%) 151 (63%) 208 (69%)	27 (36 if Gleason 7 or higher)	96 (94)	93	37	Yes	Not tested	
De la Taille [8]	319 (1993–1998)	Present 77 (24%) Absent 242 (76%) Total	40 (52%) 61 (25%) 101 (32%)	40	83	52[b]	75*	Yes	Yes[b]	PSA, Gleason score
Sebo [9]	454 (1995–1998)	Present 103 (23%) Absent 351 (76%) Total	NA NA 106 (23%)	NA	NA	NA	NA	Yes	Yes	Gleason score > 7
Ukimura [11]	84 (1987–1996)	Present 22 (26%) Absent 62 (74%) Total	14 (64%) 23 (37%) 37 (44%)	38[b]	74[b]	63[b]	63[b]	Yes	No	Ca contact length, PSA

PNI, perineal invasion; PPV, positive predictive value; NPV, negative predictive value; NA, not available; Multiv., multivariate; Univ., univariate; PSA, prostate-specific antigen; Ca, carcinoma; PNB, prostate needle core biopsy.

[a] Recalculated by Oyasu.
[b] Calculated by Oyasu.
[c] No when PSA is in consideration.

When you look at the data in Table 1-3-1, it is obvious that the sensitivity of PNI observed in PNB specimens for predicting the presence of EPE is poor, ranging from 16% to 51%. Likewise, the specificity of PNI is, at best, 91% except for the 96% reported by Bastacky's group [5] (see comments that appear later). As a result, the positive predictive values (PPV) (probability of PNI present in PNBs of predicting the presence of EPE) is low, ranging from 30% to 63%, except for the 93% reported by Bastacky's group (see comments). Similarly, the negative predictive values (NPV) (probability of the absence of PNI in PNBs of predicting the absence of EPE in the radical prostatectomy specimens) are not high enough to be informative. For example, the 37% NPV reported by the Bastacky group means that despite the absence of PNI in the PNB prostatectomy specimens revealed the presence of EPE in 63% of cases.

The frequency of EPE in prostatectomy specimens ranges from 21% to 44%. The higher frequency of 69% reported by the Bastacky group may be due to the fact that their patient population was from the late 1980s, when sextant biopsy was not in use and the patients were in a more advanced disease stage despite the clinical stage B label.

In all articles, univariate logistic analysis showed that the presence of PNI was significantly associated with EPE. However, when multivariate logistic regression analysis (used to assess the independent predictive value) was applied, the results were variable: Egan et al. [6] concluded that PNI had no value, whereas three other articles [7–9] reported significance. Nevertheless, when the preoperative PSA was considered in the statistical analysis, PNI was no longer an independent predictor [7, 8]. Thus, it is reasonable to conclude that PNI is a common event that is related to other prognostic features (e.g., a high Gleason score [6, 8, 9]), the number of cores involved by cancer [7, 10], the proportion of biopsies involved by cancer [6, 10], and the preoperative PSA [6–8, 11].

This leads us to the final question: "Shall pathologists continue reporting the presence of PNI in prostate needle core biopsy specimens?" The answer is that it is up to the individual pathologist. We routinely report this finding in the pathology report.

However, the finding should be interpreted with caution.

References

1. Wieder JA, Soloway MS (1998) Incidence, etiology, location, treatment of positive surgical margins after radical prostatectomy for prostate cancer. J Urol 160: 299–315.
2. Rodin AE, Larson DL, Roberts DK (1967) Nature of the perineural space invaded by prostate carcinoma. Cancer 29:1772–1779.
3. Li R, Wheeler T, Dai H, Ayala G (2003) Neural cell adhesion molecule is upregulated in nerves with prostate cancer invasion. Hum Pathol 34:457–461.
4. Villers A, McNeal JE, Redwine EA, Freiha FS, Stamey TA (1989) The role of perineural space invasion in the local spread of prostatic adenocarcinoma. J Urol 142: 763–768.
5. Bastacky SI, Walsh PC, Epstein JI (1993) Relationship between perineural tumor invasion on needle biopsy and radical prostatectomy capsular penetration in clinical stage B adenocarcinoma of the prostate. Am J Surg Pathol 17:336–341.
6. Egan AJM, Bostwick DG (1997) Prediction of extraprostatic extension of prostate cancer based on needle biopsy findings: perineural invasion lacks significance on multivariate analysis. Am J Surg Pathol 21:1496–1500.
7. Vargas SO, Jiroutek M, Welch WR, Nucci M, D'Amico AV, Renshaw AA (1999) Perineural invasion in prostate needle biopsy specimens: correlation with extraprostatic extension at resection. Am J Clin Pathol 111:223–228.
8. De la Taille A, Katz A, Bagiella E, Olsson CA, O'Tool KM, Rubin MA (1999) Perineural invasion on prostate needle biopsy: an independent predictor of final pathologic stage. Urology 54:1039–1043.
9. Sebo TJ, Cheville JC, Riehle DL, Lohse CM, Blute ML, Zincke H (2002) Perineural invasion and MIB-1 positivity in addition to Gleason score are significant preoperative predictors of progression after radical retropubic prostatectomy for prostate cancer. Am J Surg Pathol 26:431–439.
10. Bismar TA, Lewis JS, Vollmer RT, Humphrey PA (2003) Multiple measures of carcinoma extent versus perineural invasion in prostate needle biopsy tissue in prediction of pathologic stage in a screening population. Am J Surg Pathol 27:432–440.
11. Ukimura O, Troncoso P, Ramirez EI, Babaian RJ (1998) Prostate cancer staging: correlation between ultrasound determined tumor contact length and pathologically confirmed extraprostatic extension. J Urol 159:1251–1259.

Question 4

What is the difference between a positive surgical margin and extraprostatic extension in pathology reports of radical prostatectomy? What is the clinical relevance of these findings?

Answer

The presence of extraprostatic extension and/or a positive surgical margin in radical prostatectomy specimens predicts an earlier return of measurable serum prostate-specific antigen (PSA) and progression of prostate cancer. Whereas a positive surgical margin often requires additional therapy, such as local irradiation, extraprostatic extension indicates a higher stage but typically does not require immediate therapy unless clinical parameters of overt disease are present.

Comments

Several issues are involved in the discussion on positive surgical margins: (1) recent changes in the patient population; (2) changes in surgical techniques; and (3) the differences in interpretation of margin status among pathologists.

Positive Surgical Margins

In terms of surgical margins, urologists must face difficult problems unique to prostatectomy. Unlike with many other organs, the anatomic location of the prostate, with its limited space, makes it difficult to obtain clean margins.

The incidence of positive surgical margins with radical prostatectomy varies from 16% to 46% [1]. A number of factors affect the difference in incidence of positive margins reported in the literature. The contributing factors have been elegantly addressed by Epstein [1] and Wieder and Soloway [2].

Patient Selection

In recent years there has been a dramatic shift in the clinical stages in men diagnosed with prostate cancer who are candidates for radical prostatectomy. With the popular use of the serum PSA assay as a screening method, more and more cancers are being detected in patients who have no palpable nodules (T1c disease). Nonpalpable tumors at radical prostatectomy are associated with a lower pathologic stage, less frequent positive resection margins, and lower tumor volume than palpable tumors [1]. Even among patients with T1c disease, the incidence of positive surgical margins may vary depending on the extent of disease. Men who have had a normal PSA value previously but now present with minimally elevated PSA have less advanced disease than men who present with an abnormal PSA value and no previous PSA screening [1]. Nowadays, many men with a very high PSA value may be advised to undergo nonsurgical therapy, thus further reducing the number of advanced-stage patients.

Technical Differences in Performing Radical Prostatectomy

The most common sites of positive surgical margins are the apex and the posterolateral aspects [2]. The apex is also the most common site of iatrogenic positive margins (i.e., a positive margin induced by inadvertent incision into prostate parenchyma at the time of radical prostatectomy). Of all apical positive margins, 9%–71% are iatrogenic [2]. Incision through the apex probably occurs because of insufficient mobilization of the distal apex. If the fibromuscular bands that tether the apex are not completely transected, the plane of dissection may violate the distal-most part of the prostate [3–5]. (Also refer to the editorial comments accompanying [3].)

The posterior (rectal) margin is the second most common positive margin. The posterior aspect of the prostate is mobilized by dissecting between Denonvilliers' fascia and the rectum (see the discussion on Question 1). If an incorrect plane is entered, Denonvilliers' fascia may be stripped from the prostate, and cancer in the extraprostatic space, if present, may be left behind.

Positive bladder neck margins are uncommon. At Northwestern University where retropubic approach is the standard, many surgeons send a slice of the bladder neck margin for intraoperative frozen section examination.

Anterior and anterolateral positive margins seldom occur. A positive margin is seen more frequently with perineal radical prostatectomy. In fact, the anterior prostate is the most common site of a positive surgical margin, which occurs in approximately 25% of cases. This is because the anterior margin is less accessible during the perineal approach [1, 2].

Nerve sparing is a practical concern in the United States. Nerves that contribute to erectile function course posterolateral to the prostate in the neurovascular bundles. During nerve-sparing prostatectomy these bundles are left intact to improve the chance of postoperative potency. Unfortunately, the region of the neurovascular bundle is the most common site of "capsular" penetration (see Fig. 1-3-3 in Question 3); cancer cells spread by way of the perineural space. This brings up the issue of how to deal with the neurovascular bundles. In general, to reduce the risk of postoperative positive margins, surgeons excise the neurovascular bundle on the side of a positive biopsy or palpable tumor. However, Eggleston and Walsh [6] reported that more than 80% of patients with unilateral palpable nodules had bilateral tumor involvement of the prostate. Furthermore, Daniels et al. [7] reported that 78% of unilateral positive biopsies had bilateral tumor involvement when the excised prostate was examined. They stated that bilateral positive biopsies suggest a large-volume tumor, greater probability of "capsular" penetration, and positive surgical margins. Thus, the ideal candidate for a nerve-sparing procedure should meet several

criteria: He is potent preoperatively (and wishes to remain so), and the biopsy should demonstrate tumor on only one side of the prostate. Patients with stages T1a/A1 and T1b/A2 cancer are good candidates for nerve sparing. However, one should keep in mind that these prostates harbor cancer foci in the peripheral zone with very high frequency (refer to Question 5). Stage T1c patients may be candidates for contralateral nerve saving if the biopsy is positive unilaterally.

Analysis of Prostatectomy Specimens by Pathologists

There are two pertinent issues related to handling prostatectomy specimens and interpreting microscopic findings. First, it is common practice to paint the entire surface of the resected prostate with dye (usually black) to mark the resection margins. After an overnight fixation in formalin solution, the specimen is transected at a right angle to the urethra (horizontally) and selected blocks (or the entire specimen) submitted for microscopic study. The chance of identifying positive surgical margins may depend on the number and thickness of the sliced blocks. Thus, partial submission of thick blocks (>3 mm in thickness) may reduce the chance of finding positive margins.

A second issue is how to interpret the presence of neoplastic glands located close to the resection margin identified by ink. Because the prostate is located deep within the pelvis surrounded by structures such as the urogenital diaphragm, bladder neck, rectum, and pelvic side wall, it is impossible to remove the prostate with an ample amount of periprostatic tissue. At many sites, the true surgical margins surrounding the prostate are no more than 1–2 mm from the prostate. Some pathologists call it a positive margin if the tumor extends close to the inked surface, whereas other pathologists interpret it as positive only if the tumor appears to be directly cut across. Epstein's group demonstrated that when a tumor extends very close to the inked margin but has not yet been cut across (Fig. 1-4-1) there was no significant difference in the distance between the inked margin and the cancer front among patients with and without progression [8, 9]. In a regression analysis, only the Gleason score was predictive of progression. Therefore, Epstein's group regarded tumor close to the inked edge as negative for tumor. This is an important observation to which pathologists should pay

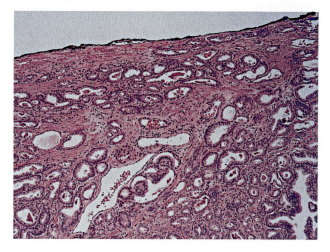

FIG. 1-4-1. Cancerous glands are present in the "capsule" and close to the inked margin, but none is cut across by the ink

attention. In our practice, we report a positive margin only in cases where cancer cells touching ink but not in cases where tumor cells are close to but not touching the ink.

Outlook of Patients with Tumor Showing Extraprostatic Extension and/or Positive Surgical Margins

Although many groups have reported data on progression following radical prostatectomy performed on patients with clinically confined cancer, it is difficult to compare their data because of different surgical technique, pathology examination technique, and different criteria of positive margins. The overall consensus is that lymph node metastasis and seminal vesicle invasion (Fig. 1-4-2) are clearly associated with a high risk of disease progression. Excluding these patients, the Gleason score, surgical margins, and EPE are independent predictors of progression by multivariate analysis [1].

We analyzed data from three groups with an extended follow-up of a large number of the patient population (Paulson group) and good clinical follow-up data supported by solid pathology examination (Epstein/Walsh group and Scardino group).

The Paulson group study from Duke University [10] has strengths in that (1) a large patient population (613 patients) was enrolled and (2) cancer-specific survival (instead of recurrence judged by a rise in PSA) was determined 13.5 years following radical prostatectomy. Their weakness is that there is

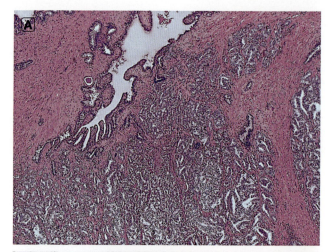

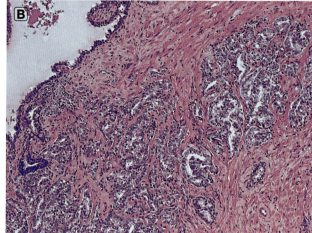

FIG. 1-4-2. **A, B** Cancerous glands infiltrate the wall of the seminal vesicle

no description of how the pathology examination was conducted. Nevertheless, their data indicate that cancer-specific survival at 13.5 years was excellent; only 10% of patients with organ-confined disease or specimen-confined disease (how many of them had EPE are not described) died of the cancer in contrast to 40% of those with margin-positive disease (presumably many, if not all, of these patients had cancer that extended to extraprostatic tissue). A second important observation was that the PSA rise preceded clinical recurrence by 3 to 5 years. Third, among 222 patients with margin-positive disease who were offered immediate adjunctive radiation therapy, 66 underwent this therapy within 6 months postoperatively. Survival curves for these patients versus those who did not undergo radiation therapy indicate that early postoperative adjunctive radiation therapy to the prostatic fossa did not enhance survival. This fact suggests that cancer had spread away from the prostatic bed at the time of the local recurrence or at the radical prostatectomy.

The Baylor group study [11] consists of 478 patients who underwent radical prostatectomy by a single surgeon for clinically localized cancer. The pathology study was conducted by one pathologist. The patients were followed for 1–126 months (median 32 months) with serum PSA assays. Progression was defined as clinical recurrence of the cancer (biopsy-proven local recurrence, evidence of distant metastasis by bone scan or other tests, or a serum PSA level of $\geq 0.4\,ng/ml$ by the Hybritech assay). Their study can be summarized as follows. At 5 years, the nonprogression rate was 64% for patients with positive surgical margins and 83% for those without positive surgical margins ($P < 0.02$). Extraprostatic extension but negative margins were associated with 84% survival at 5 years compared with 59% of patients with EPE and positive surgical margins (the difference is nearly significant, $P = 0.06$). Seminal vesicle invasion and lymph node metastasis were associated with a worse prognosis. Among these patients, margin status had no effect on the rate of progression. Positive surgical margins created by surgical incision into "intracapsular" cancer did not affect the prognosis, and the prognosis was similar to that of those with organ-confined cancer. However, this is an ill-defined group. The authors claim that all of these cases occurred because of surgical incision through the "capsule" into cancer otherwise confined to the prostate. How do they know that they are all organ-confined? To determine the effect of the Gleason score on the prognostic significance of positive surgical margins, cases without seminal vesicle invasion or lymph node metastasis were divided into two categories: those of Gleason score ≤ 6 and those of Gleason score ≥ 7. Of 53 patients in the first group with EPE and a low Gleason score for cancer, a positive surgical margin status worsened the prognosis ($P < 0.05$). Of 97 patients in the second group with EPE, the margin status had no effects. The finding confirms the results reported by the Johns Hopkins group (vide infra). Thus, margin status affected only a small proportion of patients treated with radical prostatectomy. By multivariate analysis, seminal vesicle invasion, Gleason score, and EPE were all independent prognosticators.

The study by the Johns Hopkins group [12] is based on 617 patients who did not have preoperative or postoperative radiotherapy or hormone therapy. All cases were handled by one surgeon and overseen by one expert pathologist. For those men without progression, the mean follow–up was 6.5 years. Patients with seminal vesicle invasion and lymph node metastasis were excluded. In the multivariate analysis, the Gleason score ($P < 0.0001$), surgical margins ($P < 0.004$), and EPE ($P = 0.007$) were all independent predictors of progression. Tumors with a Gleason score of 2–4 were almost invariably cured and with a 10-year progression-free risk of 96%. Thus, neither EPE nor margin status influenced the prognosis. Similarly, in patients with high Gleason scores of 8 or 9, the presence or absence of EPE or margin positivity had no influence, and the actuarial 10-year progression-free survival was 35%. For patients with a Gleason score of 5–7 (88% of cases), EPE and margin status did have effects on the progression rate. Men with a Gleason score of 5 or 6 (2 + 3 and 3 + 3) did well when their tumors were organ-confined and had a negative margin; the actuarial likelihood of being disease-free were 98.7% and 92.4% at 5 and 10 years, respectively. The intermediate-risk group consisted of two patient populations; men with focal "capsular" penetration (so defined by Epstein for a small focus of tumor extending beyond the "capsule") with either positive or negative surgical margins and men with established "capsular" penetration (so designated by Epstein for wide "capsular" penetration) but with a negative surgical margin. Interestingly, despite an apparent difference in the risk of progression, there was no statistically significant difference between the first and second patient populations. The group that carried the worst prognosis had established "capsular" penetration and a positive surgical margin. When compared with either the best or the intermediate prognostic group, the outlook was significantly worse ($P < 0.001$). Nevertheless, their outlook was optimistic, with their actuarial 5- and 10-year progression-free survivals being 84.5% and 71.7%, respectively. For Gleason score 7 tumors, the effects of "capsular" penetration and margin status were similar to those for Gleason score 5 and 6 tumors; patients whose tumors were organ-confined and had negative margins did best, with progression-free survivals of 96.6% at 5 years and 67.6% at 10 years. The intermediate group (focal "capsular" penetration with or without positive margins, or wide "capsular" penetration but negative surgical margins) had progression-free survivals of 82.8% and 47.9% at 5 and 10 years, respectively. The worst group was the one with wide "capsular" penetration and positive surgical margins. Their progression-free survivals were 50.0% and 41.6%, respectively, at 5 and 10 years. The differences between the group with the best prognosis and the intermediate- and high-risk groups were significant at $P = 0.04$ and $P = 0.0001$, respectively. The difference between the intermediate-risk and high-risk groups was likewise significant at $P = 0.0005$.

In summary, the Gleason score, EPE, and a positive margin are all significant but their influence is seen only on intermediate-risk to moderately high-risk tumors (Gleason scores 5, 6, 7). The low-grade tumors (Gleason scores 2, 3, 4) carry an excellent prognosis irrespective of the margin status. On the other hand, the high-risk tumor group (Gleason scores 8, 9) has a poor prognosis, with the margin status or EPE having little impact. The prognosis is likewise negatively affected by seminal vesicle invasion and/or lymph node metastasis.

Several questions remain unanswered. First, what is the outcome of patients with a removed prostate which has a surgeon-created (so-called iatrogenic) positive surgical margin? The study reported by the Ohori group [11] raises concerns regarding their patient population that was described as belonging to this group. A second issue is how to deal with the case in which carcinoma has invaded the muscle group in the anterior wall. Because there is no "capsule" in the anterior border, it remains unresolved how to stage such cases. Should we regard them as pT3? Our view is that we should, because invasion of this muscle group suggests that the tumor has potential for aggressive behavior. What about the case in which tumor invaded the sphincter skeletal muscle (along the distal half of the urethra) or the smooth muscle of the preprostatic sphincter of the proximal urethra? We regard these cases as pT2 tumors inasmuch as these structures are integral components of the prostate.

References

1. Epstein JI (1996) Incidence and significance of positive margins in radical prostatectomy specimens. Urol Clin North Am 23:651–663.
2. Wieder JA, Soloway MS (1998) Incidence, etiology, location, prevention, and treatment of positive surgical margins after radical prostatectomy for prostate cancer. J Urol 160:299–315.
3. Stamey TA, Villers AA, McNeal JE, Link PC, Freiha FS (1990) Positive surgical margins at radical prostatectomy:importance of the apical dissection. J Urol 143:1166–1173.
4. Catalona WJ, Bigg SW (1990) Nerve-sparing radical prostatectomy: evaluation of results after 250 patients. J Urol 143:538–544.
5. Walsh PC (1992) Radical retropubic prostatectomy. In: Das S, Crawford ED (eds) Campbell's Urology, 6th ed. Marcel Decker, New York, pp 189–223.
6. Eggleston JC, Walsh PC (1985) Radical prostatectomy with preservation of sexual function: pathological findings in the first 100 cases. J Urol 134:1146–1148.
7. Daniels GF Jr, McNeal JE, Stamey TA (1992) Predictive value of contralateral biopsies in unilaterally palpable prostatic cancer. J Urol 147:870–874.
8. Epstein JI (1990) Evaluation of radical prostatectomy capsular margins of resection: the significance of margins designated as negative, closely approaching, and positive. Am J Surg Pathol 14:626–632.
9. Epstein JE, Sauvageot J (1997) Do close but negative margins in radical prostatectomy specimens increase the risk of postoperative progression? J Urol 157:241–224.
10. Paulson DF (1994) Impact of radical prostatectomy in the management of clinically localized disease. J Urol 152:1826–1830.
11. Ohori M, Wheeler TM, Kattan MW, Goto Y, Scardino PT (1995) Prognostic significance of positive surgical margins in radical prostatectomy specimens. J Urol 154:1818-1824.
12. Epstein JI, Partin AW, Sauvageot J, Walsh PC (1996) Prediction of progression following radical prostatectomy: a multivariate analysis of 721 men with long-term follow-up. Am J Surg Pathol 20:286–292.

Question 5

What is the clinical significance of prostate cancer incidentally discovered in tissue removed to relieve urinary tract obstruction mostly by transurethral resection (stage T1a and T1b cancers)?

Answer

The concept of stage T1a and T1b (stage A) cancers applies to the prostatic adenocarcinoma discovered incidentally in a specimen removed by transurethral resection of the prostate (TURP). Stage T1a (stage A1) is defined as prostate cancer with a tumor volume ≤5% of tissue chips. Stage T1b (stage A2) cancer is defined as prostate cancer present in TURP specimens with a Gleason score ≥7 and/or tumor volume greater than 5%. Stage T1a prostate cancer may not require special treatment as it is considered indolent, whereas T1b prostate cancer requires standard treatment for prostate cancer as it is often associated with cancer in other parts of the prostate. Stage T1c prostate cancer is defined as cancer diagnosed by needle core biopsy. Therefore, in a pathology report of a TURP specimen, the pathologist should include the Gleason score and percentage of tumor involvement if present. In addition, we recommend specifying T1a or T1b in the pathology diagnosis.

Comments

Prostate cancer identified as stage T1a or T1b has declined because of less frequent use of TURP and more frequent identification of cancer of the periph-eral zone by elevated prostate-specific antigen (PSA)-driven transrectal prostate needle core biopsy (PNB). However, the concept of stage A cancer remains viable, and you may encounter it in your daily practice. There are probably two reasons why stage A cancer diagnosis has declined in the recent past; the first is due to the decrease in TURPs since pharmacologic agents have become available to ease obstructive symptoms. The second is the routine use of serum PSA assays for screening prostate cancer and an increased number of PNBs performed.

In practice, a diagnosis of stage A cancer may be rendered under one of the following three circumstances: (1) in patients who have undergone TURP with a normal preoperative PSA level; (2) in patients with elevated PSA but negative PNB prior to TURP; and (3) in patients who underwent TURP without a preoperative PSA check. The expected pathology in the prostate may differ among these three types of patient. Detailed studies on radical prostatectomy specimens were conducted in several laboratories. Their data indicate that most of these cancers found in TURP specimens are of transition zone (TZ) origin. A variable amount of residual cancer is found in the TZ, but an important finding was that a significant number of carcinomas are detected in the peripheral zone (PZ) in radical prostatectomy specimens.

Carcinoma (stage A cancer) is incidentally found in approximately 10% of specimens removed to relieve urinary obstructive symptoms [1]. In 1974, Correa et al. [2] found that the prognosis is much better if cancer is "limited or focal" than if it is diffuse. Jewett [3] in 1975 proposed to subclassify stage A disease into focal stage A1 and diffuse stage A2 disease, depending on the number of foci of carcinoma and their grade in TURP chips. Cantrell et al. [1] better characterized A1 and A2 stage cancer based on a multivariate analysis of data. Gleason grade and extent of the disease (estimated percentage of tumor) were the two factors that most accurately defined stage A2 disease, and these two parameters correlated very well. Thus, none of the 14 patients with low-grade lesions (Gleason score 2–4) showed progression of their disease, and only 1 of 48 patients whose tumor occupied <5% of the TURP specimen showed disease progression. Based on these data, cases were defined as stage A1 when the TURP specimen contained ≤5% of tumor and/or a "low" histologic grade (Gleason score <4) and as stage A2 when cancer occupied more than 5% of the resected tissue or with a "high" grade (Gleason score ≥5). Subsequently, however, the cut-point used for substaging varied among investigators; some allowed a Gleason score up to 7 [4, 5] for stage A1 if the tumor volume was <5%. Despite some variation in defining disease, stage A1 cancer, so defined, is not as aggressive as stage A2. Most studies suggest that stage A2 cancer is an aggressive form of the disease, but this is not true for all patients. Left untreated, approximately 30% of patients are free of progression after an average 10-year follow-up [6], clearly indicating that stage A2 disease consists of a heterogeneous group of tumors.

To assess the clinical significance, several groups of investigators made a detailed study of prostates removed from stage A patients. In the Mayo study reported by Zincke et al. [7], 4 of 32 stage A1 and 34 of 116 stage A2 cancers were found to be in pathology stage C (T3) or higher. According to Christensen et al. [8] of the Johns Hopkins group, residual tumors were found in all 39 cases of clinical stage A2 cancer. In 23 cases (59%) the tumors were predominantly central to anterior in location (suggesting TZ origin), whereas in 8 cases (21%) the tumors were posterior (suggesting PZ origin). The remaining 8 cases showed the tumor to be diffuse throughout the prostate gland. Of the 10 cases where tumor had extended beyond the gland, 10 had extraprostatic extension (EPE), 6 had a positive resection margin, 4 had seminal vesicle invasion, and 2 had metastasis in pelvic lymph nodes. There was, in general, a good correlation between the tumor grade of the TURP and the grade of the radical prostatectomy. The percentage of tumor in the TURP specimens was the best single predictor of pathologic stage. The combination of tumor extent and grade provided the best multivariable prediction of pathologic stage.

Larsen et al. [5], also from the Johns Hopkins Hospital, reported their experience with stage A1 cancer, which was defined as tumors occupying <5% of specimens and of low to intermediate grade (Gleason

score 2–7). At radical prostatectomy, 6% (4/64) of specimens had no residual cancer, 74% had minimal cancer, and 20% had "substantial" cancer, which was defined as a tumor with ≥1 ml total volume, "capsular" penetration, or a high Gleason score of ≥8. (According to Stamey et al. [9], tumors of >1 ml have an increased risk of EPE, seminal vesicle invasion, and lymph node metastasis.) Five cases had EPE, and two of them had positive surgical margins. In all cases, seminal vesicles and lymph nodes were negative for tumor. The location of the tumors was heterogeneous; the central (periurethral) region was predominantly involved in 25 cases (39%), and peripheral tumors predominated in 39 cases (61%). An important observation was that in 16 cases the tumor involved the apical region, and that in an additional 25 cases (39%) the tumor focally extended toward the apex. These data suggested that a substantial number of prostates removed for stage a1 tumor had clinically important cancer involving the PZ. Altogether, 28% of cases had Gleason score of 4 or less, 70% had a Gleason score of 5–7, and 2% had a Gleason score of 9. Another important observation was, unlike stage A2 tumor, the correlation between the percentage of tumor in the TURP specimen and the extent of tumor in the radical prostatectomy specimen was poor. Similarly, there were poor correlations between Gleason grade in the TURP specimen and tumor extent in the prostate. These studies suggest that a good number of both stage A1 and A2 patients have clinically significant cancers that occupy not only the TZ but also the PZ.

It was, however, the Baylor group who surveyed the location of tumors critically. Their study [4] consisted of radical prostatectomy specimens from 13 stage A1 and 29 stage A2 patients. Cancer was present in 41 prostates (98%). Tumors were multifocal (76%), peripheral (81%), and distal to the verumontanum (66%). Of the 13 stage a1 patients, 4 (30%) had significant cancer of >1 ml volume, "extracapsular" extension, or seminal vesicle invasion. When stage A1 and A2 cases were combined, residual cancer was found in the TZ in 67% and in the PZ in 90% of the patients. Eight of thirteen cases of EPE and all five cases of seminal vesicle invasion were directly attributable to PZ cancer. To determine the characteristics of TZ and PZ cancer, the Baylor group reexamined the specimens to determine the number of foci of carcinoma, zone of their origin, volume and Gleason grade of each focus, presence of high-grade prostatic intraepithelial neoplasia (HGPIN), EPE, and seminal vesicle invasion associated with the cancer in each zone. The data were compared with similarly collected data from 54 stage B radical prostatectomy specimens [10]. The results are summarized in Tables 1-5-1 and 1-5-2.

As is clear from these tables, there is a significant difference between stage A and stage B carcinomas. In total, 81% of stage A prostate specimens contained tumors of TZ origin, but 93% of them also had tumors of PZ origin (Table 1-5-1). Based on the microscopic evaluation of the TURP and prostatectomy specimens, it was shown that:

- TURP sampled TZ cancer in 77% and PZ cancer in 31% (8% had both types). All stage B prostate specimens contained a PZ cancer, and 63% also had a TZ cancer. The palpable or index cancer was of TZ origin in only one stage B cancer patient (although a separate PZ tumor was present).
- In both stage A and B tumors, PZ tumors were less well-differentiated (median Gleason scores of 6 and 7, respectively) than TZ tumors (5 and 5,

respectively) ($P < 0.01$ for each comparison) and more likely to have EPE (44% [41/93] vs. 11% [6/57]) (no statistical comparison reported). Seminal vesicle invasion was associated with PZ tumors (19% [18/93]) but none with TZ tumors (0/57) (no statistical comparison described).

Another notable finding was that HGPIN was closely associated with the PZ cancer and not with the TZ carcinoma. (A similar observation was also reported by Epstein et al. [11] and Quinn et al. [12], suggesting that HGPIN is a precursor of PZ cancer.) They concluded that cancer that arises in the TZ appears to have a different histogenesis, has an association with more favorable pathologic features, and may have less malignant potential than tumors that arise in the PZ.

What have we learned from these four groups? First, unlike stage B cancer, both stage A1 and A2 cancers consist of a heterogeneous group of tumors ranging from minimal to substantial tumors that are capable of invading the seminal vesicles and metastasizing to pelvic lymph nodes. Clearly, the risk is greater with a stage A2 tumor than with a stage A1 tumor. Second, although tumors detected in TURP specimens are overwhelmingly of TZ origin [13], a substantial number of tumors are of probable PZ origin invading the TZ (21%) [8] and a significant number of "incidental" cancers coexist in the PZ and are capable of taking an aggressive course [4].

A couple of inevitable questions arise: Is stage A PZ cancer less aggressive than stage B PZ cancer? When you look at Greene's data [10] on the frequency of seminal vesicle invasion, there is no statistically significant difference between the two groups (χ^2 1.18). A second question is whether the aggressive behavior of the coexisting PZ cancers (EPE in 21%

TABLE 1-5-1. Number of separate cancers per patient and number of stage A and B cancer patients with disease in each zone

Clinical stage	No. pts.	Mean no. of separate tumors/pt. (range)	TZ Ca. (no. pts.)	PZ Ca. (no. pts.)
A1	13	2.5 (1–4)	11 (85%)	12 (93%)
A2	29	3.3 (1–5)	23 (79%)	27 (92%)
A, total	42	3.1 (1–5)	34 (81%)	39 (93%)
B	54	2.3 (1–5)	34 (63%)	54 (100%)

From Greene et al. [10], with permission.
TZ, transition zone; PZ, peripheral zone.

TABLE 1-5-2. Frequency of associated high-grade PIN, "extracapsulr" extension, and seminal vesicle invasion of cancers found in the TZ and PZ

Site	No. of pts.	Gleason score	High-grade PIN[a] (no.)	"Extracapsular" extension	Seminal vesicle invasion
Stage A					
TZ Ca	34	5	0	5 (15%)	0
PZ Ca	39	6	35 (90%)	8 (21%)	5 (13%)
Stage B					
TZ Ca	23	5	0	1 (4%)	0
PZ Ca	54	7	50 (93%)	33 (61%)	13 (24%)

From Greene et al. [10], with permission.
PIN, prostate intraepithelial neoplasia.
[a] High-grade PIN present in close association with carcinoma foci.

and seminal vesicle invasion in 13% in Table 1-5-2) is unique to stage A carcinoma. Citing data from the McNeal group [13], who showed that none of the incidental cancers found in cystoprostatectomy specimens had "extracapsular" extension or seminal vesicle invasion [14], Greene et al. [10] concluded that "incidental" PZ cancers in stage A patient are "not insignificant," [4] suggesting that the PZ cancer observed in association with stage A cancer is aggressive.

What is the "take home" message? Although prostate cancer identified as stage A (T1a and T1b) cancer has decreased because of the decreasing practice of TURP and the increasing practice of PSA-driven needle core biopsy, if stage A cancer is diagnosed an effort should be made by pathologists to determine the percentage of tumor involvement and the Gleason score of the prostate cancer in TURP specimens for further treatment recommendations.

References

1. Cantrell BB, Deklerk DP, Eggleston JC, Boitnett JK, Walsh PC (1981) Pathological factors that influence prognosis in stage A prostatic cancer: the influence of extent versus grade. J Urol 125:516–520.
2. Correa RJ Jr, Anderson RJ, Gibbons RP, Mason JT (1974) Latent carcinoma of the prostate: why the controversy? J Urol 111:644–646.
3. Jewett HJ (1975) The present status of radical prostatectomy for stage A and B prostatic cancer. Urol Clin North Am 2:105–124.
4. Greene DR, Egawa S, Neerhut G, Flanagan W, Wheeler TM, Scardino PT (1991) The distribution of residual cancer in radical prostatectomy specimens in stage A prostate cancer. J Urol 145:324–329.
5. Larsen MP, Ballentine H, Epstein JI (1991) Can stage A1 tumor extent be predicted by transurethral resection tumor volume percent or grade? A study of 64 stage A1 radical prostatectomies with comparison to prostates removed for stage A2 and B disease. J Urol 146:1059–1063.
6. Epstein JI, Oesterling JE, Walsh PC (1988) Tumor volume versus percent involved by tumor correlated with progression of stage A prostate cancer. J Urol 129:980–984.
7. Zincke H, Blute ML, Fallen MJ, Farrow GM (1991) Radical prostatectomy for stage A adenocarcinoma of the prostate: staging errors and their implications for treatment recommendations and disease outcome. J Urol 146:1053–1058.
8. Christensen WN, Partin AW, Walsh PC, Epstein JI (1990) Pathologic findings in clinical stage A2 prostate cancer: relation of tumor volume, grade, and locations to pathologic stage. Cancer 65:1021–1027.
9. Stamey TA, McNeal JE, Freiha FS, Redwine E (1988) Morphometric and clinical studies on 68 consecutive radical prostatectomies. J Urol 139:1235–1241.
10. Greene DR, Wheeler TM, Egawa S, Dunn JK, Scardino PT (1991) A comparison of the morphological features of cancer arising in the transition zone and in the peripheral zone of the prostate. J Urol 146:1069–1076.
11. Epstein JI, Cho KR, Quinn BD (1990) Relationship of severe dysplasia to stage A (incidental) adenocarcinoma of the prostate. Cancer 65:2321–2327.
12. Quinn BD, Cho KR, Epstein JI (1990) Relationship of severe dysplasia to stage B adenocarcinoma of the prostate. Cancer 65:2328–2337.
13. McNeal JE, Redwine EA, Freiha ES, Stamey TA (1988) Zonal distribution of prostate adenocarcinoma: correlation with histologic pattern and distribution of spread. Am J Surg Pathol 12:897–906.
14. Kabalin JN, McNeal JE, Price HM, Freiha FS, Stamey TA (1989) Unsuspected adenocarcinoma of the prostate in patients undergoing cystoprostatectomy for other causes: incidence, histology, and morphometric observations. J Urol 141:1091–1094.

Question 6

What are the characteristics of transition zone cancer? Is it less aggressive than the non-transition-zone cancer?

Answer

Transition zone (TZ) cancer is commonly detected in transurethrally resected specimens but also radical prostatectomy specimens. According to a recent study, as many as 14% of stage T1c cancers are exclusively in the TZ. In general, they are small and are of low Gleason score (commonly <6). Because of their anatomic location (away from the "capsule") and fewer penetrating nerves than in the peripheral zone, they are less likely to behave aggressively than those arising in non-TZs. As the volume increases, however, they may become more aggressive and can invade the anterior fibromuscular stroma, seminal vesicles, and pelvic lymph nodes. Microscopically, most transition zone carcinomas consist of well-differentiated glands of widely variable size and contour lined by tall columnar cells with clear cytoplasm.

Comments

The TZ consists of two independent small, balloon-shaped lobes whose ducts leave the posterolateral recess of the urethral wall just proximal to the urethral angulation and at the lower border of the preprostatic sphincter (refer to Question 2). Anteriorly, the balloons are bounded by the thick fibromuscular stroma, which covers the anterior surface of the prostate. Posteriorly and laterally, it is bounded by the peripheral zone (PZ). Superiorly, the TZ faces the central zone (CZ). The TZ is covered by a "capsule" only in a small area bordering on and anterior to the PZ.

Microscopically, the TZ can be identified as a compact collection of clear cells, and it is separated from the PZ by a curved fibromuscular layer (called the "transition boundary" by McNeal et al.) [1, 2]. Frequently, the TZ histology is altered by benign prostate hyperplasia (BPH) (Fig. 1-6-1).

Most stage A cancers are of TZ origin and are detected in frequent association with BPH. Because of their central location, TZ cancers are seldom detectable by prostate needle core biopsy (PNB) unless they are of large volume [1]. Nowadays, most radical prostatectomy specimens are derived from stage T1c patients. According to a recent study, as many as 14% of T1c lesions are exclusively in the TZ zone [3].

We cite here three articles that focused on the biologic potential of TZ carcinoma as detected as an index cancer (incidentally found cancer in a prostatectomy specimen is not considered here) (Table 1-6-1).

The first study is from the Stanford group reported by McNeal et al. [1]. The series consisted of 104 cases of clinically localized cancer collected during the 1984–1987 period, the era before prostate-specific antigen (PSA) testing became available. Of the 104 prostates, the origin of the index cancer was confirmed in 88; 7 tumors were of CZ origin, 21 tumors were of TZ origin, and 60 tumors were of PZ origin. The origin could not be determined in the remaining 16 cases. Of 21 TZ tumors, 11 were diagnosed by transurethral resection of the prostate (TURP). An additional four tumors were palpable rectally because of their large size. The remaining six tumors were nonpalpable and were discovered fortuitously; they were situated anterior to a BPH nodule and were detected by PNB. Of 21 TZ carcinomas, 16 invaded the anterior fibromuscular stroma, including 11 tumors that were <1.3 ml in volume. By contrast, only

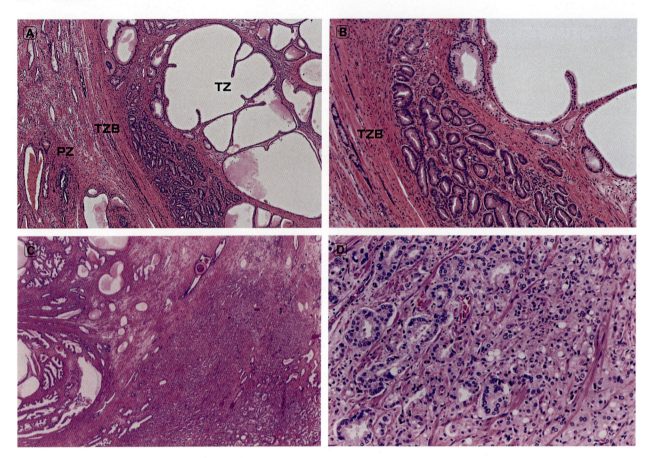

FIG. 1-6-1. The transition zone (*TZ*) shows benign prostatic hyperplasia. It is delineated from the periopheral zone (*PZ*) by the curved fibromuscular layer (*TZ* boundary, or *TZB*) (**A, B**). Along the outer border of the *TZ* but inside the *TZB* is a narrow zone of a well-differentiated adenocarcinoma (Gleason score 2 + 2 = 4), an incidental tumor. This prostate was removed because of the CT1c *PZ* cancer located just outside the *TZ* boundary (**C, D**). It is a Gleason score 4 + 4 = 8 carcinoma

TABLE 1-6-1. Aggressiveness of TZ and PZ cancer evaluated as the index cancer[a]

Study	Total cases	Gleason score (mean)	Tumor volume (mean) (ml)	"Extracapsular" extension[b] (or anterior fibromuscular invasion)[c]	Positive surgical margin	Seminal vesicle invasion	Lymph node metastasis
McNeal [1]	104						
TZ	21[d]	NA	Mostly < 1.3	16 (76%)[c]	NA	NA	NA
Non-TZ[c]	83[d]	NA	Predominantly 1.3–7.3	15 (18%)[c]	NA	NA	NA
Van de Voorde	107						
TZ	24[d]	4.5	5.3	8 (33%)[b]	7 (29%)	4 (17%)	1 (4%)
Non-TZ	83[d]	6.2	4.1	48 (58%)[b]	40 (48%)	17 (20%)	5 (6%)
Greene	88						
TZ	34[d]	5	2.5	5 (15%)[b]	NA	0	NA
Non-TZ	54[d]	7	4.0	33 (61%)[b]	NA	13 (24%)	NA

[a] Incidentally discovered cancer not considered.
[b] It is unknown if "extracapsular" extension includes anterior fibromuscular invasion in Van de Voorde's and Greene's studies.
[c] McNeal only refers to anterior fibromuscular invasion. The frequency of "extracapsular" extension is not mentioned.
[d] Index cases.

15 of the non-TZ carcinomas invaded the anterior fibromuscular stroma, and all of them were >3.7 ml in volume. In this article, however, there is no mention how many of the non-TZ carcinomas extended beyond the "capsule" or invaded the seminal vesicles or lymph nodes.

In the study by Greene et al. [4] of the Baylor group, among 34 stage A (TZ) carcinomas, "extra-capsular" extension (presumably invasion of the fibromuscular stroma included) was observed in 5 (15%), in contrast to 33 of 54 stage B (non-TZ) carcinomas (61%) ($P < 0.001$, Fisher's exact test). None of the TZ cancers invaded the seminal vesicles, whereas 24% of the PZ cancers did.

In contrast to the Greene group's report, Van de Voorde et al. [5] from Belgium argued that TZ cancer can be more aggressive and is capable of metastasizing to pelvic lymph nodes. Their study was based on 107 radical prostatectomy cases of clinically localized carcinoma (they failed to state how many of them are of clinical stage A). The entire specimen was sectioned serially and was submitted for examination. The index tumor was defined as the tumor with the largest volume; and for each cancer the zone of origin was determined by relating tumor location to the TZ boundary [1]. An index tumor was considered a PZ carcinoma when the bulk of the tumor or the complete tumor was located within the PZ, including any cancer not of TZ origin. A carcinoma was designated a TZ carcinoma when it was completely or predominantly situated in the TZ. In all, 83 cases (78%) and 24 cases (22%), respectively, were judged to be of PZ (CZ origin included) and TZ origin. There was no significant difference in the volume of the index tumor, but a Gleason score of the PZ tumors (6.2 ± 1.0) was significantly higher than that of the TZ tumors (4.5 ± 1.6) ($P < 0.0001$). "Capsular" transgression occurred in 58% (48/83) and 33% (8/24) of the PZ and TZ cancers, respectively. (They did not specify whether transgression involves the "capsule" or the fibromuscular stroma.) Positive surgical margins were found in 48% (40/83) and 29% (7/24) of the PZ and TZ cancers, respectively. Seminal vesicle invasion was observed in 20% (17/83) of the PZ cancers and 17% (4/24) of the TZ cancers. For both TZ and PZ origins, tumors invading the "capsule", seminal vesicles, and showing a positive surgical margin tended to be greater in volume than those confined to the prostate. Pelvic lymph node metastasis occurred in 6% (5/83) of the PZ group and 4% (1/24) of the TZ group.

The data presented above may be summarized as follows: (1) TZ carcinomas have a Gleason grade no higher than 3. (2) TZ carcinomas' biologic characteristics largely depend on how they are discovered. If discovered as stage A carcinomas, they are less aggressive than stage B carcinomas largely because they are small and are of low Gleason grade [1]. Because of their central location, it is unlikely that they invade the "capsule," whereas they can invade the anterior fibromuscular stroma. (3) TZ cancer is usually not detectable by sextant needle core biopsies because of their inner location. However, it may become palpable and detectable by needle core biopsy alone when it attains a large volume. As TZ carcinomas increase in size, they become capable of invading surrounding structures. To invade the PZ posteriorly, however, cancer cells must travel across the transition boundary of McNeal. Therefore, they are more likely to expand anteriorly, invading the fibromuscular stroma. TZ cancers rarely spread through the "capsule" (recall that the TZ is bounded by a capsule only in a small area bordering the PZ); but as they enlarge they may have access to the capsule and therefore perineural spaces. (4) Although generally of low grade, it may contain high-grade components (Gleason grade 4 or 5) [2, 6] as the tumor volume increases (>4 ml). Now that most of these large-volume tumors are detectable as stage B carcinomas, it is understandable why they are more aggressive. This indeed appears to be the case when Van de Voorde et al. reported that 22% of the index tumors defined as TZ cancers (mean tumor volume of 5.3 ml) are as aggressive as PZ carcinomas.

In conclusion, TZ cancer comprises a heterogeneous group of tumors, many of which are of small volume and low Gleason grade and behave as indolent tumors. Some of them, however, as their volume increases behave more aggressively accompanied by emergence of high-Gleason-grade carcinoma. Because most of these tumors become palpable and detectable by PNB, they are dealt with as stage B cancer.

References

1. McNeal JE, Redwine EA, Freiha ES, Stamey TA (1988) Zonal distribution of prostate adenocarcinoma: correlation with histologic pattern and distribution of spread. Am J Surg Pathol 12:897–906.

2. McNeal JE (1992) Cancer volume and site of origin of adenocarcinoma in the prostate: relationship to local and distant spread. Hum Pathol 23:258–266.

3. Jack GS, Cookson MS, Coffey CS, Vader V, Roberts RL, Chang SS, Smith JA Jr, Shappell SB (2002) Pathological parameters of radial prostatectomy for clinical stages T1c versus T2 prostate adenocarcinoma: decreased pathological stage and increased detection of transition zone tumors. J Urol 168:519–524.

4. Greene DR, Egawa S, Neerhut G, Flanagan W, Wheeler TM, Scardino PT (1991) The distribution of residual cancer in radical prostatectomy specimens in stage A prostate cancer. J Urol 145:324–329.

5. Van de Voorde WM, Van Poppel HP, Verbeken EK, Oyen RH, Baert LV, Lauweryns JM (1995) Morphologic and neuroendocrine features of adenocarcinoma arising in the transition zone and in the peripheral zone of the prostate. Mod Pathol 8:591–598.

6. McNeal JE, Villers AA, Redwine RA, Freiha FS, Stamey TA (1990) Histologic differentiation, cancer volume, and pelvic lymph node metastasis in adenocarcinoma of the prostate. Cancer 66:1225–1233.

Question 7

Is there a significant difference in prognosis between Gleason score 3 + 4 and 4 + 3 prostate cancers in radical prostatectomy specimens? What is the prognostic implication of Gleason score 3 + 4 versus 4 + 3 prostate cancer assigned to prostate needle core biopsy specimens?

Answer

Gleason score 3 + 4 signifies tumors with Gleason 3 component greater (>50%) than Gleason 4 component. In a Gleason 4 + 3 tumor, Gleason grade 4 component is dominant. In prostatectomy specimens, Gleason score 4 + 3 cancer is associated with a worse clinical outcome than Gleason score 3 + 4 cancer. Dividing a Gleason score 7 tumor to 3 + 4 and 4 + 3 on prostate needle core biopsy is useful only for predicting the final Gleason score in radical prostatectomy specimens. The score, however, does not necessarily correlate with Gleason 3 + 4 or 4 + 3 in the final diagnosis because of sampling issues. Nevertheless, pathologists should attempt to specify Gleason score 7 as either 4 + 3 or 3 + 4 to provide clinically relevant information.

Comments

There are several reasons for a worse prognosis being associated with Gleason 4 + 3 cancer. First, Gleason score 4 + 3 is significantly associated with seminal vesicle (SV) invasion and pelvic node metastasis, both of which are well known parameters associated with a poor prognosis. However, Gleason 4 + 3 is not an independent predictor of prognosis in men with advanced-stage cancer. Second, among patients with localized prostate cancer without SV invasion or lymph node metastasis, Gleason 4 + 3 is a significant independent predictor of survival and PSA recurrence.

Because of its clinical relevance, the Gleason grading system has been accepted throughout the world as the gold standard for histologic grading of prostate cancer. Many reports have confirmed that the Gleason score is a stronger predictor of disease-free survival than other factors, such as tumor volume or stage (excluding patients with SV invasion and lymph node metastasis) [1, 2]. Gleason score 7 cancer as the final diagnosis accounts for the largest group in prostatectomy specimens [3, 4]. In his original analysis, Gleason found that patient survival fell somewhere between that expected with the primary pattern and that expected with the secondary pattern. Thus, he combined these patterns to create the Gleason scoring system [5, 6]. Over the years questions have remained whether there was difference in prognosis between Gleason 3 + 4 and Gleason 4 + 3 cancers.

In consideration of the possible significance of subdividing Gleason score 7, several issues must be addressed. First, the pathologist in charge must be familiar with the Gleason grading system. Second, determination of the volume ratio of Gleason grade 3 and 4 that affects assignment depends on the judgment of the pathologist in charge. Third, although the Gleason pattern has been repeatedly demonstrated to influence the prognosis, it is unclear if a small difference in the volume ratio (>50% vs. <50%) could meaningfully affect the ultimate prognosis unless the ratio is either significantly high or low. For example, if more than 80% of a tumor area is made up of Gleason pattern 4, the outcome might be significantly different from that of a tumor more than 90% of which is composed of Gleason pattern 3. There are no articles that have addressed this issue. The Epstein group [7] stated that the assessment of the percentage of pattern 4 at radical prostatectomy is not likely to be reproducible, but it should be easier for pathologists to distinguish between Gleason score 3 + 4 and 4 + 3.

Gleason Score 3 + 4 Versus 4 + 3 on Prostatectomy Specimens

Several reports in the literature have dealt with the significance of Gleason score 3 + 4 versus 4 + 3 observed in radical prostatectomy specimens. The results are tabulated in Table 1-7-1. As is common with this type of study, the features evaluated and presented are not always the same from one study to the another, which makes comparison difficult. Invasion of the SV and metastasis to a regional lymph node are well-established independent risk factors. In three of the four studies, pT3c and lymph node-positive cases are included.

Common in all of these studies are several observations: (1) Gleason pattern 3 cancer is more prevalent as a predominant type than Gleason pattern 4 cancer. However, the reported ratios vary (see comment on this subject that appears later). (2) Gleason score 4 + 3 cancers exhibit a significantly higher frequency of extraprostatic extension (EPE), SV invasion, and lymph node metastasis.

In the Sakr group study [8] from Wayne State University (Detroit), 534 radical prostatectomy cases that included SV invasion and lymph node metastasis were used for comparison. Overall, patients with Gleason score 3 + 4 tumors experienced a lower incidence of PSA recurrence than did those with Gleason score 4 + 3 tumors ($P = 0.0067$). In the multivariate analysis, controlling for all other variables, Gleason pattern 4 was not a significant indicator for PSA recurrence ($P = 0.42$). However, multivariate analysis directed to patients with organ-confined tumors, accounting for preoperative PSA level, age, race, and tumor volume, revealed that Gleason score 4 + 3 is a significant predictor of survival ($P = 0.012$) and PSA recurrence ($P = 0.0021$) when compared with Gleason score 3 + 4.

In the study by Chan et al. [7] from Johns Hopkins University, only patients without SV invasion, lymph node metastasis, or tertiary Gleason pattern 5 were analyzed. The Kaplan-Meier progression-free curves for patients with Gleason score 3 + 4 and 4 + 3 are illustrated in Fig. 1-7-1. Univariate analysis showed that Gleason score 3 + 4 versus 4 + 3 was significant in predicting the prognosis ($P < 0.0001$). Gleason score 4 + 3 tumors had an increased risk of progression independent of stage and margin status ($P < 0.001$).

The multivariate analysis also showed that surgical margin status ($P < 0.0001$) and EPE ($P = 0.015$) had a significant influence in predicting progression (this has also been demonstrated in another study reported from the same group). Gleason score 4 + 3 tumors had an increased risk of metastatic disease ($P = 0.002$) independent of the surgical margin status and EPE. In essence, in the group of patients without lymph node metastasis or SV invasion, distinguishing cases of Gleason score 3 + 4 from 4 + 3 is significant in predicting the outcome of patients. However, margin status as well as the presence of EPE, are likewise important independent factors for predicting progression.

The study reported by the Mayo group [9] is based on 263 patients operated on for clinically localized cancer and diagnosed with Gleason score 7 after pathology examination. Prostates with Gleason score 4 + 3 were more likely than those with score 3 + 4 to have SV invasion (34% vs. 18%, $P = 0.006$), a higher pathologic stage (pT3, 55% vs. 41%, $P = 0.035$), node positivity (12% vs. 3%, $P = 0.047$), EPE (58% vs. 38%, $P = 0.001$), and higher median preoperative PSA (13.5 vs. 9.0 ng/ml, $P < 0.001$). Overall, by univariate analysis, the Gleason score 4 + 3 group was worse in the progression-free survival time than the Gleason score 3 + 4 group. After multivariate analysis, however, it was not an independent predictor of prognosis; only preoperative PSA ($P < 0.001$), SV invasion ($P < 0.001$), and DNA ploidy ($P = 0.002$) were associated with progression-free survival. Thus, the Mayo group concluded that Gleason scores 4 + 3 and 3 + 4 were different in regard to pathologic parameters and prognosis, but the primary Gleason pattern did not provide any additional information other than the other known prognostic factors listed above.

Lastly, Herman et al. [6] from Baylor College of Medicine reported on their experience based on 823 cases that included patients with SV and lymph node involvement (the number of pT2 and pT3a,b cases were not available). They reached the same conclusions as did the Mayo group: There was a significant difference between Gleason score 3 + 4 and 4 + 3 groups in terms of progression-free survival, but the

TABLE 1-7-1. Effect of Gleason score 3+4 versus 4+3 on various parameters including progression-free survival

Investigator groups	Total case no.	Organ confined (%)	EPE (%)	SM pos.	SV pos.	LN pos.	Tumor vol.	Follow-up (years) (mean)	Outcome progression-free survival	Additional comments
Sakr [8] (1991–1999), 2.0*	534[a]									
G3+4	356	178 (50%)	65 (18%)	95 (27%)	17 (5%)	1 (<1%)	**	2.9	$P = 0.021$ (organ-confined cases only, multivariate analysis	Two uropathologists reviewd.
4+3	178	59 (33%)	48 (27%)	31 (17%)	30 (17%)	10 (6%)	**			
		$P = 0.001$	$P = 0.001$	NS	NS	NS	$P = 0.003$			
Chan [7] (1982–1998), 4.1*	570[b]									
G3+4	458	162 (35%)	175[c] (38%)	NA	—	—	NA	4.0–4.6	Overall, $P < 0.0001$ Univariate analysis risk of metastasis, $P = 0.002$, independent of the SM status and extent of EPE	Supervised by a uropathologist Positive SM is also significant by multivariate analysis
4+3	112	36 (32%)	59 (53%)	NA	—	—	NA			
		$P = 0.001$	$P = 0.008$	NS						
Lau [9] (1986–1993), 2.0*	263[a]									
G3+4	174	97 (56%)	66 (38%)	74 (43%)	32 (18%)	5 (3%)	NA	7.1	$P = 0.02$, univariate analysis; NS by multivariate analysis	Supervised by a uropathologist Preoperative PSA, SV invasion, and tumor DNA ploidy are significant by multivariate analysis
4+3	89	29 (33%)	52 (58%)	43 (48%)	30 (34%)	11 (12%)	NA	6.7		
		$P = 0.001$	$P = 0.001$	NS	$P = 0.006$	$P = 0.047$				
Herman [6] (1983–1997), 3.6*	823[a]									
G3+4	643	321 (50%)	322 (50%)	133 (21%)	87 (14%)	38 (6%)	NA	2.7	$P < 0.001$, univariate analysis; NS by multivariate analysis	One pathologist reviewed Preoperative PSA, EPE, positive SM, and LN metastasis are all significant by multivariate analysis
4+3	180	56 (31%)	124 (69%)	45 (25%)	52 (29%)	25 (14%)	NA			
		$P = 0.001$	$P = 0.001$	NS	$P = 0.001$	$P = 0.001$				

EPE, extraprostatic extension; SM, surgical margin; SV, seminal vesicle; LN, lymph node.
[a] Cases showing seminal vesicle invasion and metastasis to lymph node included.
[b] Cases showing SV and lymph node involvement not included.
[c] So-called established extraprostatic extension (a greater degree of extension than focal extension) cases only considered.
* Gleason score 3+4/4+3 ratio.
**

	Tumor volume			
	0–2 ml	2–4 ml	4–10 ml	≧10 ml
G3+4	87 (24%)	126 (35%)	114 (32%)	29 (8%)
G4+3	31 (17%)	49 (28%)	77 (43%)	21 (11%)

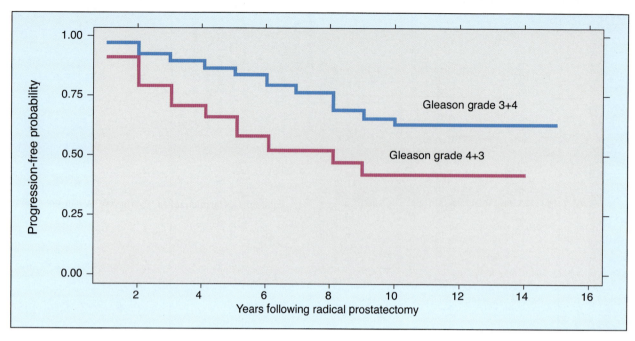

FIG. 1-7-1. Acturarial risk of progression in men with Gleason score 3 + 4 and 4 + 3 tumors without lymph node or seminal vesicle involvement. From Chan et al. [7], with permission

primary Gleason pattern was not an independent predictor with consideration of the preoperative PSA, SV invasion, lymph node metastasis, total tumor volume, and surgical margin status.

Most recently, Rubin et al. [10], based on a study of 1613 consecutive cases of radical prostatectomy conducted from 1994 to 2002, recommended that Gleason score 3 + 4 be separated from 4 + 3 because separation leads to a substantial improvement in staging accuracy (ROC curve = 0.817).[1]

Looking at data in Table 1-7-1, one notices some difference in the numbers of cases assigned to Gleason scores 3 + 4 and 4 + 3. The ratio varied from 2 to 4 (column 1). In each institution, cases were evaluated by one to several uropathologists or under the supervision of a uropathologist. The wide range in the ratio suggests either how difficult it is to assess volume ratio even in experts' hand or possibly it reflects the difference in diagnostic criteria and/or in patient population selected for prostatectomy. It is interesting to note that the wide range in the ratio did not affect the statistical comparison of pathologic par-

ameters on stage and surgical margin status. This suggests that dividing Gleason score 7 cases into two categories is effective for assessing pathologic parameters.

Gleason Score 3 + 4 Versus 4 + 3 on Prostate Needle Core Biopsy

The literature on Gleason 3 + 4 versus 4 + 3 on prostate needle core biopsy (PNB) specimens is scarce. One of the existing problems is how to assess pattern 3 and 4 among the cores involved with cancer (Fig. 1-7-2). Should one rely on the number of cores of each pattern? If the two patterns coexist in a single focus and in a blended fashion, how does one assess the percentage? Despite these potential difficulties, a comprehensive study was reported from the Johns Hopkins group. A total of 537 cases of Gleason score 7 on PNB evaluation was divided into 389 cases of 3 + 4 and 148 cases of 4 + 3 [4]. The overall ratio of the two patterns was then estimated. Other variables considered were preoperative PSA, the number of cores involved with cancer, age, and the digital rectal examination. These parameters were used to predict the pathologic findings in the radical prostatectomy specimens, including stage (organ-confined, focal and nonfocal EPE, SV/lymph node involvement), overall Gleason score, and surgical margin status. The patho-

---

[1] Receiver operating characteristics (ROC) is a statistical analysis method. The area under the ROC curve is an indication of the quality of a diagnostic test. The higher (close to 100%) the number is, the better is the test.

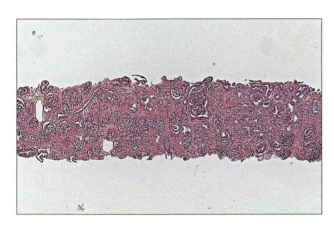

FIG. 1-7-2. Gleason score 4 + 3 adenocarcinoma on prostate needle core biopsy. This 3.8 × 0.8-mm cancer focus is predominantly composed of pattern 4 carcinoma (60%) and the rest is of pattern 3 carcinoma (40%). Note that both types exist in an intricate configuration, which makes assessment of pattern ratio difficult

logic stage correlated with the preoperative PSA ($P < 0.001$), Gleason score 4 + 3 disease ($P = 0.016$), positive digital rectal examination ($P < 0.001$), and three or more positive cores ($P = 0.016$). Positive surgical margins were predicted only by preoperative PSA ($P = 0.001$). Whether a tumor on biopsy is 3 + 4 or 4 + 3 is influential on the pathologic stage, even after accounting for the other clinical and pathologic parameters, including the number of cores involved. Thus, they concluded that future nomograms predicting pathologic stage would benefit from separating a Gleason score 4 + 3 group from a Gleason score 3 + 4 group.

Two conclusions may be drawn from these studies. First, Gleason score 4 + 3 cancer carries a worse prognosis than Gleason score 3 + 4 cancer primarily because the former is significantly associated with a higher frequency of SV and lymph node involvement, both of which are known predictors of a worse outcome. Thus, it is not an independent predictor. When comparison is limited to the cases free of SV/lymph node involvement, Gleason score 4 + 3 is a significant predictor of survival after PSA recurrence. For prostate needle core biopsy, dividing Gleason score 7 to 3 + 4 and 4 + 3 is useful for predicting the final Gleason score in the prostate but does not necessarily correlate well with Gleason 3 + 4 or Gleason 4 + 3 in the final diagnosis because of the sampling issue.

We believe that it is important to provide Gleason score 3 + 4 versus 4 + 3 on prostate needle core biopsy, TURP, and prostatectomy specimens. If assigned properly, the score provides useful information, and particularly suggests a risk of SV involvement and/or lymph node metastasis. However, further studies may be needed to determine the sensitivity and specificity of Gleason 3 + 4 versus Gleason 4 + 3 tumors on needle core biopsy.

References

1. Epstein JI, Carmichael M, Partin AW, Walsh PC (1993) Is tumor volume an independent predictor of progression following radical prostatectomy? A multivariate analysis of 185 clinical stage B adenocarcinoma of the prostate with 5 years of follow-up. J Urol 149: 1478–1481.
2. Epstein JI, Pizov G, Walsh PC (1993) Correlation of pathologic findings with progression after radical retropubic prostatectomy. Cancer 71:3582–3593.
3. Tefilli MV, Gheiler EL, Tiguert G, Sakr W, Grignon DJ, Banerjee M, Pontes JE, Wood DP (1999) Should Gleason score 7 prostate cancer be considered a unique grade category? Urology 53:372–377.
4. Makarov DV, Sanderson H, Partin AW, Epstein JI (2002) Gleason score 7 prostate cancer on needle biopsy: is the prognostic difference in Gleason score 4 + 3 and 3 + 4 independent of the number of involved cores? J Urol 167:2440–2442.
5. Gleason DF (1977) Histologic grading and clinical staging of prostate cancer. In: Tannenbaum M (ed) Urologic Pathology: The Prostate. Lea & Febiger, Philadelphia, pp 171–198.
6. Herman CM, Kattan MW, Ohori M, Scardino PT, Wheeler TM (2001) Primary Gleason pattern as a predictor of disease progression in Gleason score 7 prostate cancer: a multivariate analysis of 823 men treated with radical prostatectomy. Am J Surg Pathol 25: 657–660.
7. Chan TY, Partin AW, Walsh PC, Epstein JI (2000) Prognostic significance of Gleason score 3 + 4 versus Gleason score 4 + 3 tumor at radical prostatectomy. Urology 56:823–827.
8. Sakr WA, Tefilli MV, Grignon DJ, Banerjee M, Dey J, Gheiler El, Tiguert R, Powell IJ, Wood DP Jr (2000) Gleason score 7 prostate cancer: a heterogeneous entity? Correlation with pathologic parameters and disease-free survival. Urology 56:730–734.
9. Lau WK, Blute ML, Bostwick DG, Weaver AL, Sebo TJ, Zincke H (2001) Prognostic factor for survival of patients with pathological Gleason score 7 prostate cancer: difference in outcome between primary Gleason grades 3 and 4. J Urol 166:1692–1697.
10. Rubin MA, Dash A, Wei JY, Dunn R, Sanda MG (2004) Prostate cancer staging: recommendation for modifying pathology staging system based on accuracy in reflecting prognosis. Mod Pathol 17(suppl):174A.

Question 8

A positive surgical margin associated with an extraprostatic extension of prostate carcinoma is a significant risk for disease progression. What, then, is the risk of a positive margin created by an inadvertent surgical incision into cancerous prostate parenchyma?

Answer

In our daily practice there are several situations in which positive surgical margins are questioned. The first is a positive margin that has resulted because a tumor extending outside the prostate reaching the inked periprostatic tissue margin. A second situation is a positive margin created by an accidental surgical incision into cancerous prostate parenchyma. The third is an equivocal "positive" margin created when the surface of the pathology specimen had a disrupted appearance and the tumor reached the inked edge of the prostate. The third incidence may occur in association with either of the first two situations.

Several articles in the literature concluded that in case of clinically organ-confined disease, an inadvertently induced "capsular" incision without tumor or an inadvertent surgical incision into cancerous prostate parenchyma does not have a significant adverse effect on the clinical outcome. However, this conclusion requires further investigation simply because it was based on studies that utilized different specimen-submission techniques, varied diagnostic criteria, and relatively short follow-up periods.

Comments

A positive surgical margin is defined as neoplastic cells in contact with ink applied on the prostate external surface. To avoid the issue of "extracapsular" extension (refer to Question 1), the term "extraprostatic" extension (EPE) has been accepted at a recent consensus conference [1]. Extension of cancer beyond the edge, or "capsule," of the prostate is diagnostic of EPE [2]. According to the EPE concept, there are three circumstances in which EPE is to be considered: (1) cancer in adipose tissue (in any part of the periprostatic location); (2) cancer in fibromuscular tissue (in the anterior and basal parts); and (3) cancer in inked prostatic tissue (Fig. 1-8-1). The last margin is created when the surgeon opened a plane of resection within the prostate. Although this inadvertent separation of the plane could occur at any place, in practice it occurs almost exclusively at the apex, where a "capsule" is not clearly definable. At a recent consensus conference, participants agreed that these foci should be considered T2+ rather than T3 [2] because at these foci cancer may be outside the prostate. Because EPE occurs most frequently at the apex, it is highly desirable to determine the significance of an incision-induced positive margin.

In the study reported by Watson et al. [3], 215 patients with clinically localized carcinoma underwent a radical prostatectomy and lymph node dissection. The apex and bladder neck portions were amputated and sectioned perpendicular to the inked margin. The remainder of the specimen was serially sectioned and submitted at 2- to 3-mm intervals (Fig. 1-8-2A-1 and A-2). A positive surgical margin was defined as neoplastic cells in contact with ink. A positive surgical margin was observed in 73 patients. Progression occurred in 34% of margin-positive and 7% of margin-negative patients. Of 99 positive margin sites, 40 were

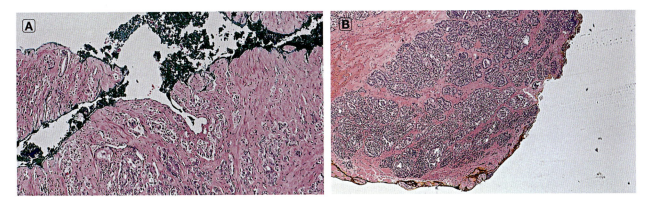

FIG. 1-8-1. **A** Medium-power view of a lateral margin in a prostatectomy specimen. It consists of smooth muscle bundles infiltrated by Gleason 4 + 3 carcinoma. There is no "capsular" tissue along the resection margin (*painted green*), and carcinomatous glands are exposed to the inked margin (iatrogenic positive margin). **B** Anterior apical margin positive for Gleason score 4 + 4 cancer. *Yellow dye* is attached to a carcinomatous gland

at the apex. In their study, an "equivocal" positive margin was synonymous with an incisional positive margin and was defined as "tumor cells in contact with ink in the absence of periprostatic tissue where a 'capsular' incision into the prostate could be identified." There were nine incision-induced positive margins, six of which involved the apex. Progression occurred in two of nine patients. Multivariate analysis of margin-positive patients identified tumor volume and Gleason score as the only significant predictors of progression.

Ohori et al. [4] from the Scardino group reported their experience based on 478 clinically localized cancer patients who underwent radical prostatectomy and lymph node dissection by one surgeon. The entire prostate was serially sectioned and submitted for examination. The transverse apical section was cut radially into pie-shaped pieces, which were sectioned longitudinally (Fig. 1-8-2B). One expert pathologist examined all of the cases. Excluding cases with lymph node metastasis or seminal vesicle (SV) invasion, 56 prostates had positive margins. If a positive surgical margin occurred in an area without periprostatic tissue, it was designated "a positive surgical margin in cancer confined to the prostate," indicating that the plane of dissection entered the prostatic "capsule" [5]. There were 23 such cases (sites not specified). None of these patients showed evidence of progression at 5 years compared to 41% of those with positive margins and "extracapsular" extension ($P < 0.03$). The data are impressive, but some concerns remain: (1) How do they know that patients with equivocal positive margins indeed have their

cancer confined to the prostate? (2) It is inappropriate to use the word "capsule" in the apical area where the capsule is not clearly defined. Although the sites of positive margin(s) were not specified, it is plausible that most of the incision-induced positive margins involved the apical area.

The study reported by the Mayo group [6] was based on 377 radical prostatectomy cases that were free from SV and lymph node involvement. The entire specimen was submitted. The apex and base were amputated and serially sectioned at 3- to 5-mm intervals in the vertical parasagittal plane (Fig. 1-8-2A-1). Instead of the word "extracapsular" extension, "extraprostatic" extension (EPE) was used when the tumor extended into extraprostatic tissue. In their study, a positive margin due to inadvertent incision into the prostate was defined as negative EPE/positive surgical margin (SM). Overall 109 cases had positive surgical margins (29%), and in 72 patients (19%) the positive margins were at the apex. The number of negative EPE/positive SM by sites is not available. The 5-year progression-free survival is shown in Table 1-8-1. The survival frequency of the negative EPE/positive SM group (surgical incision into parenchyma) was not significantly different from that of the negative EPE/negative SM group or the positive EPE/negative SM group. By overall comparison, however, there was a significant difference ($P < 0.001$) between the SM-positive groups and SM-negative groups. As in other studies, the negative EPE/positive SM group is an ill-defined group. It is uncertain how many of them are indeed organ-confined cases.

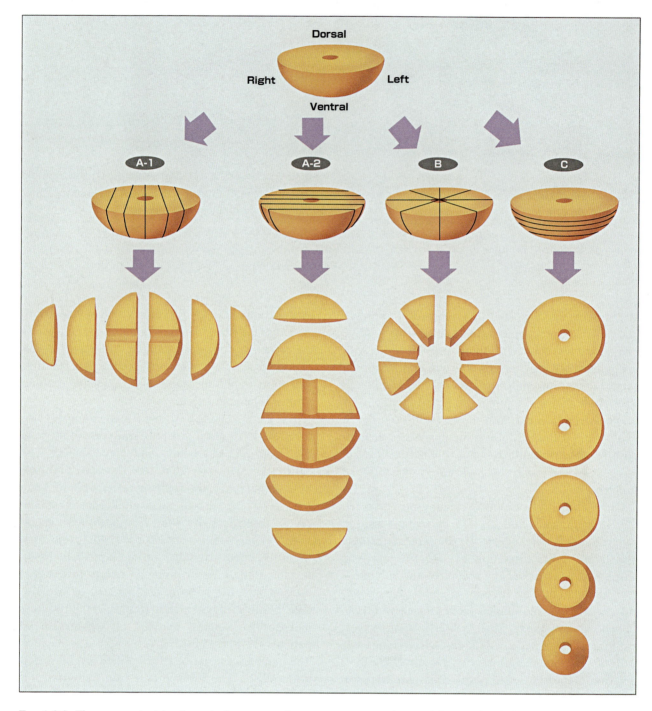

FIG. 1-8-2. Three ways to trim the apical segment of prostatectomy specimens. After cutting it into multiple pieces, the pieces are embedded sidewise with the side of interest down so that sections are taken from that side for histologic examination

The Johns Hopkins group has two reports related to incision-positive cases [7, 8]. "Capsular penetration" was defined as a tumor extending out of the prostate into the periprostatic soft tissue. Penetration was further divided into those cases in which only a few neoplastic glands were present exterior to the prostate (focal capsular extension) and cases with more extensive extraprostatic tumor spread (established capsular penetration). Equivocal margins of resection were diagnosed when the surface of the prostate had a disrupted appearance, and the tumor reached the inked edge of the prostate. In their

Table 1-8-1. 5-Year progression-free survival of 377 patients with various surgical margin status in radical prostatectomy specimens

Margin category	No.	5-Year progression-free survival (%)
EPE–/SM+	72 (19%)	78
EPE+/SM–	53 (14%)	90
EPE+/SM+	37 (10%)	55
EPE–/SM–	215 (57%)	90

Data from Cheng et al. [6].
EPE, extraprostatic extension; SM, surgical margin.

studies, the submission technique of the basal and apical portions is different from that of other groups; the thin shaved margins were taken as cross sections with the urethra running through the center (Fig. 1-8-2C). With this method, a positive circumferential margin can be defined readily when tumor cells are on the inked margins but the deep (very apical) margin cannot be assessed. Thus, the distal shave-margin was designated as positive if: (1) the distal margin showed only skeletal muscle without benign prostatic glands and contained any tumor; (2) the distal margin contained some nonneoplastic prostate glands and high-grade tumor of any quantity; and (3) the distal margin contained some nonneoplastic glands and extensive tumor of any grade. An equivocal positive margin was diagnosed when the distal margin showed nonneoplastic prostate glands and a small focus of low-grade adenocarcinoma. Margins were designated negative when the distal margin showed no evidence of tumor. This is an awkward way of examining margins.

Keeping this potential problem in mind, the study by Epstein et al. demonstrated that 42 of 507 prostates had an equivocal distal margin as the only positive margin. Patients with equivocal distal margin, as defined, were statistically neither different in their progression rate from those with negative or positive distal margins. Based on Kaplan-Meier curves, they suspected that patients with equivocal positive distal margins had a progression rate similar to that of patients with negative margins of resection. In contrast, 44 (9%) of the 507 men had equivocal "capsular" margins of resection at other sites. Here, patients with equivocal margins had progression rates similar to those with positive "capsular" margins. Patients with equivocal "capsular" margins had a significantly different progression rate compared to those with negative "capsular" margins ($P = 0.0072$). When pro-

gression was defined as local recurrence, patients with equivocal margins were again similar to those with positive margins and differed significantly from those with negative capsular margins ($P = 0.007$).

The study reported by Barocas et al. [8] of the same group is based on 92 patients selected from their file. These prostates were diagnosed with "capsular incision" (CI) in otherwise organ-confined carcinomas. CI was defined as an event that occurred in a prostate in which an iatrogenic incision was made during the operation, exposing benign or malignant glands to the inked surgical margin without evidence of extraprostatic extension or other extraprostatic disease. The sites of CI were not specified. The cases were matched one to one with prostate specimens, entirely organ-confined cases (E–M–), extraprostatic extension with negative surgical margins (E+M–), or positive surgical margins (E+M+). The actuarial 3-year likelihood of freedom from disease progression was 87.8% for the CI group, 96.4% for the E–M– group, 91.3% for the E+M– group, and 73.9% for the E+M+ group. Comparison between the CI and the E+M+ groups was significantly different ($P < 0.01$). No other comparisons with the CI group were statistically significant. Incision into benign versus malignant glands made no difference in the outcome. Barocas et al. concluded that patients with isolated CI have a significantly lower likelihood of early recurrence than patients with positive surgical margins due to extraprostatic extension regardless of whether the CI is into benign or malignant glands. Because their follow-up period was short (at least 6 months and a mean of 30 months), they cautioned that long-term follow-up is necessary to confirm the findings.

Discussion related to incisional positive margins has inherent problems. (1) By definition, it is likely that cancer-bearing prostate parenchyma remains with the patient. (2) No one is sure if the tumor has not made EPE. Despite these unsolved problems it is curious to know that patients in these studies do well, and their progression rate is no different from that of patients with organ-confined carcinoma. Does this mean that residual tumor cells were destroyed during the dissection procedure? Or does it mean that residual tumor remains dormant for a longer period of time than the tumor that has extended into periprostatic tissue? Or does the tumor residue after iatrogenic incision have a different biologic potential in a way that requires an extended period of follow-up before it manifests itself clinically? It is pertinent to point out that an incision-induced positive margin is most common at the apical area, where the "capsular" structure is ill-defined. Our unpublished study suggests that the "capsule" extends close to the apical end. If this observation is substantiated further, we must recommend that urologic surgeons revise their surgical approach and attempt to remove the prostate with an intact apical "capsular" structure. Only with such prostates can one determine the extent of cancer spread.

We need to touch briefly on the appropriate way to examine the apical margin for cancer (Fig. 1-8-2). As described above, there are three ways reported in the literature to prepare tissue for microscopic examination. None of them is perfect, and all carry some inherent problems. The most popular method is to cut the apical segment into multiple segments along either the parasagittal or frontal plane (Fig. 1-8-2A-1 and A-2). With this method, examination of the most lateral (or frontal/dorsal) segments may be inadequate. The second method is to cut the apical segment radially around the clock (Fig. 1-8-2B). This method is used to examine cervical cones from the uterus. Although theoretically it is the best method among the three, a potential technical problem is that the center portion of each piece (which represents the distal urethral margin) may not be adequately demonstrated in histology sections because the blocks are triangular. The problem can be avoided if all pieces are placed firmly, with the plane of interest down. Furthermore, the histology technician should be instructed not to trim the paraffin block aggressively, which might cause the urethral margin tissue to be lost. The third method is to embed the apical stump en bloc and take many serial sections for histologic examination (Fig. 1-8-2C). Unless exhaustive efforts are made on a routine basis, examination of the very apical margin could be inadequate. Each laboratory should select the method with which it is most comfortable.

Based on data reported in the literature, we conclude that an incisional positive margin does not appear to affect the prognosis adversely—which is a blessing to patients. However, a longer follow-up is needed to reach a definitive conclusion. When a wider excision and complete removal of the prostate apex becomes feasible, pathology examination will give us the final answer.

References

1. Sakr WA, Wheeler TM, Blute M, Bodo M, Callee-Rodrique R, Henson DE, Mostofi FK, Seiffert J, Wojno K, Zincke H (1996) International consultation on prostatic intraepithelial neoplasia and pathologic staging of prostate cancer; Work Group 2: staging and reporting of prostate cancer-sampling of radical prostatectomy specimen. Cancer 78:366–368.
2. Bostwick DG (1997) Staging prostate cancer—1997: current methods and limitation. Eur Urol 32(suppl): 2–14.
3. Watson RB, Civantos F, Soloway MS (1996) Positive margins with radical prostatectomy: detailed pathological analysis and prognosis. Urology 48:80–90.
4. Ohori M, Wheeler TM, Kattan MW, Goto Y, Scardino PT (1995) Prognostic significance of positive surgical margins in radical prostatectomy specimens. J Urol 154:1818–1824.
5. Rosen MA, Goldstone L, Lapin S, Wheeler T, Scardino PT (1992) Frequency and location of extracapsular extension and positive surgical margins in radical prostatectomy specimens. J Urol 148:331–337.
6. Cheng L, Darson MF, Bergstrahl EJ, Slezak J, Meyers RP, Bostwick DG (1999) Correlation of margin status and extraprostatic extension with progression of prostate cancer. Cancer 86:1775–1782.
7. Epstein JI, Pizov G, Walsh PC (1993) Correlation of pathologic findings with progression after radical retropubic prostatectomy. Cancer 71:3583–3593.
8. Barocas DA, Han M, Epstein JI, Chan DY, Trock BJ, Walsh PC, Partin AW (2001) Does capsular incision at radical retropubic prostatectomy affect disease-free survival in otherwise organ-confined prostate cancer? Urology 58:746–751.

Question 9

What are the neuroendocrine cells in prostate cancer? From where are these cells derived? What is the clinical implication of neuroendocrine differentiation in prostate cancer?

Answer

Neuroendocrine cells are the third type of prostatic epithelial cells in addition to secretory cells and basal cells in normal prostate glands. Neuroendocrine cells in prostate cancer are believed to derive from neuroendocrine cells or their stem precursors.

Prostate cancer with a neuroendocrine phenotype exists in two forms: (1) as a tumor composed entirely of neuroendocrine-type malignant cells; and (2) as a tumor that is a conventional-type cancer but has neuroendocrine-differentiated tumor cells as an integral component. The former encompasses small cell (neuroendocrine) carcinoma and large cell neuroendocrine carcinoma. Both of these tumors behave in an aggressive fashion. They are rare. It is more common to see a conventional-type prostate carcinoma that contains a variable number of neuroendocrine-type tumor cells. They may not readily be recognized in hematoxylin-eosin (H&E)-stained sections, but they can be identified by histochemical and immunohistochemical stainings for neuroendocrine markers.

The histogenesis and clinical significance of neuroendocrine cell differentiation remain controversial. Although neuroendocrine cell differentiation occurs in a majority of prostate carcinomas after hormonal therapy, the levels of differentiation vary markedly from patient to patient and even in a same individual among metastasis foci. Neuroendocrine cells may develop as a result of conversion of androgen receptor-negative/chromogranin-negative cells to androgen-receptor negative/chromogranin-positive cells. Though a paracrine role has been suggested for neuroendocrine cells, it is minor at best in our view. Some other mechanisms must be involved in supporting growth of androgen-independent prostate cancer cells.

Comments

The number of neuroendocrine (NE) cells in conventional adenocarcinoma may increase after hormone ablation therapy. This may be due to conversion of androgen receptor-negative tumor subclones to cells expressing the NE phenotype. The prognostic significance of NE cell differentiation has been controversial. Some studies suggest a poor prognosis, whereas others do not. A recent autopsy study based on patients dying after hormonal ablation therapy demonstrated that NE cell differentiation at metastases varies widely among patients and among metastatic bone sites [1], indicating that a paracrine stimulatory role on nonendocrine carcinoma cells may exist but is minor at best. Available data suggest that androgen-independent growth is supported by some other mechanism(s).

There is a variant that is a composite tumor made up of a conventional adenocarcinoma component and a small cell carcinoma component in the primary and/or metastasis sites. This variant may also occur sequentially in time with the initial pattern of a conventional carcinoma and with recurrence as a NE carcinoma. This variant has biologic potential similar to that of a pure NE (small cell) carcinoma.

What are prostatic neuroendocrine cells?

In addition to secretory (columnar) cells and basal cells, NE cells represent the third epithelial cell type in normal prostatic glands. A subpopulation of cells known by various names—endocrine/paracrine (EP) cells, NE cells, amine-precursor-uptake-and-decarboxylation (APUD) cells—has been known to exist in the prostate since the 1940s [2]. Their presence was identified initially by silver stains (argyrophil and argentaffin stains) and more recently by immunohistochemical methods. They are found not only in normal glands but also in benign prostatic hyperplasia and most adenocarcinomas. The prostatic NE cells have been discussed in a review by Taupenot et al. [3].

The NE cells in prostate adenocarcinoma have recently attracted considerable interest in light of the suggestion that tumors exhibiting marked NE differentiation may survive androgen deprivation therapy. Literature suggests a link between NE differentiation, tumor progression, and androgen-independent prostatic cancer growth [4, 5].

Where are neuroendocrine cells located in the normal prostate?

Most NE cells are basally oriented and scattered in the epithelium of the acini and ducts (Fig. 1-9-1). They may be more abundant in the ducts than in acini [6–8]. There are two types. The first is the "closed" type. The cells of this type do not have a luminal border. Many of them have multiple dendritic processes extending between nearby epithelial cells (Fig. 1-9-1B, arrow). A few cells are of the "open" type,

reaching the luminal surface. NE cells are more numerous in normal or atrophic prostates than in hyperplastic nodules [2]. Electron microscopy reveals these cells to contain numerous granules of various sizes and shapes [2, 9].

What is the function of normal neuroendocrine cells?

The most predominant product of NE cells is chromogranin A (chrA). It is a member of a family of acidic secretory proteins found in the secretory granules of a wide variety of endocrine cells and neurons. It is stored together with many different peptide hormones and neuropeptides [5]. Chromogranin A is a prehormone, giving rise to bioactive peptides as a result of proteolytic processing by endopeptidases; and it has autocrine, paracrine, and endocrine activities. Other secretory products commonly associated with prostatic NE cells are serotonin (5-hydroxytryptamine, a biogenic amine derived from trytophan) and neuron-specific enolase (an isoenzyme of the glycolytic enzyme enolase). The function of NE cells is unknown; but by analogy to the function of NE cells in the respiratory and gastrointestinal systems and the pancreas, they appear to be essential for growth, differentiation, and homeostatic regulation of the secretory processes in the prostate [5].

What are precursors of neuroendocrine cells in the prostate?

Before answering this question, it is necessary to touch on the histogenesis of prostate epithelial cells. According to the hypothesis proposed by the

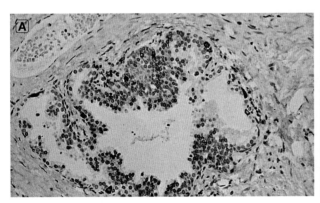 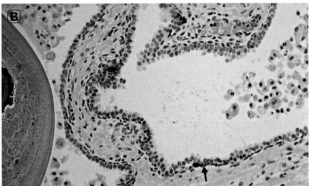

FIG. 1-9-1. **A, B** Chromogranin A (chrA)-positive cells scattered within normal prostatic acini. Most of them are located adjacent to the basal cell layer and between basal cells and secretory columnar cells. Note a dendritic chrA-positive cell (*arrow*) in **B**

Bonkhoff group [10], Xue et al. [11], and Isaacs and Coffey [12], NE cells are derived from the stem cell population residing in the basal cell layer through the stage of an intermediate cell. The hypothesis postulates the existence of at least three cell types, although the names assigned vary among investigators. According to Bonkhoff and Remberger [10], they are stem cells, intermediate cells, and luminal cells. Their presence is suggested by sequential expression of various markers: androgen receptor (AR); cytokeratins 5, 8, 14, and 18 [11, 13, 14]; prostate-specific antigen (PSA); and proliferation-associated markers (Ki-67, PCNA, MIB-1). In the model proposed by Bonkhoff and Remberger, the basal cell layer contains a small stem cell population that gives rise to all epithelial cell lineages via intermediate phenotypes. The prostate epithelium is composed of two functional compartments [10, 15]. The first is a proliferative compartment localized in the basal cell layer; it is androgen-independent but contains androgen-responsive cells. The differentiating process from basal cells to secretory luminal cells via intermediate phenotypes is induced by circulating androgens and largely depends on the presence of androgen-responsive cells in the basal layer. The second compartment is secretory (columnar) cells that express AR and PSA consistently.

The NE cells in general do not express AR (except in the report by Nakada et al. [16]). This indicates that they are derived from AR-negative cells in the proliferative cell compartment [17]. NE cells generally do not express PSA [18] but do express the columnar cell-type cytokeratin (CK18) more frequently (91%) than the basal cell marker 34βE12 (20%) [11]. Therefore, available data indicate that they are derived from an AR-negative basal cell population retaining some features of, but distinct from, the secretory cells. However, to complicate the discussion, there is a minor population of cells that exhibit hybrid features of NE cells and secretory cells (chrA+/PSA+) [18]. Evidence of synchronous expression of exocrine (PSA+) and endocrine (chrA+) markers in subsets indicates a high degree of phenotypic plasticity exhibited by basal cells and provides a support to the hypothesis by Bonkhoff and Remberger that basal cells give rise to all epithelial cell lineages of the human prostate; the differentiation pathway from basal cells to secretory columnar cells is an androgen-dependent process (mediated by AR-positive basal cells) and the pathway to NE cells is mediated by AR-negative cells present in the basal layer [17, 19]. Using a double-labeling technique, Xue et al. [11, 14] reached the same conclusion by demonstrating that NE cells and secretory cells share a common keratin phenotype. By immunostaining for proliferation markers, NE cells are terminally differentiated cells (i.e., unable to divide) [10, 20].

Based on these studies, a cell differentiation model is depicted in Fig. 1-9-2, and key marker expressions by the normal gland and adenocarcinoma are shown in Table 1-9-1.

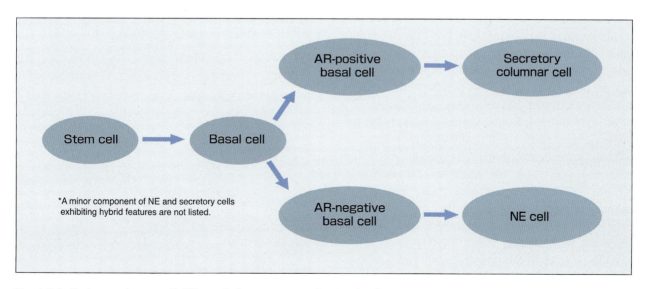

FIG. 1-9-2. Pathway of stem cell differentiation to neuroendocrine (*NE*) and secretory cells in normal prostate

TABLE 1-9-1. Major markers expressed by columnar, basal, and NE cells in normal prostate gland and adenocarcinoma

Cell type	AR	34β 12E (basal)	CK18 (secretory)	PSA (secretory)	chrA (neuroendocrine)
Normal gland					
Secretory cell	+	−	+	+	−
Basal cell	+/−	+	−	−	−
NE cells	−	−/+	+/−	−	+
Adenocarcinoma					
Most cells	+	−	+	+	−
Few cells I (non-NE cells)	−	−	+	−	−
Few cells II (NE cells)	−	−	+/−	−	+

AR, androgen receptor; chrA, chromogranin A; PSA, prostate-specific antigen; NE, neuroendocrine.

What is the histogenesis of neuroendocrine cells in prostate cancer?

Neuroendocrine cell differentiation is a common feature in prostate carcinoma, occurring in 30%–100% of tumors studied [5]. The number of NE cells in prostatic adenocarcinoma varies from case to case. Some may not show any differentiation (Fig. 1-9-3), whereas others exhibit a few scattered cells (Fig. 1-9-4) or many (Fig. 1-9-5). NE cell differentiation is independent of the Gleason pattern.

NE cells exist more commonly as scattered individual cells than as clusters among a predominant population of non-NE malignant cells [21]. Contradictory results have been reported on whether NE cells increase after hormonal therapy or in advanced-stage prostatic carcinomas. Because this issue is relevant to the discussion on NE cell effects on prognosis, it is discussed first.

The best marker of NE cell differentiation is chrA followed by serotonin. According to Aprikian et al. [22] of Memorial Sloan-Kettering Cancer Center, chrA is expressed in most NE cells when tested by a combination of various markers. It is expressed more intensely and frequently than other markers. NE cells in tumors are found typically dispersed throughout the tumor, and no specific pattern of distribution could be identified. NE cells were identified in 77% of primary untreated adenocarcinomas, and the frequency did not differ significantly by pathologic stage. NE cells were identified in 7 of 11 lymph node metastases and 2 of 5 bone metastases examined. No significant differences in frequency were noted from primary tumors. Androgen ablation therapy did not appear to increase or decrease NE cell numbers according to this study.

Ahlgren et al. of the Abrahamsson group, in contrast, reported different observations. They examined the effect of 3 months of neoadjuvant therapy prior to radical prostatectomy on NE cell appear-

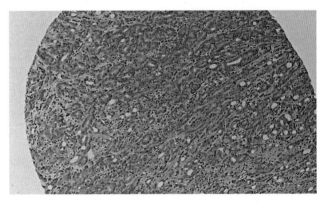

FIG. 1-9-3. Adenocarcinoma of the prostate without NE cell differentiation (chrA stain)

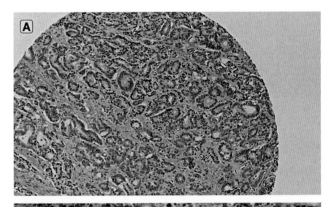

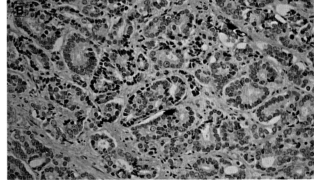

FIG. 1-9-4. **A, B** Adenocarcinoma of prostate with a few scattered chrA-positive cells

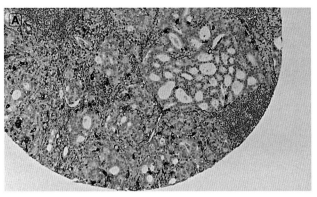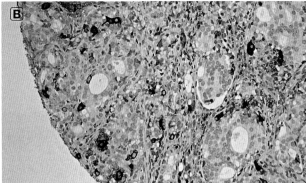

FIG. 1-9-5. **A, B** Metastatic prostate carcinoma in lymph node with numerous chrA-positive cells. Note that positively stained cells are scattered without clustering

ance. Both the number of chrA-positive cells/cm^2 tumor area ($P < 0.003$) and the proportion of NE-positive tumors ($P = 0.07$) were greater in the neoadjuvant group than in the control group. However, they observed no correlation between NE cell differentiation and the histologic degree of the hormone treatment effect.

Jibron et al. [23] from the same Abrahamsson group examined the effects of androgen ablation (by orchiectomy or hormonal treatment) on advanced-stage carcinomas by repeated biopsies (two to four per patient). All 53 cases contained chrA+ cells at varying degrees. A total of 21 carcinomas (40%) displayed increased NE cell differentiation concomitant with the progression in histologic grade, whereas 29 carcinomas (55%) showed no change in their NE cell differentiation status. However, most of the histologically unchanged tumors had many NE cells in the first transurethral resection of the prostate specimens. They concluded that androgen ablation therapy may, with time, contribute to the increase in NE differentiation.

At this point, we discuss some in vivo studies in animal models. The androgen-dependent human prostate cancer xenograft PC-310 contains cells expressing the NE phenotype. Therefore, it is a suitable model for studying the mechanism of NE cell development after androgen withdrawal [24]. Following castration the tumor mass shrank quickly within several days, apparently due to apoptotic loss of androgen-dependent cells [25]. At the same time, however, there was a sharp rise in chrA mRNA in the remaining tumor mass associated with an increase in chrA-positive cells reaching the peak 14 days after castration. This occurred without evidence of active cell proliferation. By 21 days after castration, the tumor volume was down to 30%–40% of the original. An immunohistochemical double-labeling study of the resected tumors revealed that approximately 50% of tumor cells were AR+/chrA–, and the rest were AR–/chrA+. Based on these results, they concluded that part of the initially androgen-dependent tumor cells (AR+) differentiated into NE cells after androgen withdrawal. This conclusion was reached because the increase in NE cells was not accompanied by evidence of active cell replication. They further concluded that the remaining cancer cells are surviving as androgen-sensitive (AR+/chrA–) cells in an androgen-deprived environment and could become androgen-independent after extended androgen depletion. Unfortunately, the study was terminated at 21 days. Inevitable questions arise from this report. (1) What would be the makeup of the subsequent regrowth of the xenograft? With time, do AR+/chrA– cells increase and make up the bulk of the regrowth accompanied by a relative decrease in AR–/chrA+ cells? (2) They postulated that the AR–/chrA+ cells originate from AR+/chrA– cells, but no data were provided to support their contention. It is difficult for us to accept that androgen withdrawal silenced *AR* gene expression in AR-positive cells, as *AR* gene expression is not known to be under the control of androgen. Thus, it must be concluded that the AR–/chrA+ phenotype has occurred (by an unknown mechanism) by conversion of AR–/chrA– cells (without cell proliferation). An important message from this study is that androgen withdrawal is followed by an increase in the NE cell phenotype. It is unknown if this is transient or what would become of the makeup in the subsequently regrown xenograft.

By this time, readers may be confused regarding whether endocrine therapy results in an increase in NE cells. We believe that endocrine therapy may elevate the NE cell number by two mechanisms: an apparent increase due (1) to the loss of nonendocrine androgen-dependent cells; and (2) to an actual increase by conversion of the AR–/chrA– phenotype to the AR–/chrA+ phenotype (when androgen support is removed) [25]. However, the rise in NE cells may be transient, and the NE cell/nonendocrine cell ratio will eventually be determined by the inherent ability of the tumor to induce NE cells. Our reasoning is based on the following observations: (1) Various groups have reported that NE cells are dispersed diffusely among nonendocrine carcinoma cells both before and after hormonal therapy except for a small number of high-grade carcinomas in which NE cells may occur in clusters. This suggests that NE-differentiated cells in general do not replicate. Bonkhoff demonstrated that NE cells lack markers of cell proliferations, such as Ki-67 and MIB-1 [10, 20]. (2) NE cells are also found in metastatic foci and again in dispersed fashion. This suggests that carcinoma cells, irrespective of the sites of growth, are capable of inducing NE cell differentiation [22] albeit limited.

The histogenesis of neoplastic NE cells has not been clarified. Most NE cells are reportedly AR-negative, and unequivocal expression of AR by NE cells is rare in prostate carcinoma regardless of whether it is treated [17]. This implies that (1) the AR–/chrA+ subclone(s) is inherently present in a prostate tumor mass, and (2) conversion of the AR–/chrA– subclone(s) to the AR–/chrA+ phenotype [25] is either induced spontaneously or after androgen withdrawal. We believe the latter is more likely inasmuch as NE cells, either normal or neoplastic, are reportedly terminally differentiated [20].

What is the clinical significance of neuroendocrine cell differentiation in prostate cancer? Does the presence of these cells affect prognosis adversely?

There are two opposing views reported in the literature. Adverse effects of NE cell differentiation on survival were reported by several groups, and the results are tabulated in Table 1-9-2A. Reports on the opposing view are summarized in Table 1-9-2B. The reports by Cohen et al. [26] and Glezerson et al. [27] are from the same group. Clinical information is poorly described in these papers. However, most of the patients were in an advanced stage and were treated with either radiation or hormone. They concluded that there was a significant correlation between the (prolonged) survival and the absence of NE cells ($P < 0.0001$). The study by McWilliams et al. [28] was unique in that patients ranging from clinical stages T1a and T1b to T3, including 19 M1 patients were followed without treatment other than palliative TURP to relieve obstructive symptoms. They concluded that the worse outcome significantly correlated with tumor grade, presence of NE cells, and bone metastasis at presentation. However, the presence of NE cells was not an independent marker of prognosis. The patients reported by Krijnen et al. [29] were initially at clinical stages T1b, T2, T3, and T4. After the diagnosis was established by transurethral resection, all patients received hormonal therapy. The investigators concluded that the Gleason score ($P = 0.005$) and NE cells/mm^2 tumor area ($P = 0.022$) were independent predictors of disease progression.

Of the four articles reporting negative correlation between NE cell differentiation and worse outcomes, two [22, 30] are based on patients in advanced stages treated with hormonal therapy, whereas the other two [8, 31] are based on patients in early clinical stages and treated by radical prostatectomy.

What seem to be the factors leading to the opposing conclusions? It is difficult to reconcile. Recently, an autopsy study on patients who died of prostate cancer was reported from the University of Washington [1]. It was based on immediate autopsies (within 4h after death) of 14 patients. The median survival after androgen independence was 1 year (ranging from 1 month to 3.6 years). Up to 20 bone sites were systematically sampled in each patient. Although more than 70% of tumor cells expressed PSA immunohistochemically, the fraction of PSA-positive cells varied widely in separate metastatic sites. Likewise, the fraction of NE cells (chrA) varied widely by bone sites. For example, in one patient the fraction of chrA+ cells varied from 0 to 95% of tumor cells. This study clearly demonstrated marked heterogeneity in terms of histology and immunophenotype of metastatic prostate carcinoma. This autopsy finding was also associated with a wide range in terminal serum PSA values ranging from 18 to 7402 ng/ml. The marked variation in the frequency in chrA+ cells at various bone sites (0%–100%) seems to indicate that NE cell differentiation is not a universally inevitable

TABLE 1-9-2A. NE cell differentiation is correlated with worse outcome

Investigator	Year reported	No. cases	Diagnosed by and treated with	Cancer status at presentation	Marker used	Criteria for NE cell differentiation	Frequency of NE cell-positive cases	Follow-up period	Conclusions	Comments
Cohen [26]	1991	31	TUR, hormone, or irradiation	Stage B, C, or D	chrA, NSE	Present or absent	52%	7 Years	A significant correlation between survival and absence of NE cells ($P < 0.0001$)	Clinical information insufficient Patients in stages B, C or D, without further detail
Glezerson [27] (Cohen group as above)	1991	82	Not stated	"Advanced" stage	chrA, NSE	Present or absent	50%	>5 Years	Highly significant correlation between survival and absence of NE cells ($P < 0.0001$)	Not a full length report (abstract) No detailed description
McWilliams [28]	1997	92	TUR or PNB No treatment other than TUR to relieve obstructive symptoms	M0 = 73 T1a + b, 2, and 3, M1 = 19	chrA, NSE	Positive if >10% of tumor cells stained for NE marker	52%	>132 Months	Outcome significantly correlated to tumor grade ($P = 0.005$), NE positivity ($P = 0.036$), and bone metastasis ($P < 0.001$) at presentation. NE positivity, however, not an independent marker	
Krijnen [29]	1997	72	TUR, hormonal treatment	Stage T1b (12), T2 (3), T3 (36) and T4 (21)	chrA	NE cells present/ mm^2 tumor area	55%		Gleason score ($P = 0.005$) and scattered NE cells/mm^2 ($P = 0.022$) are independent predictors of disease progression	

chrA, chromogranin A; NSE, neuron-specific enolase; TUR, transurethral resection; PNB, prastate needle core biopsy; NE, neuroendocrine.

TABLE 1-9-2B. NE cell differentiation is not correlated with worse outcome

Investigator	Year reported	No. cases	Diagnosed by and treated with	Cancer status at presentation	Marker used	Criteria for NE cell differentiation	Frequency of NE cell-positive cases	Follow-up period	Conclusions	Comments
Paul [30]	1993	53	TUR and PNB, hormonal treatment for all	Stage D1 (4) Stage D2 (49)	chrA, NSE, serotonin	Absent or present	49%	Until death, >5 years	NE cell differentiation has no significance on survival	Report in abstract form. All cases in advanced stages and treated with hormonal therapy
Aprikian [22]	1994	41	Metastasis in lymph node (41) and bone (21) All treated with hormonal therapy once bone involved	Stage D1 (N+, M0)	chrA	Absent or present	46%	Median 61 months	No significant difference in median estimated disease-specific survival	chrA-positive cells coexpress PSA
Cohen [31]	1994	38	Radical prostatectomy	cT2, node-positive and seminal vesicle-positive cases excluded	chrA	4-Tier system (−,+,++,+++)	29%	7 Years (at least 4 years)	NE cell differentiation does not predict progression in clinical stage B patients	Strength: all in clinical stage B; two pathologists blinded examined Weakness: staining criteria difficult to follow
Noordzij [8]	1995	90	Radical prostatectomy	cT1-3, node-positive cases not included	chrA	5-Tier system (−,±,+,++,+++) chrA scores used	78%	Mean 86 months	chrA scores have no prognostic value Gleason score and pT stage are independent prognostic factors for progression	chrA scores not related to Gleason score or TNM classification

consequence of hormonal therapy but, rather, can be seen as a marker of a carcinoma of androgen independence. They found no correlation between the average percentage of NE cells in the metastasis and survival.

The article cited above strongly suggests that different conclusions on the effect of NE cell differentiation on the outcome (Tables 9-2A,B) may be due to sampling of specimens on which they drew their conclusions.

Based on the above studies, we conclude as follows: (1) NE cell differentiation occurs in most prostate carcinomas after hormonal therapy and is unrelated to the Gleason score [8, 22, 29, 32]. (2) The levels of NE cell differentiation observed after hormonal therapy may vary among subclones. In some subclones, NE cells may develop as a result of conversion of AR–/chrA– to AR–/chrA+ phenotype. (3) NE cells may have a growth-stimulatory paracrine role on non-NE (androgen-independent) carcinoma cells. The haphazard expression of NE phenotype suggests that some other mechanism(s) must operate in supporting androgen-independent growth. Data from our previous study indicate that one of mechanisms is the activation of hepatocyte growth factor/c-met signal [33, 34]. An immunohistochemical study on the advanced-stage prostate carcinomas showed expression of c-met and its ligand, hepatocyte growth factor at high frequency [35]. (4) Although NE cells may play a minor role in support of the growth of androgen-independent prostate carcinomas, they nevertheless may serve as markers of presence of androgen-independent prostate cancer. Clinically, these patients can be monitored by their chrA serum levels.

References

1. Roudier MP, True LD, Higano CS, Vesselle H, Ellis W, Lange P, Vessella RL (2003) Phenotypic heterogeneity of end-stage prostate carcinoma metastatic to bone. Hum Pathol 34:646–653.
2. Di Sant'Agnese PA, de Mesy Jensen KL (1984) Endocrine-paracrine cells of the prostate: an ultrastructural study. Hum Pathol 15:1034–1044.
3. Taupenot L, Harper KL, OConner DT (2003) Mechanisms of disease: the chromogranin-secretogranin family. N Engl J Med 348:1134–1149.
4. Kadmon D, Thompson TC, Lynch GR, Scardino PT (1991) Elevated plasma chromogranin-A concentration in prostatic carcinoma. J Urol 146:358–361.
5. Abrahamsson, P-A (1999) Neuroendocrine differentiation in prostatic carcinoma. Prostate 39:135–148.
6. Di Sant'Agnese PA, de Mesy Jensen KL, Chrukian CJ, Agarwal MK (1985) Human prostatic endocrine-paracrine (APUD) cells. Arch Pathol Lab Med 109:607–612.
7. Di Sant'Agnese PA (1995) Neuroendocrine differentiation in prostatic carcinoma. Cancer (suppl) 75:1850–1859.
8. Noordzij MA, van der Kwast TH, van Steenbrugge GJ, Hop WJC, Schroeder FH (1995) The prognostic influence of neuroendocrine cells in prostate cancer: results of a long-term follow-up study with patients treated with radical prostatectomy. Int J Cancer 62:252–258.
9. Di Sant'Agnese PA (1992) Neuroendocrine differentiation in carcinoma of the prostate. Cancer 70:254–268.
10. Bonkhoff H, Remberger K (1996) Differentiation pathways and histogenetic aspects of normal and abnormal prostatic growth: a stem cell model. Prostate 28:98–106.
11. Xue Y, Verhofstad A, Lange W, Smedts F, Debruyne F, de la Rossette J, Schalkan J (1997) Prostate neuroendocrine cells have a unique keratin expression pattern and do not express Bcl-2. Am J Pathol 151:1759–1765.
12. Isaacs JT, Coffey DS (1989) Etiology and disease process of benign prostatic hyperplasia. Prostate 2(suppl):33–50.
13. Verhagen APM, Raemaker FCS, Aalders TW, Shaafsma HE, Debruyne MJ, Schalken JA (1992) Colocalization of basal and luminal cell-type cytokeratins in human prostate cancer. Cancer Res 52:6182–6187.
14. Xue Y, Smedt F, Debruyne FMJ, de la Rosette JJMDH, Shalkan J (1998) Identification of intermediate cell types by keratin expression in the developing human prostate. Prostate 34:292–301.
15. Bonkhoff H, Stein U, Remberger K (1994) The proliferative function of basal cells in the normal and hyperplastic human prostate. Prostate 24:114–118.
16. Nakada SY, di Sant'Agnese PA, Moynes RA, Hiipakka RA, Liao S, Cockett TK, Abrahamsson P-A (1993) The androgen receptor status of neuroendocrine cells in human benign and malignant prostatic tissue. Cancer Res 53:1967–1970.
17. Bonkhoff H, Stein U, Remberger K (1993) Androgen receptor status in endocrine-paracrine cell types of the normal, hyperplastic, and neoplastic human prostate. Virchows Arch A Pathol Anat 423:291–294.
18. Bonkhoff H, Stein U, Remberger K (1994) Multidirectional differentiation in the normal, hyperplastic, and neoplastic human prostate: simultaneous demonstration of cell-specific epithelial markers. Hum Pathol 25:42–46.
19. Bonkhoff H, Remberger K (1993) Widespread distribution of nuclear androgen receptors in the basal layer of the normal and hyperplastic human prostate. Virchows Arch A Pathol Anat 422:35–38.

20. Bonkhoff H, Wernert N, Dhom G, Remberger K (1991) Relation of endocrine-paracrine cells to cell proliferation in normal, hyperplastic, and neoplastic human prostate. Prostate 19:91–98.

21. Ahlgren G, Pedersen K, Aus G, Hugosson J, Abahamsson P-A (2000) Progressive changes and neuroendocrine differentiation in prostate cancer after neoadjuvant hormonal treatment. Prostate 42:274–279.

22. Aprikian AG, Cordon-Cardo C, Fair WR, Zhang Z-F, Bezinet M, Hamdy SF, Reuter VE (1994) Neuroendocrine differentiation in metastatic prostatic carcinoma. J Urol 151:914–919.

23. Jibron T, Bjartell A, Abrahamsson P-A (1998) Neuroendocrine differentiation in prostatic carcinoma during hormonal treatment. Urology 51:585–589.

24. Jongsma J, Oomen MH, Noordzij MA, Van Weerden WM, Martens GJM, van der Kwast TH, Schroeder FH, van Steenbrugge GJ (1999) Kinetics of neuroendocrine differentiation in an androgen-dependent human prostate xenograft model. Am J Pathol 154:543–551.

25. Jongsma J, Oomen MH, Noordzij MA, Van Weerden WM, Martens GJM, van der Kwast TH, Schroeder FH, van Steenbrugge GJ (2000) Androgen deprivation of the pro-hormone convertase-310 human prostate cancer model system induces neuroendocrine differentiation. Cancer Res 60:741–748.

26. Cohen RJ, Glezerson G, Haffejee Z (1991) Neuroendocrine cells: a new prognostic parameter in prostate cancer. Br J Urol 68:258–262.

27. Glezerson G, Cohen RJ (1991) Prognostic value of neuroendocrine cells in prostatic adenocarcinoma. J Urol 145(suppl):296A.

28. McWilliams LJ, Manson C, George NJR (1997) Neuroendocrine differentiation and prognosis in prostatic adenocarcinoma. Br J Urol 80:287–290.

29. Krijnen JL, Bogdanowicz JAFT, Seldenrijk CA, Mulder PGH, van der Kwast TH (1997) The prognostic value of neuroendocrine differentiation in adenocarcinoma of the prostate in relation to progression of disease after endocrine therapy. J Urol 158:171–174.

30. Paul R, Chang P, di Sant'Agnese PA, Cockett TK, Abrahamsson P-A (1993) Prognostic significance of neuroendocrine differentiation in biopsy specimens from patients with metastatic prostate cancer. J Urol 149(suppl):480A.

31. Cohen MK, Arber DA, Coffield S, Keegan GT, McCLintock J, Speights Jr VO (1994) Neuroendocrine differentiation in prostate adenocarcinoma and its relationship to tumor progression. Cancer 74:1899–1903.

32. Bubendorf L, Sauter G, Moch H, Schmid HP, Gasser TC, Jordan P, Miihatch MJ (1996) Ki67 labelling index: an independent predictor of progression in prostate cancer treated by radical prostatectomy. J Pathol 178:437–441.

33. Nakashiro K, Okamoto M, Hayashi Y, Oyasu R (2000) Hepatocyte growth factor secreted by prostate-derived stromal cells stimulates growth of androgen-independent human prostatic carcinoma cells. Am J Pathol 157:795–803.

34. Nakashiro K, Hara S, Shinohara Y, Oyasu M, Kawamata H, Shintani S, Hamakawa H, Oyasu R (2004) Phenotypic switch from paracrine to autocrine role of hepatocyte growth factor in an androgen-independent human prostatic carcinoma cell line, CWR22R. Am J Pathol 165:533–540.

35. Humphrey PA, Zhu X, Zarnegar R, Swanson PE, Ratliff TL, Vollmer RT, Day ML (1995) Hepatocyte growth factor and its receptor (c-MET) in prostatic carcinoma. Am J Pathol 147:386–396.

Question 10

What is prostatic ductal adenocarcinoma? How is it clinically and pathologically different from the conventional (acinar) adenocarcinoma?

Answer

Most adenocarcinomas of the prostate are composed of cuboidal cells characteristic of prostate acini. Therefore, they are defined as acinar adenocarcinoma. Prostate adenocarcinoma characterized by tall columnar cells resembling prostatic ductal cells is defined as ductal adenocarcinoma. Tumor cells are arranged in papillary, complex glandular (cribriform), comedo or solid architectures. Ductal adenocarcinomas usually behave more aggressively than acinar-type adenocarcinoma. They may be periurethral in location and present with hematuria and obstructive symptoms. Ductal adenocarcinoma may occur peripherally without obstructive symptoms and be discovered by prostate needle core biopsy performed for elevated prostate-specific antigen (PSA) levels.

Comments

Prostatic ductal adenocarcinoma is a distinct morphologic variant of prostatic adenocarcinoma. It was originally described by Melicow and Pachter [1] as endometrioid adenocarcinoma of the prostate. These authors suggested that the tumors were from the Müllerian (female) remnant, the utriculus masculinus. However, subsequent studies using immunohistochemical technique have decisively determined that ductal adenocarcinoma is a histologic variant of adenocarcinoma of the prostate. Ductal adenocarcinoma is rare, accounting for 0.2%–0.8% of prostate adenocarcinomas [2, 3].

What is ductal adenocarcinoma of the prostate, and where is it located in the prostate?

Ductal adenocarcinoma is characterized by tall columnar cells with abundant cytoplasm. The tumor cells often display amphophilic cytoplasm and form a pseudostratified layer resembling endometrial adenocarcinoma [4].

Unlike acinar adenocarcinoma, which is mostly peripheral in location, most of reported ductal adenocarcinomas are central and are distributed around the prostatic urethra. Back in the early 1970s, Dube et al. [5] from the Mayo Clinic reported a large series of adenocarcinomas of ductal type. After reviewing 4286 cases of prostatic adenocarcinoma (1950–1970), they were divided into three groups: group 1, ordinary acinar adenocarcinomas; group 2, pure ductal adenocarcinomas (55 cases, or 1.3%); and group 3, mixed acinar and ductal adenocarcinomas (207 cases, or 4.8%). The ductal adenocarcinomas were divided into two subgroups: adenocarcinoma of the primary prostatic ducts (major ducts draining into the prostatic urethra) and adenocarcinoma of the secondary prostatic ducts (duct portions more distal to primary ducts) depending on the primary site of growth. Most of these studies, however, were based on transurethral resection material before the radical prostatectomy era. Therefore, the tumors in the peripheral zone may not have been represented in the study.

What are the histologic features of ductal adenocarcinoma?

According to Dube et al. [5], primary duct adenocarcinomas were composed of exuberant papillary fronds supported by a complex, branching fibroconnective tissue cores lined by a single layer of tall columnar epithelial cells. These papillary fronds projected freely into a dilated central prostatic ductal space (Fig. 1-10-1). The tumor cells had elongated nuclei in a basal position and ample apical pale eosinophilic (basophilic) cytoplasm. In some tumors, cells were piled up in multiple layers. The neoplasms were graded 1 to 4 by the Dube group according to the degree of differentiation. There were one grade 1, five grade 2, and two grade 3 carcinomas; none were judged grade 4. Four of the eight cases showed focal extension into the secondary ducts and in small areas the features merged histologically with those of the secondary ducts.

The secondary duct adenocarcinoma was characterized by multicentric involvement and growth confined within intermediate and small ducts. The

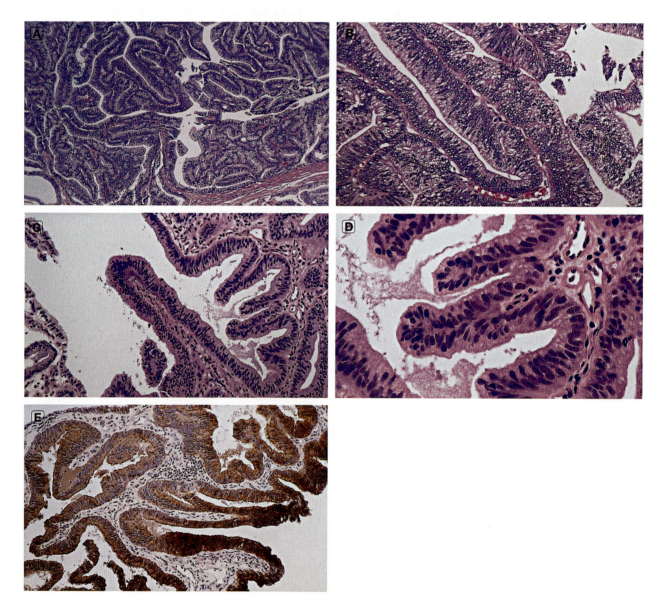

FIG. 1-10-1. The patient presented with frequent episodes of hematuria. Endoscopic examination revealed papillary fronds at the level of the verumontanum. A Transurethral resection (TUR) specimen revealed a typical papillary (ductal) adenocarcinoma projecting into the urethral lumen. The papillae were lined by pale tall columnar cells with basally placed elongated nuclei and prominent nucleoli and are supported by a delicate fibrovascular stroma (**A, B**). Three years later, the patient returned with obstructive symptoms. A second TUR revealed a well-differentiated papillary (ductal) adenocarcinoma (**C, D**) similar to that of the original tumor. The tumor cells are prostate-specific antigen (PSA)-positive (**E**)

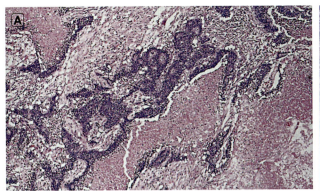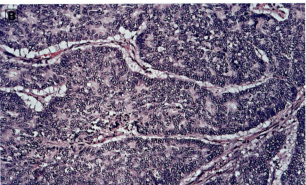

Fɪɢ. 1-10-2. Ductal adenocarcinoma showing extensive coagulative (comedo) necrosis (**A**). In other areas glandular fronds are fused creating a cribriform appearance (**B**)

neoplastic cells varied from a single layer to multilayered and usually had small papillary projections. Many of the lumens were filled with eosinophilic debris of comedo-like appearance (Fig. 1-10-2A). The cells had eosinophilic cytoplasm and large nuclei. In other areas, a combined papillary and cribriform pattern was found (Fig. 1-10-2B). The cells lining the papillae are generally tall and columnar and had eosinophilic and sometimes clear cytoplasm. Invasion of the stroma was noted in every case. Two of the 47 cases were classified as grade 1, 18 cases as grade 2, 21 cases as grade 3, and 6 cases as grade 4.

There are several notable findings on ductal adenocarcinomas: (1) Ductal adenocarcinoma may spread along the urethra or prostatic ducts. Frequently, basal cells may be retained in a discontinuous or continuous manner, which can be demonstrated immunohistochemically by basal cell marker 34β12E [6]. Consequently, the distinction from prostatic intraepithelial neoplasia is important but may be difficult. The differential diagnosis depends on the fact that the ductal adenocarcinomas are architecturally more complex and cytologically different (tall columnar cells with elongated nuclei instead of round to oval nuclei of the acinar type). In the papillary type of ductal adenocarcinoma, the papillae are supported by a fibrovascular core (Fig. 1-10-1B–D). It is absent in the papillae of the prostatic intraepithelial neoplasia. (2) The assessment of invasion is sometimes difficult when the tumor mass invades in an expansible manner. (3) In all cases, ductal adenocarcinoma cells are strongly positive for PSA (Fig. 1-10-1E). (4) Many reports describe a frequent association of ductal adenocarcinoma with acinar adenocarcinoma,

either sequentially or simultaneously (Fig. 1-10-3); 13 of the 15 cases in the Christensen series [7] had a component of standard acinar carcinoma with a Gleason score of 6–9.

In summary, characteristic microscopic features of ductal adenocarcinomas are tall cells, elongated nuclei, and frequent mitotic figures. They grow in a papillary pattern supported by a fibrovascular core or in solid, or cribriform, nests. Using these features the pathologist should be able to make a diagnosis of ductal rather than acinar adenocarcinoma. Those arising from the secondary ducts are more widespread than those arising in the primary ducts and are in more advanced stages [5, 8].

How does ductal adenocarcinoma present clinically?

In contrast to the acinar (conventional) type, which typically produces no symptoms (until having reached an advanced stage), most ductal adenocarcinomas produce hematuria and/or symptoms of obstruction because of their central (periurethral) location.

Digital rectal examination reveals most commonly prostatic enlargement but also nodularity and firmness. Because of hematuria/obstruction, cystoscopic examination is performed and reveals friable, exophytic white fronds of tumor protruding into the urethral lumen at or near the prostatic utricle [2].

In contrast to the centrally located (primary) ductal adenocarcinomas, which were regarded as "benign" in half of the cases by the examining urologists in one study, those arising in the secondary ducts were judged "malignant" in 43 of 47 cases [5].

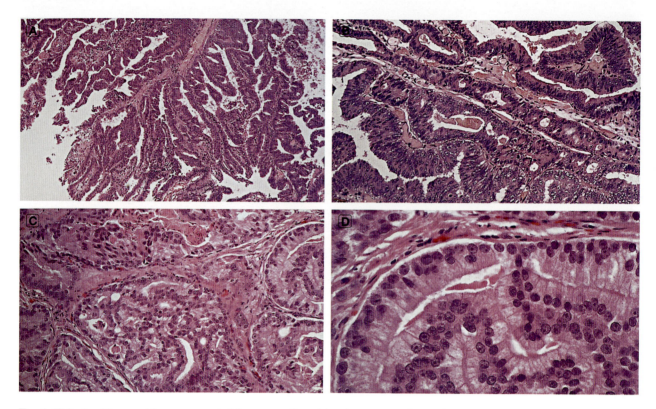

FIG. 1-10-3. An 85 year-old man presented 8 years earlier with urinary tract obstruction. At that time, cystoscopic examination revealed an exophytic mass in the prostatic urethra. Following TUR of the mass, the patient remained well until 8 years later, when a recurrent mass was noted and resected. The two specimens showed an identical microscopic pattern, consisting of papillary (ductal) adenocarcinoma (**A, B**). In some areas of both specimens, however, acini showing cribriform patterns consisting of low columnar cells consistent with acinar-type adenocarcinoma. Gleason score 4 + 4 (**C**) was found, blending imperceptibly with ductal-type adenocarcinoma (**C, D**)

More recently, however, ductal adenocarcinomas located in the peripheral zone may remain entirely silent, being discovered only by needle core biopsy performed because of an elevated PSA level. According to Brinker et al. [8], of 57 patients with ductal adenocarcinomas and available clinical data, 12 (21%) were stage cT1, 24 (42%) were cT2, 8 (14%) were cT3, and 1 was cT4. Six patients had evidence of metastasis at diagnosis.

Does ductal adenocarcinoma carry a worse prognosis than acinar adenocarcinoma?

There have been conflicting reports on the prognosis of ductal adenocarcinoma. Some groups noted the prognosis to be comparable to that of acinar adenocarcinoma [9–11]. Most studies have reported, however, that ductal adenocarcinoma is more aggressive [2, 5, 7, 12, 13]. Metastasis is evident at the time of diagnosis in 25%–40% of cases [3, 7]. It is true,

however, that these figures are based on cases reported by the early 1990s. Microscopically, these tumors exhibited high-grade histology with areas of necrosis and frequent mitotic figures. An improved prognosis could be expected if the disease is discovered in earlier stages that are amenable to radical prostatectomy and if the tumor is of low histologic grade [5, 8, 12]. Christensen et al. [7] from the Johns Hopkins Hospital reported their experience of 15 cases of both pure ductal (2 cases) and mixed acinar/ductal (13 cases) adenocarcinomas in clinical stage B with palpable prostatic lesions. By comparing them with data on acinar adenocarcinomas reported previously from the same group [14], they found that ductal adenocarcinomas were typically greater in volume, occupying a large proportion of the prostate, and at advanced pathologic stages: 93% with "capsular" penetration, 47% with positive margins, 40% with seminal vesicle invasion, and 27% with pelvic lymph node involvement.

More recently, the Johns Hopkins group reported that ductal carcinomas involving the peripheral zone are detected by needle core biopsy [8]. Therefore, these carcinomas are different from those located more centrally and present as an asymptomatic disease. Two years after treatment, the actuarial risk of PSA-evidenced progression was 42% for all patients and 34% for patients who underwent radical prostatectomy. Compared with 721 patients who underwent radical prostatectomy for acinar adenocarcinoma [15], patients with ductal adenocarcinoma showed a shorter time to progression ($P < 0.00001$). The 5-year progression-free survival was 50% for ductal adenocarcinomas, whereas it was 95% for Gleason score 5–6, 66% for Gleason score 7, and 35% for Gleason score 8–9 acinar adenocarcinomas [8, 15]. In the univariate analysis, the actuarial risk of the progression of ductal adenocarcinoma was dependent on the number of positive cores (≤ 3 vs. ≥ 4) in the biopsy ($P = 0.016$). They concluded that ductal adenocarcinoma seen on prostate needle core biopsy implies more advanced cancer with a shorter time to progression. The observation is consistent with that of Dube on secondary ductal adenocarcinomas [5].

Nevertheless, it must be stated that the prognosis of ductal adenocarcinoma as well as acinar adenocarcinoma in some patients is unpredictable. We have seen patients living with the disease for more than 8 years [16] (Fig. 1-10-3).

Is ductal adenocarcinoma a distinct morphologic and clinical entity?

For a discussion of ductal adenocarcinoma, the diagnostic criteria described above must be stringently applied when cases are reviewed. This is particularly important when distinguishing ductal adenocarcinoma involving the prostate parenchyma (away from the periurethral area) from acinar adenocarcinoma. Inclusion of acinar adenocarcinoma of papillary and cribriform growth to ductal type led to the query "Does prostatic ductal adenocarcinoma exist?" by Bock and Bostwick [17]. The cribriform lesion in their Fig. 1-4 is a typical cribriform pattern seen in acinar adenocarcinoma (as they admit) and should not be considered as having "ductal" features. The cells making up cribriform ductal adenocarcinoma are tall columnar and have large elongated hyperchromatic nuclei, contrasting with the cuboidal cells with regular round to oval nuclei of the acinar cell cribriform pattern.

It is true that in many ductal adenocarcinomas extending into the parenchyma the cell morphology changes either gradually or suddenly to the acinar cell type, and these cases are reported to be a mixed acinar and ductal type adenocarcinoma. Extraprostatic extension of such cancer revealed dual features of both acinar and ductal differentiation [8]. The Bostwick group suggested that, similar to endometrial adenocarcinoma expanding into the uterine cavity, the ductal growth pattern results from growth into an open space (a large duct or urethra), and that the limited space and the stroma influence the peripheral zone [2]. It is well known that acinar adenocarcinoma of the prostate spreads along ducts and acini at a high frequency and frequently forms a cribriform pattern [18, 19]. Yet, carcinoma cells retain the cytologic characteristics of acinar cells (i.e., cuboidal cells with round nuclei). They seldom acquire the columnar cell features with increased cytologic anaplasia of ductal adenocarcinoma.

Recently, there has been some controversy as to whether some ductal adenocarcinomas should be considered intraductal carcinoma [20]. As to whether an intraepithelial growth pattern retains a basal cell layer (as evidenced by a 34βE12-positive cell layer), Epstein group proposed that these lesions be regarded as ductal adenocarcinoma because tumors with this histologic pattern progress as invasive ductal adenocarcinoma [8]. We believe this is an important message regarding the intraductal lesion exhibiting atypical ductal-cell morphology distinct from that of acinar-cell morphology, which is characteristic of prostatic intraepithelial neoplasia.

In conclusion, prostatic ductal adenocarcinoma should be regarded as a distinct morphologic and clinical entity because of its morphologic features and biologic aggressiveness, which are distinct from those of acinar adenocarcinoma, regardless of its location or the presence of a coexisting acinar-type component.

References

1. Melicow DG, Pachter MR (1971) Endometrial carcinoma of prostatic utricle (uterus masculinus). Cancer 20:1715–1721.
2. Bostwick DG, Kindrachuk RW, Rouse RV (1985) Prostatic adenocarcinoma with endometrial features:

clinical, pathological, and ultrastructural findings. Am J Surg Pathol 9:596–609.

3. Epstein JI, Wooddruff J (1986) Prostatic carcinoma with endometrioid features: a light microscopic and immunohistochemical study of 10 cases. Cancer 57:111–119.

4. Yang XJ, Cheng LB, Helpap B, Samaratunga HM (2004) Ductal adenocarcinoma of the prostate. In: Eble JN, Sauter G, Epstein JI, Sesterhenn IA (eds) WHO Classification of Tumours. Tumours of the Urinary System and Male Genital Organs. IARC Press, Lyon, pp 199–201.

5. Dube VE, Farrow GM, Green LF (1973) Prostatic adenocarcinoma of ductal origin. Cancer 32:402–409.

6. Samaratunga H, Singh M (1997) Distribution pattern of basal cells detected by cytokeratin 34betaE12 in primary prostatic duct adenocarcinoma. Am J Surg Pathol 21:435–440.

7. Christensen WN, Steinberg WN, Walsh PC, Epstein JI (1991) Prostatic duct adenocarcinoma: findings at radical prostatectomy. Cancer 67:2118–2124.

8. Brinker DA, Potter SR, Epstein JI (1999) Ductal adenocarcinoma of the prostate diagnosed on needle biopsy: correlation with clinical and radical prostatectomy findings and progression. Am J Surg Pathol 23:1471–1479.

9. Aydin F (1993) Endometrioid adenocarcinoma of prostatic urethra presenting with anterior urethral implantation. Urology 41:91–95.

10. Millar EKA, Sharma NK, Lessels EM (1996) Ductal (endometrial) adenocarcinoma of the prostate: a clinicopathologic study of 16 cases. Histopathology 29:11–19.

11. Tannenbaum M (1975) Endometrial tumors and/or associated carcinomas of prostate. Urology 6:372–375.

12. Greene LF, Farrow GM, Ravits JM, Tomera FM (1979) Prostatic adenocarcinoma of ductal origin. J Urol 121:303–305.

13. Ro JY, Ayala AG, Wishnow KI, Ordonez NG (1988) Prostatic duct adenocarcinoma with endometrioid features: immunohistochemical and electron microscopic features. Semin Diagn Pathol 5:301–311.

14. Oesterling JE, Brendler CB, Epstein JI, Kimball AW, Walsh PC (1987) Correlation of clinical stage, serum prostatic acid phosphatase, and preoperative Gleason grade with final pathologic stage in 275 patients with clinically localized adenocarcinoma of the prostate. J Urol 138:92–98.

15. Epstein JI, Partin AW, Sauvageot J, Walsh PC (1996) Prediction of progression following radical prostatectomy: a multivariate analysis of 721 men with long-term follow-up. Am J Surg Pathol 20:286–292.

16. August CZ, Oyasu R (1983) Adenocarcinoma of the prostate gland: a spectrum of differentiation. Arch Pathol Lab Med 107:501–502.

17. Bock BJ, Bostwick DG (1999) Does prostatic duct adenocarcinoma exist? Am J Surg Pathol 23:781–785.

18. Kovi J, Jackson MA, Heshmat MY (1985) Ductal spread in prostatic carcinoma. Cancer 56:1566–1573.

19. McNeal JE, Yemoto CEM (1996) Spread of adenocarcinoma within prostatic ducts and acini: morphologic and clinical correlations. Am J Surg Pathol 20:802–814.

20. Rubin MA, de La Taille A, Bagiella E, Olsson CA, O' Toole KM (1998) Cribriform carcinoma of the prostate and prostatic intraepithelial neoplasia: incidence and clinical implications. Am J Surg Pathol 22:840–848.

Question 11

What immunohistochemical markers are useful for the diagnosis of prostate cancer?

Answer

The primary purpose of using the immunohistochemical staining technique is to rule in or rule out carcinoma primarily in a prostate needle core biopsy (PNB) specimen. Two types of markers are available. The first is basal cell-specific markers including high-molecular-weight cytokeratins (34βE12) and nuclear protein p63. The use of immunohistochemical markers for basal cells is justified on the premise that cancerous acini lack basal cells. The second type of marker is cancer-specific α-methylacyl-CoA racemase (AMACR), which is overexpressed in adenocarcinoma cells and to lesser degree in high-grade prostatic intraepithelial neoplasia. This marker exhibits high sensitivity and specificity for carcinoma cells of the prostate. A cocktail of two antibodies (AMACR and 34βE12), which may increase the accuracy of the diagnosis, is recommended.

Comments

The use of serum prostate-specific antigen (PSA) as a screening test in efforts to improve the early detection of prostate cancer has resulted in an increased number of prostate needle core biopsies (PNBs). The surgical pathologist these days is often faced with an increased number of PNBs with exceedingly small foci of carcinoma. Underdiagnosis of a small focus of carcinoma or overdiagnosis of a benign lesion mimicking cancer on PNB is not uncommon [1], which may create a devastating situation for the patients because there is no other clinical measure to confirm the pathologic diagnosis before therapy.

Often the differential diagnosis includes a number of benign lesions that mimic adenocarcinoma morphologically, such as atrophy, partial atrophy, postatrophic hyperplasia [2], basal cell hyperplasia, atypical basal cell hyperplasia, atypical adenomatous hyperplasia (adenosis), sclerosing adenosis, nephrogenic adenoma, and high-grade intraepithelial neoplasia (HGPIN).

An important diagnostic criterion in the differential diagnosis is the loss of the basal cell layer in adenocarcinoma and its presence in benign conditions. In the benign lesions described above, it is not uncommon not to observe basal cells clearly on H&E-stained sections. Therefore, immunohistochemical markers may be useful for distinguishing adenocarcinoma from benign mimics.

34βE12

In 1985, Brawer et al. [3] introduced the use of the basal cell-specific monoclonal antibody 34βE12 to high-molecular-weight keratins 1, 5, 10, and 11 to discriminate benign and malignant prostatic acini. This antibody was found to be an excellent tool in a challenging biopsy specimen; the diagnosis of carcinoma can be confirmed in a highly suspicious focus on the basis of negative immunoreactivity. Because the utility of 34βE12 relies on the fact that adenocarcinoma lacks basal cells (Fig. 1-11-1) but benign glands and prostatic intraepithelial neoplasia have basal cells (Figs. 1-11-1, 1-11-2, 1-11-3), it is critical that immunostaining does not result in a false-negative reaction.

Basal cell staining by 34βE12 may be affected by the fixation time and the method of antigen retrieval. The most commonly used fixative is formalin. High-molecular-weight (HMW) keratins are sensitive to

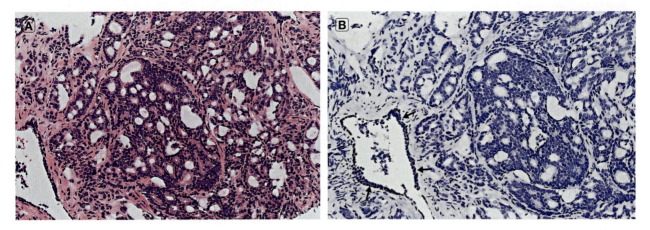

Fig. 1-11-1. **A, B** Gleason score 4 + 4 adenocarcinoma lacking basal cells as evidenced by a negative 34βE12 stain (basal cell marker) (**B**). A dilated benign gland on the left side of the photograph is decorated with a basal cell layer (*arrows*)

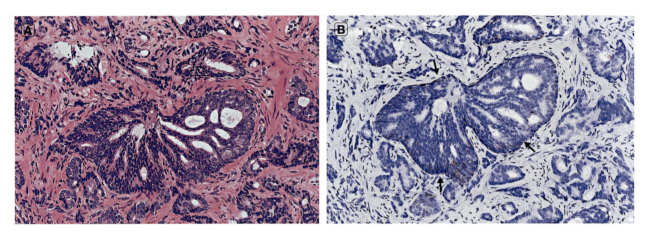

Fig. 1-11-2. **A, B** High-grade prostatic intraepithelial neoplasia in the center is supported by an interrupted basal cell layer, demonstrated by 34βE12 stain (stained brown) (*arrows*), whereas glands in the right lower corner lack a basal cell layer, indicative of invasive nests

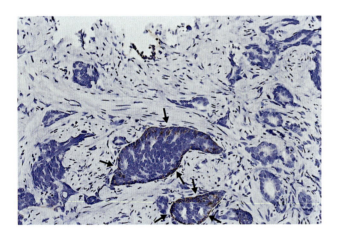

Fig. 1-11-3. High-grade prostatic intraepithelial neoplasia. The two atypical nests in the center have a basal cell layer (*arrows*) indicative of high-grade prostatic intraepithelial neoplasia

formalin. The Amin group addressed this issue and made a detailed study on the effect of formalin fixation and epitope retrieval techniques on 34βE12 staining [4]. Tested were the length in formalin fixation (ranging from 6h to 1 month) and the epitope retrieval methods. The latter were (1) predigestion with 0.4% pepsin for 60min at 37°C; (2) microwave heat-induced epitope retrieval (tissue sections placed in a Coplin jar filled with 0.2M citrate buffer at pH 6.0 and microwaved at high power for two periods of 5mins each in a 900-W microwave and then allowed to cool at room temperature for 30min; and (3) hot plate use (tissue sections placed in a beaker containing 1000ml of 0.2M citrate buffer at pH 6.0 and heated for 10min at 100°C on a hot plate and then allowed to cool at room temperature for 20min).

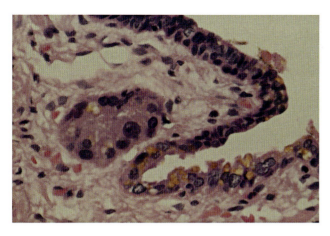

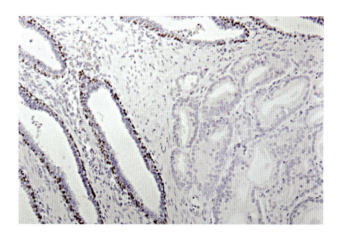

FIG. 1-11-4. Portion of ejaculatory duct. The cells are tall and contain hyperchromatic large pleomorphic nuclei and lipochrome pigment in the cytoplasm (H&E)

FIG. 1-11-5. Gleason 3 + 3 adenocarcinoma. Note that the carcinoma cells lack nuclear stain for p63, whereas the nuclei of basal cells in the adjacent normal acini (left side of photograph) are intensely stained for p63

They found that although prolonged formalin fixation resulted in a progressive decrease of staining intensity after enzymatic digestion it is significant only after formalin fixation of more than 1 week. Among the three retrieval techniques, consistently strong staining intensity was observed at all time points of formalin fixation when the hot plate method was used. They recommended that each laboratory standardize the fixation and select an appropriate antigen retrieval technique for anti-HMW keratins. They found the hot plate technique to be simple, and it produced consistently reliable results on immunostaining of HMW cytokeratins.

It should be emphasized that benign glands in the transition zone obtained by transurethral resection often have variable distribution of basal cells because of their patchy nature of distribution in some glands. It is essential that immunostaining for basal cells be used only as an adjunct to confirm the diagnosis based on the routine H&E-stained section.

The ejaculatory duct and the seminal vesicle may be sampled with transurethral resection of the prostate or PNB. Because of their cytologic atypia (nucleomegaly and hyperchromasia), the differential diagnosis from adenocarcinoma must be considered. However, lack of prominent nucleoli and the presence of yellow lipofuscin pigment in the cytoplasm are sufficiently diagnostic of an ejaculatory duct or seminal vesicle and are unlikely to need a special stain (Fig. 1-11-4). It should be noted that the basal cells of the ejaculatory duct and seminal vesicles are reactive to HMW keratin.

p63

The *p63* gene is a recently cloned homologue of the tumor-suppressor gene *p53* and was reported to be highly expressed in the basal or progenitor layers of many epithelia [5]. Both mouse and human prostate basal cells express p63 protein, suggesting that p63 may play a critical role in prostate development by maintaining a stem cell population [6]. The same group demonstrated for the first time that basal cells, but not secretory columnar or neuroendocrine cells of the prostate, expressed p63 protein in the nucleus, whereas it was not detected in human prostatic adenocarcinomas [7]. Subsequently, other laboratories tested its utility for the diagnosis of minute foci of adenocarcinoma on PNB and compared the results with those of 34βE12. In the study by the Rubin group of the University of Michigan [8], none of 67 carcinomas observed on PNB demonstrated positive staining by 34βE12 or p63 (100% specific) (Fig. 1-11-5). In most of the atypical cases ($n = 27$), the staining difference by the two methods was not significant, except in two cases in which the diagnosis of carcinoma was established based on the p63 staining results. For 12 transurethral resection cases, the mean basal cell staining in benign glands was higher with p63 than with 34βE12 (95% vs. 75%). It was concluded that both stains are highly specific for basal cells, that p63 was slightly more sensitive than 34βE12 in staining basal cells, and that p63 offered a slight advantage over 34βE12 in diagnostically challenging cases.

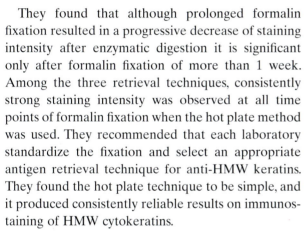

Combined Use of 34βE12 and p63

As p63 antibody stains nuclei and 34βE12 stains the cytoplasm and cell membrane, it is feasible to combine the two antibodies. Recently, the Rubin group tested if the cocktail of the antibodies could improve immunohistochemical detection of basal cells [9]. The combination of the antibodies stained the basal cell layer more intensely than either 34βE12 or p63 alone. Complete and partial strong basal cell staining was observed in 93% and 1%, respectively, of benign glands, compared with 55% and 4% with 34βE12 alone and 81% and 1% with p63 alone, respectively. They concluded that the combination of antibodies not only increased the sensitivity of basal cell detection but also reduced the staining variability and therefore rendered basal cell immunostaining more consistent. They recommend this basal cell cocktail for routine diagnostic workup.

As was mentioned above, prostatic glands of the transition zone may not reveal basal cells in areas. The combination of the antibodies reduced the frequency of benign glands lacking basal cells from 6% to 2% [9].

α-Methylacyl Coenzyme A Racemase (AMACR, P504S)

Using cDNA library subtraction and the tissue microarray technique, Xu et al. [10] isolated a gene (*P504S*) that is uniquely overexpressed in prostate carcinoma cells. It encodes a 382-amino-acid protein and was identified as human α-methylacyl-CoA racemase.

Although immunohistochemical stains for basal cells, such as 34βE12 or p63, can aid in the diagnosis of a tiny focus of carcinoma in a PNB, their use may be limited. Negative staining for basal cell markers is, by itself, not diagnostic of carcinoma, as occasional benign glands may not show immunoreactivity. A marker specific for prostate cancer by positive staining would be of considerable value in establishing a definitive diagnosis of carcinoma. Several laboratories reported their experience with the antibody made against AMACR. AMACR showed strong cytoplasmic staining in carcinomas (Fig. 1-11-6) ranging from 82% [11], 88% [12, 13], 95% [14], and 96% [12] to 100% [15], regardless of the Gleason score [11, 12, 15, 16] or the pathologic stage [12, 16]. The staining was diffuse (>77% of tumor) in 92% of cases [15]. In contrast, benign glands are only focally weakly stained, ranging from 4% [12], 8% [13], and 12% [15] to 21% [11] of cases. Expression of AMACR was not found in basal cell hyperplasia, urothelial cells/metaplasia, atrophic glands, glands with irradiation changes, or sclerosing adenosis, all of which can mimic carcinoma [15]. In addition, positive staining for AMACR was observed in 17.5% of atypical adenomatous hyperplasia (adenosis) cases [17]. Staining in HGPIN was generally positive, although the staining was more variable and often less intense than in adjacent carcinoma [12, 18] (Fig. 1-11-6A). The sensitivity in prostate adenocarcinoma ranged from 82% [11], 97% [16] to 100% [15]; and specificity was 100% [16]. The positive predictive value for cancer was 100%, and the negative predictive value was 92%

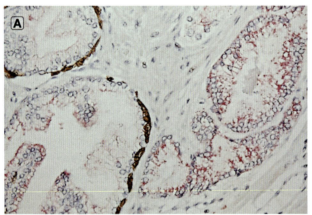
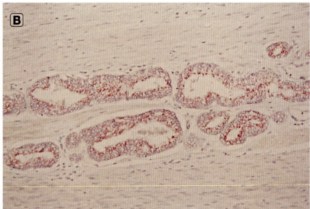

FIG. 1-11-6. Gleason 3 + 3 adenocarcinoma and high-grade prostatic intraepithelial neoplasia stained by a combination of 34βE12 and α-methylacyl coenzyme A racemase (AMACR) antibodies. The carcinomatous glands in the right half **A** and those in **B** are negative for 34βE12 and show diffuse cytoplasmic staining for AMACR. Note the columnar cells of high-grade prostatic intraepithelial neoplasia in **A** also stain weakly for AMACR

[16]. The sensitivity may be affected by the difference in antibodies used, fixation method, and immunohistochemical staining method [12].

After adjuvant hormonal therapy, the residual adenocarcinoma becomes difficult to recognize because of morphologic alterations. This is particularly true with the cancer at the excisional margins because of surgical trauma. AMACR should be useful to identify cancer cells after hormonal therapy. Sonamala et al. [19] stained adenocarcinoma for AMACR in needle core biopsies and radical prostatectomies before and after an androgen-deprivation therapy (Lupron and flutamide). The pretherapy adenocarcinoma cases were 100% positive (22/22); and after therapy 82% had positive immunostaining for AMACR. Thus, they concluded that the racemase immunostain is an effective method for identifying neoplastic cells after hormonal therapy. Our study demonstrated decreased AMACR immunoreactivity in hormonally treated prostatic adenocarcinoma [20]. Caution should be exercised when interpreting PNB findings from a patient with previous hormonal therapy.

Biologic Significance of Positive Immunohistochemical Staining of AMACR in Prostate Cancer

AMACR plays a key role in peroxisomal β-oxidation of dietary branched-chain fatty acids [12]. This pathway may have potential significance for the development of prostate cancer. First, the main sources of branched-chain fatty acids in human diet (milk, beef, dairy products) [21] have been implicated as dietary risk factors for prostate cancer [22]; and second, peroxisomal β-oxidation generates hydrogen peroxide, a potential source of carcinogenic oxidative damage [23]. One implication of the upregulation of AMACR is that prostate carcinoma cells (and their precursor HGPIN cells) have a consistently greater capacity to metabolize dietary branched-chain fatty acids than do normal epithelial cells. Although the contribution of this upregulation to prostate carcinogenesis, if any, is unclear at present, two interesting aspects of this pathway may be relevant. (1) The first step of the pathway in β oxidation of branched-chain fatty acids is an oxidation step catalyzed by acyl CoA oxidases, which leads to the generation of hydrogen peroxide. Previously, we induced a neoplastic transformation in human uro-

thelial cells by overexpression of acyl CoA oxidase [24]. (2) The primary branched-chain fatty acid is phytanic acid, a breakdown product of chlorophyll in ruminants, which is found primarily in milk and dairy products derived from milk as well as in beef but not meat from chicken or some fish [12, 25]. An interesting question is whether the increased risk for prostate cancer by consuming dairy products and red meat is related to the upregulation of AMACR and its associated pathway during the early stages of prostate carcinogenesis (i.e., in HGPIN) [12].

Expression of AMACR in Tissues and Tumors Other Than the Prostate

First, one must question whether the high expression of AMACR is specific to prostate cancer. Jiang et al. [26] addressed this question. In normal tissues, AMACR protein was detected in the liver (hepatocytes), kidney (tubular epithelial cells), lung (only bronchial epithelial cells), and gallbladder (epithelial cells). Altogether, 17 of 21 (81%) hepatocellular carcinomas and 18 of 24 (75%) renal cell carcinomas were immunohistochemically positive for AMACR. AMACR is expressed in high frequency (100%) and more intensely by papillary renal cell carcinoma than other types [27]. Also positive were 11 of 29 (38%) urothelial carcinomas, both low and high grade [26]. AMACR is detected in approximately one-half of nephrogenic adenomas of the urothelial tract [28], although nephrogenic adenoma is not considered as a true neoplasm. Thus, AMACR alone has limited value in diagnosing metastatic prostate carcinoma.

In summary, the histologic diagnosis of prostate cancer can be greatly facilitated by applying the immunohistochemical techniques described above. However, as we have emphasized repeatedly, immunostaining should be used only as an adjunct to the standard evaluation based on H&E-stained sections. Now that those antibodies for both positive (AMACR) and negative (34βE12 and p63) markers are available, it is reasonable to combine these antibodies for the diagnostic workup in difficult cases. It could decrease the diagnostic uncertainty in PNBs.

References

1. Troxel D (2000) Diagnostic errors in surgical pathology uncovered by a review of malpractice claims. Part 1. General considerations. Int J Surg Pathol 8:161–163.

2. De Marzo AM, Platz EA, Epstein JI, Ali T, Billis A, Chan TY, Cheng L, Datta M, Egevad L, Ertoy-Baydor D, Farree X, Fine SW, Iczkowski KA, Ittmann M, Knudsen BS, Loda M, Lopez-Beltran A, Magi-Galluzzi C, Mikuz G, Montironi R, Pikarsky E, Pizov G, Rubin MA, Samaratunga H, Sebo T, Sesterhenn IA, Shah RB, Signoretti S, Simko J, Thomas G, Trocoso P, Tsuzuki TT, van Leenders GJ, Yang XJ, Zhou M, Figg WD, Hoque A, Lucia MS (2006) A working group classification of focal prostate atrophy lesions. Am J Surg Pathol 30:1281–1291.

3. Brawer MK, Peehl DM, Stamey TA, Bostwick DG (1985) Keratin immunoreactivity in the benign and neoplastic human prostate. Cancer Res 45:3663–3667.

4. Varma M, Linden MD, Amin MB (1999) Effect of formalin fixation and epitope retrieval techniques on antibody 34βE12 immunostaining of prostate tissue. Mod Pathol 12:472–478.

5. Yang A, Schweitzer R, Sun D, Kaghad M, Walker N, Bronson RT, Tabin C, Sharpe A, Caput D, Crum C, McKeon F (1999) p63 is essential for regenerative proliferation in limb, craniofacial and epithelial development. Nature 398:714–718.

6. Yang A, Kaghad M, Wang Y, Gillette E, Flemming MD, Dotsch V, Andrews NC, Capu D, McKeon F (1998) p63: a p53 homolog at 3q27-29, encodes multiple products with transactivating, death-inducing, and dominant-negative activities. Mol Cell 2:305–316.

7. Signoretti S, Waltregny D, Dilkes J, Isaac B, Lin D, Garraway L, Yang A, Montironi R, McKeon F, Loda M (2000) p63 is a prostate basal cell marker and is required for prostate development. Am J Pathol 157:1769–1775.

8. Shah R, Zhou M, LeBlanc M, Snyder M, Rubin MA (2002) Comparison of the basal cell-specific markers, 34βE12 and p63, in the diagnosis of prostate cancer. Am J Surg Pathol 26:1161–1168.

9. Zhou M, Shah R, Shen R, Rubin MA (2003) Basal cell cocktail (34βE12 + p63) improves the detection of prostate basal cells. Am J Surg Pathol 27:365–371.

10. Xu J, Stolk JA, Zhang X, Silva SJ, Houghton RL, Matsumura M, Vedvick TS, Leslie KS, Badaro R, Reed SG (2000) Identification of differentially expressed genes in human prostate cancer using subtraction and microarray. Cancer Res 60:1677–1682.

11. Beach B, Gown AM, de Peralta-Ventrina MN, Folpe AL, Yaziji H, Salles PG, Grignon DJ, Fanger GR, Amin MB (2002) P504S immunohistochemical detection in 405 prostatic specimens including 376 18-gauge needle biopsies. Am J Surg Pathol 26:1588–1596.

12. Luo J, Zha S, Gage WR, Dunn TA, Hicks JL, Bennett CJ, Ewing CM, Platz EA, Ferdinandusse S, Wanders RJ, Trent JM, Isaacs WB, De Marzo AM (2002) Alpha-methylacyl CoA racemase: a new molecular marker for prostate cancer. Cancer Res 62:2220–2226.

13. Magi-Galluzzi C, Luo J, Isaacs WB, Hicks JL, De Marzo AM, Epstein JI (2003) Alpha-methylacyl-CoA racemase: a variably sensitive immunohistochemical marker for the diagnosis of small prostate cancer foci on needle biopsy. Am J Surg Pathol 27:1128–1114.

14. Jiang Z, Wu C-L, Woda BA, Dresser K, Xu J, Fanger GR, Yang XJ (2002) P504S/alpha-methyacyl-CoA racemase: a useful marker for diagnosis of small foci of prostate carcinoma on needle biopsy. Am J Surg Pathol 26:1169–1174.

15. Jiang Z, Woda BA, Rock KL, Xu Y, Savas L, Khan A, Pihan G, Cai F, Babcock JS, Rathanaswami P, Reed SG, Xu J, Fanger GR (2001) P504S: a new molecular marker for the detection of prostate carcinoma. Am J Surg Pathol 25:1397–1404.

16. Rubin MA, Zhou M, Dhanasekaran SM, Varambally S, Barrette TR, Sanda MG, Pienta KJ, Ghosh D, Chinnaiyan AM (2002) Alpha-methylacyl coenzyme A racemase as a tissue biomarker for prostate cancer. JAMA 287:1662–1670.

17. Yang XJ, Wu CL, Woda BA, Dresser K, Tretikova M, Fanger GR, Zhong J (2002) Expression of P505S/alpha-methyl Co A racemase in atypical adenomatous hyperplasia of the prostate. Am J Surg Pathol 25:921–925.

18. Wu CL, Yang XJ, Tretokova MS, Patton KY, Halpern EF, Woda BA, Young RH, Jiang Z (2004) Analysis of expression of alpha-methyl-Co A racemase in high grade prostatic intraepithelial neoplasia. Hum Pathol 35:1008–1013.

19. Sonamala AB, Swanson G, Speights VO (2004) Variable staining of AMACR (racemase) in pre and post androgen deprivation therapy of prostate adenocarcinoma. Mod Pathol 17(suppl 1):178A.

20. Suzue K, Montag AG, Tretikova M, Yang XJ, Sahoo S (2005) Altered expression of alpha-methyl-Co A racemase in prostatic adenocarcinoma following hormone therapy. Am J Clin Pathol 123:413–417.

21. Wanders RJA, Jacobs C, Skjeldal O (2001) Refsum disease. In: Scriver CR, Beaudet AL, Sly WS, Valle D (eds) The metabolic and molecular bases of inherited disease. McGraw-Hill, London, pp 3303–3321.

22. Chan JM, Stampfer MJ, Ma J, Gann PH, Gaziano JM, Giovannucci EL (2001) Dairy products, calcium, and prostate cancer risk in the Physician's Health Study. Am J Clin Nutr 74:549–554.

23. Feig DI, Reid TM, Loeb LA (1994) Reactive oxygen species in tumorigenesis. Cancer Res (suppl 54):1890s–1894s.

24. Tamatani T, Hattori K, Nakashiro K, Hayashi Y, Wu S-Q, Klumpp D, Reddy JK, Oyasu R (1999) Neoplastic conversion of human urothelial cells by overexpression of H_2O_2-generating peroxisomal fatty acyl CoA oxidase. Int J Oncol 15:743–749.

25. Flanagan VP, Ferretti A, Schwartz DP, Ruth JM (1975) Characterization of two steroidal ketones and two isopropenoid alcohols in diary products. J Lipid Res 16:97–101.

26. Jiang Z, Fanger GR, Woda BA, Banner BF, Algate P, Dresser K, Xu J, Chu PG (2003) Expression of alpha-methylacyl-CoA racemase (P504S) in various malignant neoplasms and normal tissues: a study of 761 cases. Hum Pathol 34:792–796.

27. Tretikova MS, Sahoo S, Takahashi M, Turkylmaz M, Vogelzang NJ, Lin F, Krausz T, Teh BT, Yang XJ (2004) Expression of alpha-methyl-acyl-CoA racemase in papillary renal cell carcinoma. Am J Surg Pathol 28:69–76.

28. Gupta A, Wang HL, Policarpio-Nicolas ML, Tretikova M, Yang XL (2004) Expression of alpha-methyl-acyl-coenzyme A racemase in nephrogenic adenoma. Mod Pathol 17(suppl 1):155A.

Question 12

When a basal cell-specific marker (34βE12 or p63) is negative in an atypical focus, can the diagnosis of adenocarcinoma be rendered? By the same token, if 34βE12- or p63-positive cells are present, can carcinoma be ruled out?

Answer

The loss of the basal cell layer is a hallmark of adenocarcinoma of the prostate. Generally speaking, the absence of basal cells as demonstrated by immunohistochemical technique provides strong support for the diagnosis of adenocarcinoma. If an atypical lesion contains basal cells (seen by immunostaining), the diagnosis of adenocarcinoma should be avoided.

However, recent studies indicate that on rare occasions, lesions that fully satisfy the histologic criteria for acinar adenocarcinoma may contain cells stained positive for the basal cell marker 34βE12 at both primary sites as well as at metastasis. In the event of observing 34βE12-positive cells, the diagnosis of carcinoma should be made with extreme caution. On the other hand, there are many situations where basal cells may not be obvious in the suspicious focus, and 34βE12 negativity alone may not be sufficient for the diagnosis of adenocarcinoma. The key message here is that most strong diagnostic evidence should be based on H&E-stained sections, and immunostaining is an adjunctive test providing supportive evidence.

Comments

In the discussion under Question 11, we have described the value of immunohistochemical techniques for distinguishing benign conditions from adenocarcinoma. The most commonly used is 34βE12, an antibody that stains basal cells. However, immunohistochemical technique should be used only as an adjunct to support your impression based on H&E-stained sections.

Recently, there have been a few articles in the literature reporting the rare presence of 34βE12-positive cells in lesions that are deemed cancerous by the accepted microscopic criteria. They are found in both the prostate and metastatic sites.

The study by Yang et al. [1] was based on 100 cases of metastatic prostate adenocarcinomas (67 in regional nodes, 19 in bone, 14 at other sites) and 10 cases of prostate adenocarcinomas invading the seminal vesicles. Four cases were found positive for 34βE12 staining. Two had weak staining and two others (in lymph nodes) showed strong staining. None of the positively stained cells had the morphology of basal cells. It was concluded that albeit rare, prostate cancer, even of high grade, expresses high-molecular-weight (HMW) keratin. Nevertheless, the basal cell marker is a useful adjunct in the diagnosis of prostate cancer.

The study by Oliai et al. [2] was based primarily on prostate needle core biopsies received for consultation. A total of 36 cases (1.1%) that on H&E staining were unequivocal cancer had at least focal 34βE12-positive cells in a basal cell distribution. Their basal cell nature was confirmed in selected cases by applying an antibody to p63, another basal cell marker. In 16 of 25 cases (64%) available for further studies, high-grade prostatic intraepithelial neoplasia (HGPIN) was present adjacent to infiltrating carcinomas with basal cells, the finding suggesting that these neoplastic glands could be cells outpouching from HGPIN. In the remaining nine cases, however, an absence of HGPIN foci was against this argument. One case demonstrated the basal cell marker expressed in tumor cells.

As stated earlier (Question 11), immunohistochemical staining is significantly influenced by the technique used. In the case of HMW keratin stained with 34βE12, we have already alluded that a prolonged formalin fixation time reduces the staining quality. On the other hand, false-positive staining with 34βE12 has been associated with certain antigen retrieval techniques. Focal reactivity (<1% of glands) in carcinoma was observed in 3 of 10 radical prostatectomy specimens after hot plate antigen retrieval but not with pepsin predigestion or microwave methods [3].

What have we learned from the above-cited reports? There are three points of note: (1) Basal cells may accompany carcinomatous glands on rare occasions in patchy fashion. Although the exact frequency is unknown, it is probably less than 1% of cancer in the prostate. Because HGPIN is believed to be the precursor of (invasive) carcinoma, at least in some cases, invasive carcinoma coming off PIN may be accompanied by basal cells. The picture reminds us of a newly hatched chicken with eggshell still attached to the body. (2) There are two types of HMW keratin-positive cells in prostate carcinoma. In a cancerous focus in the prostate, positively stained cells are either scattered residual basal cells admixed with cancer cells and/or cancer cells expressing HMW keratin. At extraprostatic sites, as you would expect, all stained cells are carcinoma cells. (3) Despite rare cases of basal cells accompanying carcinomatous glands that can be detected by immunohistochemical staining, 34βE12 antibody is a useful adjunct in the biopsy diagnosis of prostate cancer. Because most prostate cancers can be diagnosed with H&E-stained sections without cytokeratin stain, the true frequency is unknown. Immunohistochemistry for HMW keratin, though useful, should be used judiciously and not be performed routinely.

References

1. Yang XI, Lecksell K, Gaudin P, Epstein JI (1999) Rare expression of high-molecular-weight cytokeratin in adenocarcinoma of the prostate gland: a study of 100 cases of metastatic and locally advanced prostate cancer. Am J Surg Pathol 23:147–152.
2. Oliai BR, Kahane H, Epstein JI (2002) Can basal cells be seen in adenocarcinoma of the prostate? Am J Surg Pathol 26;1151–1160.
3. Varma M, Linden MD, Amin MB (1999) Effect of formalin fixation and epitope retrieval techniques on antibody 34βE12 immunostaining of prostatic tissue. Mod Pathol 12:472–478.

Question 13

How often is cancer detected when serum PSA is elevated? What factors affect the prostate cancer detection rate?

one-half that of the initial biopsy. Moreover, there is no difference between the cancers detected by the first and second biopsies in regard to the stage and Gleason score of the radical prostatectomy specimens.

Answer

The detection rate of prostate cancer is influenced by several factors: clinical features including the serum PSA level and an abnormal digital rectal examination (DRE); the number of biopsy cores examined; and the volume of the prostate. Among men with serum PSA < 4 ng/ml, 4–10 ng/ml, and >10 ng/ml, cancer detection rates by prostate needle core biopsy (PNB) are approximately 15%, 25%, and 60%, respectively. Men with low screening PSA (<4 ng/ml) and treated with radical prostatectomy have smaller cancers, lower Gleason scores, lower pathologic tumor stages, and lower PSA recurrence rates than men with higher PSA levels (≥4 ng/ml). If the initial serum PSA values are >10 ng/ml, cancers are pathologically in more advanced stages. Cancers detected with an abnormal DRE are more frequently in advanced stages than those discovered by PSA screening.

As compared with the standard sextant biopsy method, increasing core numbers up to 12 can significantly improve cancer detection. If the initial biopsy is negative, the detection rate in the repeat biopsy is dependent on the initial biopsy core number, interval between biopsies, clinical parameters including DRE findings, PSA level, and free fraction of PSA. After an initial negative sextant biopsy, the detection rate by a repeat sextant biopsy performed within a year is approximately

Comments

Effect of Serum PSA Cutoff Levels

Traditionally, a serum PSA level >4 ng/ml is considered abnormal, and these patients require further workup including ultimately PNB. Using this level as cutoff for screening, the cancer detection rate among subjects enrolled was 3.2% in men with a positive DRE, 4.6% for those with elevated serum PSA, and 5.8% in men with both abnormal tests [1]. Significantly more cancers were organ-confined in the prostate removed by PSA screening than those based on abnormal DRE ($P = 0.003$) [1]. Thus, PSA screening has clearly been shown to be superior to DRE.

When rise in PSA level is confirmed by repeat testing, most urologists recommend PNB. However, the usefulness of PSA determination is limited in the range of 4–10 ng/ml because of the relative lack of specificity. PNB detects cancer in only one-fourth of patients. In the study reported by Catalona et al. [2], 174 of 652 men (27%) had biopsy-proven cancer. With PSA > 10 ng/ml, however, cancer was detected in 122 of 208 men (59%); and in more than half of them, the cancer was in an advanced stage. Thus, compared with the lower PSA group (PSA 4–10 ng/ml), higher initial PSA values (>10 ng/ml) were significantly associated with the presence of carcinoma ($P < 0.0001$) and advanced pathologic stage ($P < 0.0001$) [2].

Although the cutoff at 4.0 ng/ml for serum PSA has been considered predictive of prostate cancer, it has been well recognized that there are many prostate cancer patients who have a low serum PSA level at diagnosis. Therefore, this threshold has been challenged with studies suggesting that perhaps a PSA value >2.5 ng/ml should be considered abnormal [3]. In a recent study, men with a screening serum PSA level of <4.0 ng/ml were shown to have an approximately 15% risk of needle biopsy-proven prostate cancer. Of these, approximately 15% had a Gleason score ≥7 for cancer [4]. According to another recent study [5], 3416 men diagnosed with prostate cancer by PSA screening were stratified in groups based on their serum PSA level. Altogether, 14% of men (n = 468) had PSA levels <4 ng/ml, and 4.2% (n = 142) had PSA of <2.0 ng/ml. Patients with low screening PSA (<4.0 ng/ml) treated with radical prostatectomy had smaller cancers, lower Gleason scores, lower pathologic stage tumors, and lower PSA recurrence rates than men with high PSA levels (>4 ng/ml) [5].

The decision to lower the PSA threshold for biopsy is not without controversy. Carter [6] argued that prostate cancer detected by lowering PSA levels are more likely to be of a small volume (<0.5 ml) and low grade and thus more likely to represent clinically insignificant cancer. They also stated that there is no convincing evidence that men who are treated when their cancers are detected have a better outcome than men who are treated with cancer detected when PSA is slightly >4 ng/ml. Development of high-grade cancer (Gleason score ≥7) is proportional to the serum PSA level. Yet, the fact that as many as 15% of cancers detected in men with PSA values of 3.1–4.0 ng/ml were high-grade tumors [4] is a serious concern. Punglia et al. [3] argued that 82% of prostate cancers in young men (<60 years of age) and 65% of cancers in older men would be missed if the threshold PSA value for undergoing biopsy were set at 4.1 ng/ml. Lowering the threshold for biopsy to 2.6 ng/ml in men younger than 60 years would double the cancer detection rate from 18% to 36%, and the specificity would fall from 0.98 to 0.94. They concluded that reducing the threshold PSA level to 2.6 ng/ml at which biopsy is recommended may be reasonable at least in men under 60 years of age.

Effect of Biopsy Core Numbers and Biopsy Sites

The detection rate is also influenced by the number of biopsy cores sampled. Standard sextant biopsy examines only the mid-lobe parasagittal plane halfway between the lateral border and the midline of the prostate. Therefore, the lateral aspect of the peripheral zone, where many cancers are located, is poorly sampled [7]. Recent reports clearly indicate that extended PNB technique (from 8 to 15 cores including the lateral aspects of the prostate) yields significantly higher rates of cancer detection [7–14]. In these studies, additional cores were obtained together with the standard sextant biopsy specimen. Although the core numbers and biopsy sites vary somewhat among reports, all indicate that increasing the core numbers and including the lateral aspects improve the cancer detection rate by approximately 15%–25% over that of sextant biopsy. Not only increasing detection rate of cancer, but additional systemic lateral core sampling correlated more strongly with extraprostatic extension of cancer [15].

The study reported by Naughton et al. [16] is different in that biopsy core numbers were compared between two groups of men—one group with a standard sextant biopsy and a second group undergoing standard sextant biopsy plus an additional six cores from the lateral peripheral zone. These authors failed to demonstrate a difference between the groups. It was thought, though, that the study did not have enough power to detect a difference between the two groups [17].

Effect of Prostate Volume

Another factor that affects cancer detection is the volume of the prostate [8, 10, 14, 18–20]. In the study by Rietbergen et al. [21], the mean planimetric prostate volume in the initial biopsy-positive group was 43.6 ml, whereas in the repeat biopsy-positive group it was 53.4 ml (P < 0.0001). According to Djavan et al. [19], the mean total volume measured in radical prostatectomy specimens was 34.3 ml in the first biopsy-positive group and 42.5 ml in the second biopsy-positive group (P < 0.001). This suggests that in an enlarged prostate hitting cancerous focus is more difficult. Djavan's group, however, stated that cancer in biopsy 2 was located in a more apicodorsal position and suggested that re-biopsy should be directed to this area. Eskicorapci et al. [22] suggested that the biopsy protocol be adjusted to the prostate volume.

What is the likelihood of finding cancer in subsequent biopsies after an initially negative biopsy? What are predictors of cancer on repeat prostate biopsy?

The presence of atypia, including high-grade prostatic intraepithelial neoplasia (HGPIN) and atypical foci suspicious but not diagnostic of cancer, are known to significantly increase the cancer detection rate in a subsequent biopsy. This subject is addressed in Questions 14 and 17. Here our discussion is based on a negative initial biopsy.

In the study reported by Keetch et al. [23], 1136 men with serum PSA levels >4ng/ml and either abnormal DRE or transrectal ultrasonography (TRUS) findings underwent PNB. All 204 men whose initial PSA was ≥10ng/ml underwent PNB. The 427 men who had a negative initial biopsy but persistently elevated serum PSA levels >4ng/ml and abnormal DRE or TRUS findings underwent a second biopsy; 84 (19%) of them had cancer. Of 203 men with persistent abnormalities, 16 (8%) had cancer on the third biopsy, and 6 of 91 (7%) had cancer on biopsy no. 4 or later. An additional important observation was that the initial PSA values (PSA 4.1–9.9ng/ml vs. >10ng/ml, $P = 0.0001$) and follow-up PSA values ($P = 0.002$) and the change in yearly rate of PSA levels (PSA velocity, $P = 0.0001$) were significantly higher in men in whom cancer was detected compared with those in whom cancer was not detected.

In the European Prostate Cancer Detection Study reported in 2001 by Djavan et al. [19], a total of 1051 men with PSA levels of 4–10ng/ml underwent a TRUS-guided sextant biopsy and a two-core transition zone biopsy. This study is unique in that all patients with a negative biopsy underwent a repeat biopsy after 6 weeks. If again negative, a third biopsy and even a fourth biopsy were performed at an 8-week interval. Cancer detection rates on biopsies 1, 2, 3, and 4 were 22% (231/1051), 10% (83/820), 5% (36/737), and 4% (4/49), respectively. Significant observations were drawn from the European study [19]: (1) There was no difference between cancers detected on the first biopsy and the second biopsy in terms of the Gleason score and the mean percentage of Gleason pattern 4/5 carcinoma (in both biopsy and radical prostatectomy specimens). The findings suggest that the second biopsy detected the cancer that was missed in the first biopsy. (2) Compared with cancers detected on biopsy 1, cancers detected on biopsies 3 and 4 have a lower Gleason score—in both biopsies ($P = 0.02$) and radical prostatectomy specimens ($P = 0.001$), lower tumor volume ($P = 0.001$), lower Gleason pattern 4/5 cancer percent volume ($P = 0.001$), and lower stage ($P = 0.001$). (3) The mean volume of the second biopsy-positive prostate is significantly larger than that of the first biopsy-positive prostate (42.5ml vs. 34.3ml, $P < 0.001$).

As of today, the most useful parameter for detecting cancer on repeat biopsy is the free PSA fraction. The percentage of the free PSA fraction was an independent predictor of cancer on repeat biopsy in several studies: $P < 0.001$ [24], $P = 0.0003$ [25], $P < 0.001$ [18]. Catalona et al. [24] recommend a cutoff of 25% free PSA. This level detected 95% of cancers while avoiding 20% of unnecessary biopsies.

References

1. Catalona WJ, Richie JP, Ahmann FR, Hudson MA, Scardino PT, Flanigan RC, deKernion JB, Ratliff TL, Kavoussi LR, Dalkin BL, Waters WB, MacFarlane MT, Southwick PC (1994) Comparison of digital rectal examination and serum prostate-specific antigen in the early detection of prostate cancer; results of a multicenter clinical trial of 6,630 men. J Urol 151: 1283–1290.
2. Catalona WJ, Smith DS, Ratliff TL, Basler JW (1993) Detection of organ-confined prostate cancer is increased through prostate-specific antigen-based screening. JAMA 270:948–954.
3. Punglia RS, D'Amico AV, Catalona WJ, Roehl KA, Kunz KM (2003) Effect of verification bias on screening for prostate cancer by measurement of prostate-specific antigen. N Engl J Med 349:335–342.
4. Thompson IM, Pauler DK, Goodman PJ, Tangen CM, Lucia MS, Parnes HL, Minasian LM, Ford LG, Lippman SM, Crawford ED, Crowley JJ, Coltman CA Jr (2004) Prevalence of prostate cancer among men with a prostate-specific antigen level ≤4.0ng per milliliter. N Engl J Med 350:2239–2246.
5. Datta MW, Dhir R, Dobbin K, Bosland MC, Melamed J, Becich MJ, Orenstein JM, Kajdacsy-Balla AA, Patel A, Macias V, Berman JJ (2005) Prostate cancer in patients with screening serum prostate specific antigen values less than 4.0ng/dl: results from the cooperative prostate cancer tissue resource. J Urol 173:1546–1551.
6. Carter HB (2004) Prostate cancers in men with low PSA levels—must we find them? N Engl J Med 350: 2292–2294.
7. Gore JL, Shariat SF, Miles BJ, Kadmon D, Jiang N, Wheeler TM, Slawn KM (2001) Optimal combinations of systemic sextant and laterally directed biopsies for

the detection of prostate cancer. J Urol 165: 1554–1559.

8. Eskew LA, Bare RL, McCullough DL (1997) Systemic 5 region prostate biopsy is superior to sextant method for diagnosing carcinoma of prostate. J Urol 157: 199–203.

9. Babaian RJ, Toi A, Kamoi K, Troncoso P, Sweet J, Evans R, Johnston D, Chen M (2000) A comparative analysis of sextant and an extended 11-core multisite directed biopsy strategy. J Urol 163:152–157.

10. Emiliozzi P, Scarpone P, DePaula F, Pizzo M, Federico G, Pansandoro A, Martini M, Pansandoro V (2004) The incidence of prostate cancer in men with prostate specific antigen greater than 4.0 ng/ml: a randomized study of 6 versus 12 core transperitoneal prostate biopsy. J Urol 171:197–199.

11. Presti JC Jr, O'Dowd GL, Miller MC, Masttu R, Veltri RW (2003) Extended peripheral zone biopsy schemes increase cancer detection rates and minimize variance in prostate specific antigen and age related cancer rates: results of a community multi-practice study. J Urol 165:125–129.

12. Levine MA, Ittman M, Melamed J, Lepor H (1998) Two consecutive sets of transrectal ultrasound guided sextant biopsies of prostate for the detection of prostate cancer. J Urol 159:471–476.

13. Norberg M, Egevad L, Holmberg L, Sparen P, Norlen BJ, Busch C (1997) The sextant protocol for ultrasound-guided core biopsies of the prostate underestimates the presence of cancer. Urology 50:562–566.

14. Naughton CK, Smith DS, Humphrey PA, Catalona WL, Keetch DW (1998) Clinical and pathologic tumor characteristics of prostate cancer as a function of the number of biopsy cores: a retrospective study. Urology 52:808–813.

15. Singh H, Canto EI, Shariat SF, Kadmon D, Miles BJ, Wheeler TM, Slawn KM (2004) Six additional systemic lateral cores enhance sextant biopsy prediction of pathological features at radical prostatectomy. J Urol 171:204–209.

16. Naughton CK, Miller DC, Mager DE, Ornstein DK, Catalona WJ (2000) A prospective randomized trial comparing 6 versus 12 prostate biopsy cores: impact on cancer detection. J Urol 164:388–392.

17. Lerner SP, Atkinson N (2000) Editorial comment. J Urol 164:392.

18. Djavan B, Zlotta A, Remzi M, Ghawidel K, Basharkhah A, Schulman CC, Marberger M (2000) Optimal predictors of prostate cancer on repeat prostate biopsy: a prospective study of 1051 men. J Urol 163:1144–1149.

19. Djavan B, Ravery V, Zlotta A, Dobronski P, Dobrovits M, Fakhari M, Seitz C, Susani M, Borkowski A, Boccon-Gibod L, Schulman CC, Marberger M (2001) Prospective evaluation of prostate cancer detected on biopsies 1, 2, 3, and 4: when should we stop? J Urol 166:1679–1683.

20. Levine MA, Ittman M, Melamed J, Lepor H (1998) Two consecutive sets of transrectal ultrasound guided sextant biopsies of the prostate for the detection of prostate cancer. J Urol 159:471–476.

21. Rietbergen JBW, Boeken Kruger AE, Hoedemaker RF, Bangma CH, Kirkels WJ, Schroeder FH (1998) Repeat screening for prostate cancer after 1-year follow-up in 984 biopsied men: clinical pathological features of detected cancer. J Urol 160:2121–2125.

22. Eskicorapci SY, Guliyev F, Akdogan B, Dogan HS, Ergen A, Ozen H (2005) Individualization of the biopsy protocol accounting to the prostate gland volume for prostate cancer detection. J Urol 173:1536–1540.

23. Keetch DW, Catalona WJ, Smith DS (1994) Serial prostatic biopsies in men with persistently elevated serum prostate specific antigen values. J Urol 151:1571–1574.

24. Catalona WJ, Partin AW, Slawin KM, Brawer MK, Flanigan RC, Patel A, Richie JP, deKernion JB, Walsh PC, Scardino PT, Lange PH, Subong EP, Parson RE, Gasior GH, Loveland KG, Southwick PC (1998) Use of the percentage of free prostate-specific antigen to enhance differentiation of prostate cancer from benign prostate disease: a prospective multicenter clinical trial. JAMA 279:1542–1547.

25. Fowler JE Jr, Bigler SA, Miles D, Yalkut DA (2000) Predictor of first repeat biopsy cancer detection with suspected local stage prostate cancer. J Urol 163:813–818.

Question 14

What is the clinical significance of isolated high-grade prostatic intraepithelial neoplasia discovered on a prostate needle core biopsy? How often does it occur? Does its presence predict cancer on a subsequent biopsy? Are there any specific clinical or pathologic findings that favorably predict cancer on a subsequent biopsy?

Answer

The incidence of high-grade intraepithelial neoplasia (HGPIN) depends on the study population and the number of biopsy cores examined. Among men screened for prostate cancer by the serum prostate-specific antigen (PSA) assay, the frequency of isolated HGPIN (without concomitant cancer) is 4%–10%. Traditionally, HGPIN has a high predictive value as a marker for adenocarcinoma. A repeat biopsy is generally indicated in men with HGPIN. It should not be limited to the HGPIN loci. The clinical parameters—including the initial PSA, changes in PSA, and digital rectal examination (DRE) and transrectal ultrasonography (TRUS) findings—do not appear useful. However, the number of biopsy cores involved by HGPIN is predictive. If cancer is not found on the next two follow-up biopsies, it is unlikely that cancer will be found on a subsequent biopsy. With wide application of the extended prostate needle core biopsy, the predictive value of HGPIN is decreasing as many cancers have been detected on the initial biopsy. Epstein recently suggested that no repeat biopsy is necessary during the first year for patients with isolated HGPIN diagnosed on extended initial biopsy, provided other clinical indicators of cancer are absent.

Comments

The PSA-led prostate needle core biopsy (PNB) has increased the detection rate of prostate cancer at an early stage. It also increased the chance of discovering either low- or high-grade prostatic intraepithelial neoplasia (PIN). Earlier studies showed that low-grade PIN was significantly different from HGPIN in terms of cancer risk: $P < 0.05$ [1], $P < 0.001$ [2], and $P < 0.01$ [3] and was not associated with an increased risk of cancer any more than is the initially negative biopsy [1]. Only HGPIN is considered a precancerous lesion (Fig. 1-14-1). HGPIN is often multifocal and coexists with carcinoma in high frequency in radical prostatectomy specimens [4–6].

HGPIN discovered as an isolated lesion on a PNB may signify a coexisting cancer or the development of cancer in the near future. HGPIN has a high predictive value as a marker of carcinoma, and its identification warrants repeat biopsy [7].

How often is HGPIN detected as an isolated lesion on PNB?

The reported incidence varies widely from 2.1% to 16.5%. The lowest frequency is in men participating in cancer screening with PSA, whereas men undergoing PNB because of abnormal DRE and/or abnormal TRUS tend to have higher values (Table 1-14-1). The high frequency (16.5%) reported from the Mayo Clinic by Bostwick et al. [8] may be due to inclusion of men who were referred to the academic center

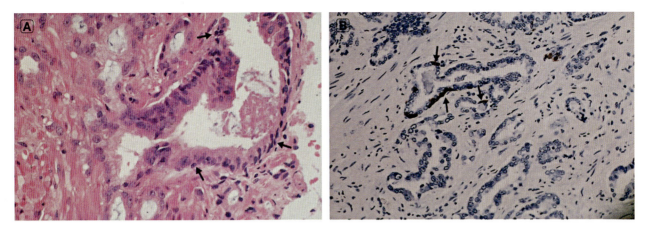

FIG. 1-14-1. **A** Focus of high-grade intraepithelial neoplasia (PIN) from which an invasive nest abuts. Basal cells are distributed sparsely (*arrows*). Around this focus are cancerous glands scattered in the stroma (Gleason score 3 + 3). **B** Most of the abnormal acini are devoid of high-molecular-weight cytokeratin (HMWK)-positive cells, indicating they are invasive cancerous glands. One acinus in the center still retains HMWK-positive cells (*arrows*), indicating that this acinus may be in transition to becoming an invasive gland

TABLE 1-14-1. Frequency of isolated high-grade prostatic intraepithelial neoplasia detection in prostate cancer screening by prostate needle core biopsy

Study	What led to PNB	Total no. biopsied	HGPIN (%)	Number of cores examined	Comments
Mettlin [12], 1991	Abnormal DRE/TRUS	396	17 (4.3%)	Biopsy directed to suspicious lesion (DRE/TRUS). Core number not stated	Multicenter study organized by the American Cancer Society National Prostate Cancer Detection Project. Biopsy recommended on abnormal DRE and/or TRUS and not by PSA value.
Bostwick [8], 1995	Not stated	Mayo 200 Glendale M. Hospital 200	33 (16.5%) 19 (9.5%)	6 or more (mean 7.1) Not stated	Most (78.5%) had unilateral palpable nodule. Glendale M. Hospital is a private practice medical center.
Langer [13], 1996	↑ PSA, abnormal DRE/TRUS	1275	61 (4.8%)	At least 6 cores	
Ramos [9], 1999	PSA > 2.5, abnormal DRE	2237	48 (2.1%)	Not stated	Men with PSA > 2.5 ng/ml were biopsied.
Borboroglu [14], 2001	Not stated	1391	137 (9.8%)	Sextant	
Lefkowitz [11], 2001	Not stated	619	103 (16.6%)	12 Cores	

PNB, prostate needle core biopsy; HGPIN, high-grade intraepithelial neoplasia; DRE, digital rectal examination; TRUS, transrectal ultrasonography; PSA, prostate-specific antigen.

because of abnormal DRE findings. This suggestion is supported by the lower frequency (9.5%) reported by the same authors as data from a nearby community hospital. The lowest frequency of HGPIN (2.1%), reported by Ramos et al. [9], is most likely due to inclusion of men whose PSA was between 2.5 and 4.0 ng/ml. Therefore, a number of men who are unlikely to have cancer/HGPIN may have been subjected to PNB.

A second reason for the variable frequency rates is the difference in the biopsy method. HGPIN is often a multifocal lesion. Thus, its detection rate (as well as that of cancer) would increase in proportion to the number of biopsy cores examined. The following two reports are exemplary in support of this notion. In the study by Rosser et al. [10] (Table 1-14-2), as many as 14 cores were removed by the technique designated the five-region method. With this method, an

TABLE 1-14-2. Follow-up rebiopsy results in men initially presenting with high-grade prostatic intraepithelial neoplasia on prostate needle core biopsy

Author/Year	What led to PNB	HGPIN cases with follow-up biopsy	Intervals between initial and repeat biopsies	Repeat biopsy findings		
				Benign	Low-grade PIN	HGPIN
Brawer [22], 1991	Abnormal DRE and/or abnormal TRUS	10	1–24 mos (mean 8.8 mos)	0	0	0
Aboseif [18], 1995	Not stated	24	Every 6 mos			5
Davidson [15], 1995	Not stated	100 Control with follow-up biopsy 112	Mean 265 days Mean 500 days	22 77		43 20
Keetch [1], 1995	Twice elevated PSA > 4.1 ng/ml and abnormal DRE and/or TRUS	37	Not stated	17		1
Raviv [2], 1996	Suspicious DRE finding or PSA > 4	48	3-6 mos If repeat biopsy is negative, third biopsy done only when abnormal DRE or ↑ PSA		25 (no cancer)	
Langer [13], 1996	↑ PSA, abnormal DRE and/or abnormal TRUS	53	Mean 101 days	30		8
Shepherd [3], 1996	PSA > 4.1 suspicious DRE	45		18		1
Park [20], 2001	Not stated	43	1–62 mos (mean 10.6 mos)			
Borboroglu [14], 2001	↑ PSA, abnormal DRE, abnormal PSA density, or PSA velocity	45	<12 mos (mean 3.9 mos)	21		4
Lefkowitz [11], 2001	Not stated	43	Within a year (median 4.2 mos)	20	1	21 (1 atypia included)

Ca	No. of biopsy cores and biopsy sites	Comments/conclusions
10 (100%)	2–8 (mean 4.2)	Initial biopsy: directed to hypoechoic lesion, but subsequently Stanford systemic biopsy. Repeat biopsy: limited to sites showing PIN.
19 (79%)	DRE/TRUS positive site (core number not stated); in others, sextant.	Repeat biopsy every 6 mos until either cancer is found or 2 years had elapsed.
35 (35%)	Mean 3.7	Controls consist of men with abnormal DRE, elevated PSA, and/or TRUS, but the initial biopsy is negative for PIN and Ca. Detection rate of cancer is significantly higher among men with HGPIN than among men with neither cancer nor HGPIN in initial biopsy ($P < 0.001$).
15 (13%)	Mean 3.2	
19 (51%)	4–6 Directed to DRE/TRUS-positive area. Otherwise biopsy quadrant biopsy.	1. HGPIN in initial biopsy is significantly associated with cancer detection in repeat biopsy than either low-grade PIN ($P < 0.05$) or negative initial biopsy ($P < 0.05$). 2. The control group consists of men with a persistently elevated PSA value after an initial negative biopsy.
23 (48%)	Biopsy of hypoechoic lesion and two other systematic biopsies. If no hypoechoic lesion, sextant biopsy done	Significant differences between cancer and noncancer groups in PSA ($P = 0.016$), TRUS appearance ($P < 0.001$), and DRE ($P = 0.008$). Only abnormal DRE and ↑ PSA are predictive of subsequent cancer by multivariate analysis. HGPIN is a strong predictor of cancer especially in men with abnormal DRE and ↑ PSA (mean 14.5).
15 (28%)	At least 6 cores obtained either from hypoechoic site or HGPIN site	No significant differences among subsequent benign, HGPIN, and cancer diagnosis groups in DRE/TRUS findings and biopsy methods used. Cancer detection sites not correlated with initial HGPIN sites.
26 (58%)	Biopsy 4–6 cores, directed to suspicious site. If no abnormality, selected quadrant biopsy	Directing repeat biopsy to the PIN side misses cancer in approximately 35% of positive cases. Systemic biopsy should be used.
22 (55%), 3/5	Biopsy core number <6	20 of 22 cancer cases diagnosed on the first rebiopsy. No significant differences between cancer and noncancer cases in age, PSA, DRE findings, and number of biopsy cores. 26% of cancer cases would have been missed if rebiopsy were to be used only at sites showing HGPIN.
16/13, 3/7	6–10 >11	
20 (44%)	Sextant initially. Repeat biopsy: extended biopsy technique or sextant + TZ sampling	Limiting rebiopsy to HGPIN site is not advised (53% would have been missed). PSA velocity is a significant predictor of cancer diagnosis.
1 (2%)	12 core biopsies, both initial and repeat	

TABLE 1-14-2. *Continued*

Author/Year	What led to PNB	HGPIN cases with follow-up biopsy	Intervals between initial and repeat biopsies	Repeat biopsy findings		
				Benign	Low-grade PIN	HGPIN
Lefkowitz [19], 2002	PSA ↑	31	3 Years	12		11
Rosser [9], 1999	PSA ↑ and/or abnormal DRE	24	Mean 9.2 mos	13		
Kronz [21], 2001	Not stated	245	Median 5.3 mos First rebiopsy (*n* = 245) Second rebiopsy (*n* = 81) Third or more rebiopsy (*n* = 15)	185 Men without cancer ↙ Benign Cancer in 3/40 Cancer in 1/10	↓ HGPIN Cancer in 7/27 Cancer in 0/3	↘ Atypia Cancer in 7/14 Cancer in 1/2
Bishara [23], 2004	Not stated	132	1–33 mos (mean 7 mos)	60		23 (11 atypical)
Roscigno [24], 2004	Not stated	47	≤6 mos (24) >6 mos (23)	18 8 7		
Singh [16], 2004	PSA > 2.5 and/or abnormal DRE	14	Median			
Herawi [17], 2006	Attempt at establishing diagnosis of cancer after HGPIN diagnosis	791	within 1 year mean 4.6 months			

For abbreviation used, refer to Table 1-14-1.

additional eight cores are biopsied together with the standard sextant biopsy cores. Because of elevated PSA and/or abnormal DRE, 50 men underwent the five region biopsies; 26 of them were diagnosed with HGPIN. HGPIN was detected in the sextant regions in only 14 patients (53%), whereas an additional 12 patients (47%) were diagnosed with HGPIN in regions not examined by the sextant biopsies ($P < 0.05$). The study by Lefkowitz et al. [11] is based on the 12-core biopsy method (double sextant biopsies). Of a total of 619 men, 208 (34%) were found to have cancer and 103 men to have HGPIN alone (17%). The HGPIN detection rate is higher than those reported for the standard sextant biopsy method. Because the sextant biopsy method was most commonly used, the frequency of HGPIN on patients with PSA-based prostate cancer screening and the standard biopsy ranges from 4% to 10%.

Ca	No. of biopsy cores and biopsy sites	Comments/conclusions
8 (26%)	12 core biopsies in all men, both initial and repeat	Changes in PSA not associated with detection of cancer. All 4 patients who subsequently underwent radical prostatectomy had organ-confined cancer.
8 (33%)	Sextant and 5-region biopsy (14 cores)	Reprospective study to compare the detection rate of HGPIN by traditional sextant biopsy technique with rate by 5-region biopsy technique. Of 50 patients, sextant biopsy technique detected HGPIN in only 14 patients (53%), whereas 5-region technique detected HGPIN in additional 12 patients ($P < 0.05$).
60 (24%) 17 (21%) 2 (13%)	Not stated	No predictive value of initial PSA, DRE, and TRUS findings or PSA change. Predictive values in histologic findings in initial biopsy: number of cores with HGPIN, ($P = 0.01$), absence of mitosis ($P = 0.009$). Very large prominent nucleoli, predominant micropapillary/cribriform HGPIN ($P = 0.002$).
38 (29%) 27 First rebiopsy 7 Second rebiopsy 4 Subsequent rebiopsy	4–15 cores. Sextant biopsy in 60% of initial and 61% of repeat biopsy.	90% of cancers identified on the second and third rebiopsies. If multiple cores are involved by HGPIN on the first rebiopsy, cancer risk on subsequent biopsy is 50%, regardless of single or multiple core involvement on the initial biopsy. Histologic subtypes not informative of subsequent cancer detection.
6 (25%) 15 (65%) $P < 0.01$	10 to 12 cores; both initial and repeat biopsy	Multivariate analysis shows multiple core (versus single core) involvement is a strong independent predictor in cancer detection. Age, PSA, DRE, and TRUS findings are not significant. PSA density is significant by univariate analysis ($P = 0.02$).
7 (50%)	12 Cores, both initial and repeat biopsy	HGPIN in initial biopsy is significantly associated with cancer detection or repeat biopsy ($P < 0.01$).
No. cores 1st biopsy / No. cores on rebiopsy / Ca/total 1. 6 / 6 / 20/142 (14.1%) 2. 6 / 8 or more / 36/113 (31.9%) 3. 8 or more / 8 or more / 37/253 (14.6%) 4. 8 or more / 6 / 4/44 (9.1%) group 2 vs 1 $P = 0.001$; 2 vs 3 $P < 0.001$; 2 vs 4 $P = 0.003$; 1 vs 3 $P = 0.93$; 1 vs 4 $P = 0.37$; 3 vs 4 $P = 0.33$	6 and 8 or more	Initial sextant biopsy misses a large number of cancers that can be detected on 8 or more cores on repeat biopsy. Initial 8 cores or more detect more cancers and therefore the detection rate on repeat biopsy is significantly lower.

How often is cancer detected on the follow-up biopsies among men with isolated HGPIN in the initial biopsy, and how aggressive should the urologist be about cancer detection if the repeat biopsy is again negative?

There are a number of studies reported in the literature. The findings [1–3, 9, 11, 13–24] are tabulated in Table 1-14-2. The cancer detection rates on a repeat biopsy range widely from 2% to 100 %. It depends on the patient population (PSA screening-based population vs. men presenting with abnormal DRE/TRUS findings), the interval between initial and repeat biopsies, the number of repeat biopsies (more than two repeat biopsies in some patients) [2, 18], the number of biopsy cores examined, and the number of cores involved with HGPIN on the initial biopsy. The lowest frequency reported by Lefkowitz et al.

[11] was for men whose HGPIN detection was based on the 12-core sampling method (two-consecutive sextant biopsy method). Of a total of 619 men who underwent initial 12-core biopsies, 208 (34%) were found to have cancer and 103 men to have HGPIN alone (17%). These detection rates are somewhat higher than those after the standard sextant biopsy method. Of the 103 men, 43 underwent a repeat 12-core biopsy after a mean of 4.2 months (all biopsies were done within a year). Only one carcinoma (2.3%) was found and 20 of the men had HGPIN again. The authors concluded that a repeat biopsy after the diagnosis of HGPIN based on the 12-core biopsy rarely results in cancer detection and that in the absence of suspicion of cancer, immediate repeat biopsy is unnecessary. To define the natural history of HGPIN, however, the same group performed biopsy 3 years later using the same biopsy method [16]. Of 31 men who underwent re-biopsy regardless of changes in the PSA or DRE, 8 had carcinoma (26%) and 11 had HGPIN (36%); the remaining 12 had a benign diagnosis. In comparison to the 2.3% incidence of cancer detected within 1 year by the same group [11], the rise in incidence to 26% after a 3-year interval was interpreted that HGPIN was a precursor to prostate cancer and repeat biopsy at a delayed interval is recommended regardless of changes in PSA.

What are predictors for carcinoma in patients diagnosed with HGPIN?

Are there clinical and pathologic parameters that are useful for predicting cancer in a follow-up biopsy? Raviv et al. [2] claimed that abnormal DRE ($P = 0.008$), abnormal TRUS ($P < 0.001$), and high PSA (14.5 vs. 8.2 ng/ml, $P = 0.016$) are predictive of carcinoma in the subsequent biopsy. These findings were refuted by others, however, [13, 19–21]. Initially high PSA levels suggest concomitant carcinoma.

In earlier studies, rebiopsy was directed to the site of the HGPIN or DRE-positive focus either exclusively or inclusively [2, 3, 13, 18, 22]. Lesion-directed biopsy would miss 26%–53% of cancers [3, 14, 20]. Rebiopsy should be taken by the systematic method because of the multifocal nature of prostate carcinoma.

Krontz et al. [21] made an extensive morphologic study looking for clues that predict cancer in the repeat biopsy. If the first repeat biopsy is benign, has HGPIN, or is atypical, the eventual cancer rates were

8%, 26%, and 50%, respectively. Of 15 patients with more than two repeat biopsies, only 2 had cancer. The following findings in the initial biopsy were predictive of cancer in the repeat biopsy: the number of cores with HGPIN ($P = 0.01$); the absence of mitosis versus its presence ($P = 0.009$); large prominent nucleoli; and a predominantly micropapillary/cribriform pattern ($P = 0.002$). Subsequently, the same group reported an updated information on HGPIN for subsequent detection of cancer. Multiple core involvement by HGPIN on both the initial and first repeat biopsy defined a subset of men who were at increased risk of harboring synchronous invasive carcinoma. They now stated that the histololgic subtypes on the initial biopsy do not appear to influence the detection rate of cancer on the subsequent repeat biopsy [23]. More recently, an Italian group came to the same conclusion: Multiple core (in contrast to single core) involvement is the only independent predictor of cancer in a repeat biopsy [24].

The extended PNB detected more prostate cancer than did the traditional sextant biopsy. As a consequence, the predictive value of HGPIN is decreasing as many cancers have been detected in the initial extended biopsy. Whether this change in clinical management will be accepted remains to be seen. Nevertheless, the clinical significance of isolated HGPIN is decreasing. The relation between the number of cores on initial biopsy and the number of cores on rebiopsy and the risk of finding cancer in the rebiopsy specimen was illustrated in a series of 791 men with HGPIN on initial biopsy who underwent re-biopsy within 1 year of the diagnosis [17]. Cancer detection rates on rebiopsy varied based on the biopsy schema: The rates were highest in men who underwent initial sextant biopsy and who then underwent an extended number of cores for rebiopsy.

Based on the recent studies by the Johns Hopkins group, some investigators suggested that for patients diagnosed with HGPIN based on extended initial core sampling a repeat biopsy within the year was unnecessary in the absence of other clinical indicators of cancer [25]. Obviously, more studies are needed for rationally adjusting the re-biopsy strategy in men who were found to have HGPIN after undergoing extended core biopsy. The most important aspect is close clinical follow-up with serum PSA assays. If there are clinical signs suspicious for prostate cancer, these patients should be re-biopsied.

It must be pointed out that the repeat biopsy should include the site of HGPIN and sites without HGPIN. If the repeat biopsy is negative again, a repeat second biopsy is indicated only in patients who continue to have other clinical findings suggestive of cancer.

The finding of HGPIN with adjacent small atypical glands indicates a situation quite different from isolated HGPIN. This subject is discussed under Question 17. The rate of finding cancer in repeat biopsies from patients with HGPIN with small atypical glands is approximately 50%, similar to the finding in men with small atypical glands suspicious but not diagnostic of carcinoma [26]. Repeat biopsy is recommended in men with HGPIN with small atypical glands [25].

References

1. Keetch DW, Humphrey P, Stahl D, Smith DS, Catalona WJ (1995) Morphometric analysis and clinical follow-up of isolated prostatic intraepithelial neoplasia in needle biopsy of the prostate. J Urol 154:347–351.

2. Raviv G, Janssen T, Zlotta AR, Descamps F, Verhest A, Schulman CC (1996) Prostatic intraepithelial neoplasia: influence of clinical and pathological data on the prediction of prostate cancer. J Urol 156:1050–1055.

3. Shepherd D, Keetch DW, Humphrey PA, Smith DS, Stahl D (1996) Repeat biopsy strategy in men with isolated prostatic intraepithelial neoplasia on prostatic needle biopsy. J Urol 156:460–463.

4. McNeal JE, Bostwick DG (1986) Intraductal dysplasia: a premalignant lesion of the prostate. Hum Pathol 17:64–71.

5. Oyasu R, Bahnson RR, Nowels K, Garnett JE (1986) Cytological atypia in the prostate gland: frequency, distribution, and possible relevance to carcinoma. J Urol 136:959–962.

6. Troncoso P, Grignon DJ, Babaian RJ, von Eschenbach AC, Ro JY, Ayala AG (1989) Prostatic intraepithelial neoplasia and invasive prostatic adenocarcinoma in cystoprostatectomy specimens. Urology 34:52–56.

7. Bostwick DG (1999) Prostatic intraepithelial neoplasia is a risk factor for cancer. Semin Urol Oncol 17:187–198.

8. Bostwick DG, Qian J, Frankel K (1995) The incidence of high-grade prostatic intraepithelial neoplasia in needle biopsies. J Urol 154:1791–1794.

9. Ramos CG, Carvahal GF, Mager DE, Haberer B, Catalona WJ (1999) The effect of high grade prostatic intraepithelial neoplasia on serum total and percentage of free prostate specific antigen levels. J Urol 162:1587–1590.

10. Rosser CJ, Broberg J, Case D, Eskew A, McCullough D (1999) Detection of high-grade prostatic intraepithelial neoplasia with the five-region biopsy technique. Urology 54:853–856.

11. Lefkowitz GK, Sidhu GS, Torre P, Lepor H, Taneja SS (2001) Is repeat biopsy prostate biopsy for high-grade prostatic intraepithelial neoplasia necessary after routine 12-core sampling? Urology 58:999–1003.

12. Mettlin C, Lee F, Drago J, Murphy GP, the Investigators of the American Cancer Society National Prostate Cancer Detection Project (1991) The American Cancer Society National Prostate Cancer Project: findings on the detection of early prostate cancer in 2425 men. Cancer 67:2949–2958.

13. Langer JE, Rovner ES, Coleman BG, Yin D, Arger PH, Malkowicz SB, Nisenbaum HL, Bowling SE, Tomaszewski JE, Wein AJ (1996) Strategy for repeat biopsy of patients with prostatic intraepithelial neoplasia detected by prostate needle biopsy. J Urol 155:228–231.

14. Borboroglu PG, Sur RL, Roberts JL, Amling CL (2001) Repeat biopsy strategy in patients with atypical small acinar proliferation or high grade prostatic intraepithelial neoplasia onn initial needle biopsy. J Urol 166:866–870.

15. Davidson D, Bostwick DG, Qian J, Wollan PC, Oesterling JE, Rudders RA, Siroky M, Stilmant M (1995) Prostatic intraepithelial neoplasia is a risk factor for adenocarcinoma: predictive accuracy in needle biopsies. J Urol 154:1295–1299.

16. Singh H, Canto EI, Shariat SF, Kadmon D, Miles BJ, Wheeler TM, Slawin KM (2004) Predictors of prostatic cancer after initial negative systemic 12 core biopsy. J Urol 171:1850–1854.

17. Herawi M, Kahane H, Cavallo C, Epstein JI (2006) Risk of prostate cancer on first rebiopsy within 1 year following a diagnosis of high grade intraepithelial neoplasia is related to the number of cores sampled. J Urol 175:121–124.

18. Aboseif S, Shinohara K, Weinder N, Parayan P, Carrol PR (1995) The significance of prostatic intra-epithelial neoplasia. Br J Urol 76:355–359.

19. Lefkowitz GK, Taneja SS, Brown J, Melamed J, Lepor H (2002) Follow-up interval prostate biopsy 3 years after diagnosis of high-grade prostatic intraepithelial neoplasia is associated with high likelihood of prostate cancer, independent of changes in prostate specific antigen levels. J Urol 168:1415–1418.

20. Park S, Shinohara K, Grossfeld GD, Carrol PR (2001) Prostate cancer detection in men with prior high-grade prostatic intraepithelial neoplasia or atypical prostate biopsy. J Urol 165:1409–1414.

21. Kronz JD, Allan CH, Shaikh AA, Epstein JI (2001A) Predicting cancer following a diagnosis of high-grade prostatic intraepithelial neoplasia on needle biopsy: data on men with more than one follow-up biopsy. Am J Surg Pathol 25:1079–1085.

22. Brawer MK, Nagle RB, Bigler SA, Lange PH, Sohlberg OE (1991) Significance of intraepithelial neoplasia on prostate needle biopsy. Urology 38:103–107.

23. Bishara T, Ramnani DM, Epstein JI (2004) High-grade prostatic intraepithelial neoplasia on needle biopsy: risk of cancer on repeated biopsy related to number of involved cores and morphologic pattern. Am J Surg Pathol 28:629–633.

24. Roscigno M, Scattoni V, Freschi M, Raber M, Colombo R, Bertini R, Montorsi F, Rigatti P (2004) Monofocal and plurifocal high-grade prostatic intraepithelial neoplasia on extended prostate biopsies: factors predicting cancer detection on extended repeat biopsy, Urology 63:1105–1110.

25. Epstein JI, Herawi M (2006) Prostatic needle biopsies containing prostatic intraepithelial neoplasia or atypical foci suspicious for carcinoma: implications for patient care. J Urol 175:820–834.

26. Kronz JD, Shaikh AA, Epstein JI (2001B) High-grade prostatic intraepithelial neoplasia with adjacent small atypical glands on prostate biopsy. Hum Pathol 32: 389–395.

Question 15

What is the clinical significance of a Gleason pattern 4 or 5 tumor found on a prostate needle core biopsy? What impact does a Gleason pattern 4 or 5 tumor have on the prognosis after radical prostatectomy?

Answer

The Gleason system of prostate cancer is based on the architectural patterns.[1] The primary (predominant) and secondary (second most prevalent) patterns are recognized and assigned a grade from 1 (most differentiated) to 5 (least differentiated). Prostate cancer is noted for its multifocal occurrence of different Gleason grades. Likewise, it is not uncommon to observe more than one histologic pattern in a single mass as a greater amount of tissue is available with a radical prostatectomy specimen than a biopsy. Each tumor is given a score as the sum of two grades of these patterns. If the third most common pattern is of a lower Gleason pattern, it can be ignored. If a higher-grade component (Gleason pattern 4 or 5) is found, its presence must be reported because the tertiary higher-grade component worsens the pathologic stage of otherwise typical Gleason scores 5, 6, and 7 carcinomas and is associated with a higher PSA recurrence rate. With regards to a pattern 4 or 5 carcinoma observed in a prostate needle core biopsy, its presence should be reported as a secondary or tertiary component. However, the percentage volume of Gleason pattern 4 or 5 tumor in the radical prostatectomy specimen cannot reliably be predicted based on its volume in the biopsy specimen.

Comments

The Gleason scoring system is a well-established prognostic parameter of prostate cancer. Historically, patients with high Gleason score carcinomas (8, 9, 10) on initial biopsy are not considered candidates for radical prostatectomy because the long-term tumor-free survival is poor and many patients are found to have a pelvic lymph node metastasis [1]. With the advent of PSA-based screening for detection of prostate cancer, more and more cases are detected in an early stage with a favorable Gleason score. As a result, tumors tend to cluster in the midrange (Gleason scores 5–7). In prostatectomy series, 79%–94% have been reported to be Gleason score 5–7 and 50%–89% have been assigned a Gleason score of 6 or 7 [2–5]. Prostate cancer is noted for its multifocality and different histologic patterns representing different Gleason grades, and it is not uncommon to observe more than two patterns in a single tumor as well as among tumors.

To improve the prognostic value of Gleason score in the midrange, McNeal et al. [6] and Stamey et al. [7] proposed the percent Gleason pattern 4 or 5 as a new prognostic parameter. Based on 379 patients with peripheral zone cancers from radical prostatectomy specimens, they [7] suggested that the cancer grade expressed as percent Gleason grade 4/5 as well as cancer volume were highly predictive of disease

---

[1] Gleason "pattern" and "grade" are frequently used interchangeably, and Gleason "score" and "sum" are synonymous.

progression. In this study, however, data were collected between 1983 and 1992, and only 96 men had clinical stage T1c. As many as 81% ($n = 307$) of the patients had a Gleason pattern 4/5 lesion, which ranged in volume from <1% to >90%. Only 19% ($n = 72$) of 379 men had no evidence of any Gleason grade 4/5 cancer. In this group of 72 men, the cumulative failure rate (as judged by PSA recurrence) was only 5.6%, in contrast to the steady rise in the failure rate in the remaining men, which was in proportion to the percent Gleason pattern 4/5 cancer, ultimately approaching 87% [7]. In this study, however, the frequency of Gleason pattern 4/5 cancers was much higher than that reported in later studies, perhaps reflecting the fact that the cases were collected before PSA screening was initiated.

Epstein et al. [8] evaluated 720 individual tumor foci in 153 radical prostatectomy specimens removed for T1c. Among them, 671 foci were located in the peripheral region (presumably in the peripheral and central zones), and 49 were in the transition zone. Of the 671 peripheral region tumors, 119 foci (17.7%) contained some elements of Gleason pattern 4/5. Thirteen foci had a high Gleason score of 8–10. An important message for urologists as well as pathologists is that 54 high-grade foci were less than 1 ml in volume, and 9% of the prostates contained foci of <1 ml in volume.

Knowing that the presence of a high-grade tumor component adversely affects the prognosis, we cannot ignore its presence (even a small focus) in either prostate needle core biopsies or radical prostatectomy specimens.

By definition, the Gleason score consists of the two most common Gleason grades of the tumor (primary and secondary patterns), and focal areas of tertiary high-grade pattern are not included. There is no consensus on how the tertiary pattern(s) should be handled. A modified Gleason score comprising the primary and the worst grade has been suggested [9].

Pan et al. [9] from the Johns Hopkins Hospital analyzed 114 radical prostatectomy cases with small tertiary higher-grade components that mostly occupied <5% of the total tumors. The results were compared with those of 2276 consecutive cases without tertiary higher-grade components collected in the same institution. Parameters compared were the frequency of organ-confined cases, "extracapsular" extension (focal vs. established), seminal vesicle invasion, and pelvic lymph node metastasis. Of the 114 cases, 47 (41%) had a typical Gleason score 5 (3 + 2 or 2 + 3) or 6 (3 + 3) adenocarcinomas with a tertiary component of Gleason pattern 4 or 5; 56 cases (49%) were typical Gleason score 7 (3 + 4 or 4 + 3) with a tertiary component of Gleason pattern 5; and 11 cases (10%) were typical Gleason score 8 (4 + 4) with a tertiary component of Gleason pattern 5. The tertiary tumor volumes ranged from <0.01 to 0.68 ml. With the exception of six cases with a volume ratio of 6%–15%, all others measured <5%. The pathologic stages were significantly more advanced when higher tertiary Gleason grade components were present in Gleason score 5–6 tumors ($P = 0.018$) or 7 tumors ($P = 0.008$) (Table 1-15-1).

As for the risk of progression, the presence of a tertiary high-grade component in a typical Gleason score 5–6 increased it significantly compared with typical Gleason score 5–6 ($P < 0.001$), but there was no difference between the former and typical Gleason score 7. When compared with typical Gleason score 7 tumors, Gleason score 5–6 tumors with high-grade components had a less advanced pathologic stage ($P = 0.021$). No difference in the progression rate was demonstrated between typical Gleason score 7 with tertiary Gleason pattern 5 and typical Gleason score 8 tumors. No difference was found between typical Gleason score 8 tumors and Gleason score 8 tumors

TABLE 1-15-1. Significant worsening of pathologic stage and progression rate in the presence of a higher tertiary Gleason grade component. p values by Chi-square analysis

Gleason score and associated tertiary grade			Pathologic stage (P)*	Progression rate (P)*
5–6 without tertiary 4/5	vs.	5–6 with tertiary 4/5	0.018	<0.0001
5–6 with tertiary 4/5	vs.	7 without tertiary 5	0.021	NS
7 without tertiary 5	vs	7 with tertiary 5	0.008	0.0003
7 with tertiary 5	vs.	8 without 5	NS	NS
8 without 5	vs.	8 with 5	NS	NS

From Pan et al. [9], with permission.
* By χ^2 analysis.

with Gleason pattern 5 component. A strong message from this study is that the presence of a high-grade component, even if it constitutes <5% of the tumor volume, has a significant adverse effect on the pathologic stage and prognosis.

The study reported by Egevad et al. [10] from Karolinska Hospital in Sweden is based on cases diagnosed at transurethral resection of the prostate (TURP) performed because of obstructive symptoms. Hormonal therapy was administered to patients with symptomatic locally progressive or metastatic disease. In 104 of the 305 cancers (34%), no Gleason pattern 4/5 was identified. The prostate cancer was the cause of death in proportion to Gleason pattern 4/5 cancer in the resected tumor tissue—8% (0% in volume), 28% (up to 5%), 38% (5%–50%), 65% (51%–100%)—at a median follow-up of 7.3 years. Patients with Gleason grade 4/5 tumor of any amount did significantly worse than those without grade 4/5 disease ($P < 0.001$). Gleason score 3 + 3 tumors with focal pattern 4/5 (<5% of the lesion) had a worse prognosis than pure Gleason 3 + 3 tumors ($P = 0.008$).

There have been a few studies that focus on the relation between high-grade cancers observed on a prostate needle core biopsy (PNB) and the extent of high-grade cancer in the prostatectomy specimens. Stamey [11] reported on the percent Gleason pattern 4/5 on sextant biopsies from 120 men who subsequently underwent radical prostatectomy. The sensitivity of the biopsies for predicting the percent Gleason pattern 4/5 cancer on prostatectomy specimens was 62%, and the specificity for indicating the absence of any pattern 4 in the prostate was 46 of 47 (98%). He emphasized that each biopsy report should state the total millimeters of cancer and the percentage of Gleason pattern 4/5 tumor in that cancer. He further stated that the prognostic difference between a tumor composed of 95% Gleason pattern 3 and 5% Gleason pattern 4 and a tumor composed of 95% Gleason grade 4 and 5% Gleason pattern 3 is huge. In the first instance a cancer is likely to be confined in the prostate, whereas in the latter instance it is a cancer with a much higher probability of being incurable by radical prostatectomy. Reporting that the cancer observed in the biopsy specimens contains no Gleason pattern 4/5 component is clinically significant (although it does not guarantee its absence in the radical prostatectomy specimens; see a later comment).

The Stamey group also studied the effect of multifocal cancer on PSA failure [12]. Secondary cancers (which are smaller than the primary or index tumor) in multiple prostate cancers did not adversely influence the results of preoperative clinical parameters, including PSA and needle biopsy findings. The percent Gleason pattern 4/5 cancer in needle core biopsies and prostatectomy specimens was the most powerful predictor of PSA recurrence in men with stage T1c prostate cancer.

Rubin et al. [13] of the University of Michigan conducted a similar study with 101 consecutive radical prostatectomies performed for clinically localized prostate cancer. Their conclusions are not as optimistic as Stamey's. They used ≥10% of Gleason pattern 4/5 in the prostatectomy specimens as a cutoff. Their decision was based on the observation by Stamey et al. [7] that PSA recurrence began to increase dramatically at ≥10%. Thus, using the logistic regression models for predicting any or >10% Gleason pattern 4/5 carcinoma in prostatectomy specimens, an area of pattern 4/5 disease >0.01 cm^2 on biopsy was the best single predictor. [Assuming that the full width of an 18-gauge needle core is involved, a tumor area that is 2 mm long would make up a 0.01 cm^2 specimen (Fig. 1-15-1) [14].] The sensitivity and specificity for a biopsy area of >0.01 cm^2 were 34% and 88%, respectively. They concluded that due to high false-negative rates, their models had limited predictive value on an individual basis.

What have we learned from these studies? First, Gleason pattern 4/5 cancer in any amount discovered in radical prostatectomy specimens worsens the prognosis as judged by PSA recurrence, and it becomes progressively worse in proportion to a pattern 4/5 component. Second, the presence of Gleason pattern 4/5 carcinoma in a biopsy tumor predicts a worse prognosis than its absence, but an estimate of the percentage pattern 4/5 carcinoma in a PNB appears to be a poor predictor of its volume in the radical prostatectomy specimen due to low sensitivity. In the study by Rubin et al. [13], despite a strong statistical correlation between biopsy and prostatectomy Gleason pattern 4/5 ($P = 0.0001$), as many as 30% of the radical prostatectomy specimens had a significant amount (>10% in volume) of pattern 4/5 cancer. These findings demonstrate that sampling errors significantly affect the reliability of the PNB findings on predicting the tumor grade in the radical prostatectomy specimens.

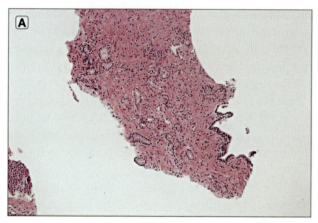
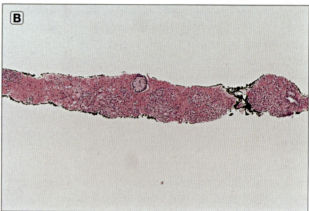

FIG. 1-15-1. These photographs are intended to demonstrate cancer size observed in a prostate needle core biopsy. **A** Small focus of a Gleason score 3 + 3 adenocarcinoma measuring 0.6×0.5 mm (0.003 cm^2). Photograph taken with a 10× objective. For a minute focus of low-grade carcinoma of this type, the likelihood of carcinoma to be pT2 is about 90% according to Bismar et al. [14] **B** A large focus of Gleason score 4 + 4 adenocarcinoma, occupying the entire field of photograph taken with 4× objective. It measures 0.47×3.56 mm (0.016 cm^2). According to the Rubin criteria [13], this patient is unlikely to have a localized cancer

In conclusion, If a tertiary high grade lesion (Gleason pattern 4/5) is found in the radical prostatectomy specimen, irrespective of its location, its presence and percent volume estimate (<10% or >10% of the total tumor) should be reported because according to the Stanford group 10% is a significant cutoff point influencing PSA recurrence. With a needle biopsy, if a Gleason grade 4/5 component is found as a tertiary element, its presence should be stated. However, the percentage volume of Gleason pattern 4/5 tumor in the radical prostatectomy specimen cannot reliably be predicted based on its volume observed in the biopsy specimen. Thus, reporting its volume ratio is not recommended.

References

1. Gleason DF, Mellinger GT, Veterans Administrative Cooperative Urological Research Group (1974) Prediction of prognosis for prostatic adenocarcinoma by combined histologic grading and clinical staging. J Urol 111:58–64.
2. Garnett JE, Oyasu R, Grayhack JT (1984) The accuracy of diagnostic specimens in predicting tumor grades by Gleason's classification of radical prostatectomy specimens. J Urol 131:690–693.
3. Bostwick DG (1994) Gleason grading of prostatic needle biopsies: correlation with grade in 316 matched prostatectomies. Am J Surg Pathol 18:796–803.
4. Rubin MA, Dunn R, Kambham N, Misick CP, O'Toole KM (2000) Should a Gleason score be assigned to a minute focus of carcinoma on prostate biopsy? Am J Surg Pathol 24:1634–1640.
5. Steinberg DM, Sauvageot J, Piatadosi S, Epstein JI (1997) Correlation of prostate needle biopsy and radical prostatectomy Gleason grade in academic and community settings. Am J Surg Pathol 21:566–576.
6. McNeal JE, Villers AA, Redwine EA, Freiha ES, Stamey TA (1990) Histologic differentiation, cancer volume, and pelvic lymph node metastasis in adenocarcinoma of the prostate. Cancer 66:1225–1233.
7. Stamey TA, McNeal JE, Yemoto CM, Sigal BM, Johnstone IM (1999) Biological determinants of cancer progression in men with prostate cancer. JAMA 281:1395–1400.
8. Epstein JI, Carmichael MJ, Partin AW, Walsh PC (1994) Small high grade adenocarcinoma of the prostate in radical prostatectomy specimens performed for nonpalpable disease: pathogenetic and clinical implications. J Urol 151:1587–1592.
9. Pan C-C, Potter SR, Partin AW, Epstein JI (2000) The prognostic significance of tertiary Gleason patterns of higher grade in radical prostatectomy specimens: a proposal to modify the Gleason grading system. Am J Surg Pathol 24:563–569.
10. Egevad L, Granfors T, Karlberg L, Bergh A, Stattin P (2002) Percent Gleason grade 4/5 as prognostic factor in prostate cancer diagnosed at transurethral resection. J Urol 168:509–513.
11. Stamey TA (1995) Making the most out of six systematic sextant biopsies. Urology 45:2–12.
12. Noguchi M, Stamey TA, McNeal JE, Nolley R (2003) Prognostic factors for multifocal prostate cancer in radical prostatectomy specimens: lack of significance of secondary cancer. J Urol 170:459–463.

13. Rubin MA, Mucci NR, Manley S, Sanda M, Cushenberry E, Strawderman M (2001) Predictors of Gleason pattern 4/5 prostate cancer on prostatectomy specimens: can high grade tumor be predicted preoperatively? J Urol 165:114–118.

14. Bismar TA, Lewis JS, Vollmer RT, Humphrey PA (2003) Multiple measures of carcinoma extent versus perineural invasion in prostate needle biopsy tissue in prediction of pathologic stage in a screening population. Am J Surg Pathol 27:432–440.

Question 16

What clinically useful information should be included in the pathology report on a prostate needle core biopsy? Are there specific microscopic findings useful when assessing cancer staging?

Answer

Prostate needle core biopsy (PNB) can generate a great deal of information that is useful for assessing the prognosis of prostate cancer and providing essential guidance for successful therapeutic interventions such as radical prostatectomy. If a PNB is positive for adenocarcinoma, the following information should be provided in the pathology report: (1) location of the carcinoma, usually indicated in each part (location); (2) Gleason score (not a single grade) in each core (even for a small focus); (3) the number of positive cores of the total cores examined for each part or side; (4) the percentage of adenocarcinoma in each core and the highest percentage of a single core; (5) the presence of perineural invasion or extraprostatic extension; (6) special features of adenocarcinoma, such as neuroendocrine differentiation and ductal differentiation; and (7) immunohistochemical staining results if available. All these measures can be obtained on visual inspection without a micrometer.

Comments

Serum PSA levels, the biopsy Gleason score, and clinical staging are used by clinicians to predict prostatectomy pathology results for men with localized prostate cancer. When cancer is found on a PNB, pathologists try to provide the most information to predict the stage of cancer. We have listed several key findings that should be included in the biopsy pathology report.

Location of Carcinoma in Biopsy Cores

Badalament et al. [1] reported that involvement of more than 5% of a base and/or apex core biopsy predicts extraprostatic extension. Submitting each core in separate containers is costly. Many institutions submit biopsy cores in two containers, one from the left side and one from the right side. As a compromise, Epstein and Potter [2] recommend that each core obtained from one side be marked with different colors.

Gleason Score to Be Assigned to Each Core

The Epstein group recommended that a Gleason score be assigned to each cancer-bearing core even when the cancer focus is small. Kunz and Epstein [3] demonstrated that a high Gleason score in one core dictated the pathologic stage in prostatectomy specimens. For example, a Gleason score of $4 + 4 = 8$ with a grade 3 focus in other cores had a more advanced stage than a pure Gleason score $4 + 3 = 7$ ($P = 0.008$). If one had assigned an overall Gleason score, a biopsy with Gleason score $4 + 4 = 8$ on one core or more cores and some foci of Gleason grade 3 in other cores would be designated a Gleason score of $4 + 3 = 7$. In such cases, these patients are more likely to have a higher stage and grade on radical prostatectomy. This is more important in cases with a high Gleason score cancer in at least one core.

Positive Cores/Total Cores for Each Part or Side; Percentage of Cancer in Each Core; Highest Percentage of a Single Core

According to Bismar et al. [4], the total percentage of carcinoma was significantly related to pathologic

T stage (pT3) by multivariate ($P = 0.003$) and univariate ($P = 0.003$) analysis. The same group demonstrated that the greatest percentage of carcinoma in a single core is significantly related to pT3 stage and a positive surgical margin by univariate analysis. A similar positive correlation was reported by Rubin et al. [5]. The risk of stage T3 disease by the greatest percentage of cancer on a single core was 18% if <40%, 33% if 40%–60%, 50% if 60%–80%, and 63% if >80% ($P = 0.001$). The risk of stage T3 disease by the total percentage of cancer over all cores was 18% if <40%, 36% if 40%–60%, 41% if 60%–80%, and 54% if >80% ($P = 0.001$).

Perineural Invasion and Extraprostatic Extension

The significance of perineural invasion in needle biopsy specimens was discussed in detail in Question 3. Several groups have reported that the presence of perineural invasion by adenocarcinoma on needle biopsy is a significant predictor of extraprostatic extension but that it is not an independent factor. Its importance is that perineural invasion and the greatest percentage in any single core involved are highly correlated [5].

It is uncommon to observe extraprostatic extension of cancer by needle biopsy. However, if observed, it is clear evidence of pT3 disease.

References

1. Badalament RA, Craig MM, Peller PA, Young DC, Bahn DK, Kochie P, O'Dowd GJ, Veltri RW (1996) An algorithm for predicting nonorgan confined prostate cancer using the results obtained from sextant core biopsies with prostatic specific antigen level. J Urol 156: 1375–1380.
2. Epstein JI, Potter SR (2001) The pathological interpretation and significance of prostate needle biopsy findings: implications and current controversies. J Urol 166:402–410.
3. Kunz GM, Epstein JI (2003) Should each core with prostate cancer be assigned a separate Gleason score? Hum Pathol 34;911–914.
4. Bismar TA, Lewis JS Jr, Vollmer RT, Humphrey PA (2003) Multiple measure of carcinoma extent versus perineural invasion in prostate needle biopsy tissue in prediction of pathologic stage in a screening population. Am J Surg Pathol 27:432–440.
5. Rubin MA, Bassily N, Sanda M, Montie J, Strawderman MS, Wojno K (2000) Relationship and significance of greatest percentage of tumor and perineural invasion on needle biopsy in prostatic adenocarcinoma. Am J Surg Pathol 24:183–189.

Question 17

What is the meaning of "atypical glands suspicious but not diagnostic of adenocarcinoma" in a pathology diagnosis? Is "atypical small acinar proliferation" a pathologic entity?

Answer

Atypical glands suspicious but not diagnostic of carcinoma indicate that the pathologic findings are not sufficient for a definitive diagnosis of cancer but suspicious enough for further investigation. Therefore, a rebiopsy should be recommended. Only a definitive diagnosis of carcinoma is an indication for therapy; a suspicious diagnosis should not lead to therapy for prostate cancer such as surgery, irradiation, or hormonal therapy.

"Atypical glands suspicious but not diagnostic of adenocarcinoma"—known also as "atypical small acinar proliferation (ASAP)"—is not a pathologic entity but a diagnostic term used when uncertainty is encountered on prostate needle core biopsy.

Comments

When a prostate needle core biopsy (PNB) is performed, a definite pathologic diagnosis is expected for the purpose of clinical management. Unfortunately, a definitive diagnosis is not always possible [1]. For the diagnosis of prostatic adenocarcinoma, there must be absolutely no doubt on the part of the surgical pathologist who renders such a diagnosis. To establish a diagnosis of prostate cancer on limited needle core biopsy is one of the most challenging situations in surgical pathology. The histologic features of prostatic adenocarcinoma are complex and may be subtle. An error during any step of tissue processing including tissue fixation, dehydration, embedding, or even staining may interfere with a proper diagnosis. Even if tissue processing is perfect, a definitive diagnosis of cancer may still be difficult for even experienced pathologists [2]. One of the common problems hindering our ability to make a definitive diagnosis is the size of the suspicious lesion. Most pathologists are not comfortable making a diagnosis of malignancy when the focus of concern contains only two or three atypical glands or acini.

In the situation where the pathologist suspects, but is not totally convinced of a diagnosis of prostate cancer, the term "atypical glands suspicious for but not diagnostic of prostatic adenocarcinoma" is often applied [3]. Other pathologists prefer the diagnostic term "atypical small acinar proliferation" (ASAP) [4]. This phrase, however, has been heavily criticized because it may be interpreted as a defined pathologic entity [5, 6].

It is important to point out that ASAP does not represent a disease or a definable lesion. Studies have shown that these ASAP cases eventually become either malignant or benign lesions when additional studies are done [7]. The term ASAP has never been used in the diagnosis of radical prostatectomy specimens. Regardless of the use of ASAP, all experts agree that there is a high risk of finding cancer on a repeat biopsy in these suspicious cases. The pathologist who is making such a noncommittal diagnosis should communicate with the clinician responsible for the management of this patient. His risk of being diagnosed with cancer on a repeat biopsy is as high as 50%.

Between 1% and 23% of needle core biopsy specimens (average 5%) carry a diagnosis of atypical foci suspicious for carcinoma. This is a subjective term, heavily depending on the experience of the pathologist. It is used only when there is suspicion of, but not sufficient evidence for, making a definitive diagnosis of cancer. Because the average risk of subsequently documented cancer diagnosis following an atypical or suspicious focus of cancer is approximately 40%–50% [8, 9], repeat biopsy is necessary within 3–6 months in all cases. Repeat biopsy should include more sampling of the initial atypical site as well as other areas. To enhance the detection rate for these men, some pathologists prefer the saturation biopsy method during which more than 24 cores are obtained.

The incidence of an uncertain atypical diagnosis could be reduced when immunohistochemical staining for high-molecular-weight (HMW) keratin (34βE12), p63, and AMACR is applied [10]. The significance of finding ASAP associated with high-grade prostatic intraepithelial neoplasia (HGPIN) in a needle biopsy specimen is essentially the same as ASAP alone but quite different from HGPIN as discussed previously (see answer for Question 14).

The following options are available for cases with diagnostic uncertainty.

1. Examine multiple deeper tissue sections. Typically, a total of 30 sections can be generated from a 1-mm prostate core for better evaluation. In daily practice, at least three deeper recut levels should be ordered. On the deeper levels, a minute suspicious lesion might show sufficient evidence to permit a diagnosis of carcinoma.

2. Perform immunohistochemical study for 34βE12, p63 (negative for prostatic adenocarcinoma), and AMACR (positive for prostatic adenocarcinoma) (see answer for Question 11). However, immunohistochemical stains may be falsely positive or falsely negative, and the diagnosis of prostatic adenocarcinoma should always be primarily based on the histologic features from H&E-stained slides rather than immunohistochemical stains alone.

3. Consult with other pathologists with greater experience with prostate biopsy, particularly expert genitourinary pathologists who review difficult prostate cases on a regular basis to avoid an unnecessary second biopsy.

4. Rebiopsy the prostate if clinically indicated. Approximately one-half of men with atypical or suspicious foci have cancer identified on repeat biopsy [3, 8, 9, 11].

References

1. Kisner HJ (1998) The gray zone. Clin Lab Manage Rev 12:277–280.
2. Epstein JI (1998) Atypical small acinar proliferation of the prostate gland. Am J Surg Pathol 22:1430.
3. Chan TY, Epstein JI (1999) Follow-up of atypical prostate needle biopsies suspicious for cancer. Urology 53:351–355.
4. Iczkowski KA, MacLennan GT, Boswick DG (1997) Atypical small acinar proliferation suspicious for malignancy in prostate needle biopsy: clinical significance in 33 cases. Am J Surg Pathol 21:1489–1495.
5. Murphy WM (1999) ASAP is a bad idea: atypical small acinar proliferation. Hum Pathol 30:601.
6. Epstein JI (1999) How should atypical prostate needle biopsies be reported? Controversies regarding the term "ASAP." Hum Pathol 30:1401–1402.
7. Iczkowski KA, Cheng L, Qian J, Shanks J, Gadaleanu V, Bostwick DG, Ramnani DM (1999) ASAP is a valid diagnosis: atypical small acinar proliferation. Hum Pathol 30:774.
8. O'Dowd GL, Miller MC, Orozco R (2000) Analysis of repeated biopsy results within 1 year after a noncancer diagnosis. Urology 55:553–559.
9. Epstein JI, Herawi M (2006) Prostate needle biopsies containing prostatic intraepithelial neoplasia or atypical foci suspicious for carcinoma: implications for patient care. J Urol 175:820–834.
10. Jiang Z, Iczkowski KA, Woda BA, Tretiakova M, Yang XJ (2004) P504 immunostaining boosts diagnostic resolution of "suspicious" foci in prostatic needle biopsy specimens. Am J Clin Pathol 121:99–107.
11. Kronz JD, Shaikh AA, Epstein JI (2001) High-grade prostatic intraepithelial neoplasia with adjacent atypical glands on prostate biopsy. Hum Pathol 32:389–395.

Part 2. Kidney

Question 1

What are the essential features of renal neoplasms based on the current (2004) WHO classification system? What is the clinical implication of the new classification? How does the Fuhrman grading system work? What are the factors affecting survival of renal cell carcinoma patients?

Answer

Renal cell neoplasms are classified histologically into several types (Table 2-1-1). The four most common types of renal cell neoplasms are clear cell (51%–83%), papillary (11%–20%), and chromophobe (4%–6%) renal cell carcinomas (RCCs) and (benign) oncocytoma (4%–8%). Uncommon tumors, which account for 5%–10% of renal neoplasms, include collecting duct carcinoma, renal medullary carcinoma, mucinous tubular and spindle cell carcinoma, and unclassifiable carcinoma, which does not fit any defined category. Unclassifiable RCCs and collecting duct carcinoma are the most aggressive followed by, in descending order of aggressiveness, clear cell carcinoma, papillary carcinoma, and chromophobe carcinomas. Factors significantly affecting the cancer-specific survival are pathologic stage, nuclear grade, the presence of tumor necrosis, the histologic tumor type, and the presence of sarcomatoid differentiation.

Comments

The current (2004) World Health Organization (WHO) classification system of renal tumors [1], incorporating our recent knowledge of molecular and genetic mechanisms and clinicopathologic features, provides a standard for diagnosing kidney tumors. This system is still primarily based on well-defined morphologic characteristics.

2004 WHO Classification of Renal Neoplasms

Currently, RCCs, as defined, adopted, and recommended by the International Consensus Conference on Renal Cell Carcinomas sponsored by the Union Internationale Contre Cancer (UICC) [2] and the American Joint Committee on Cancer (AJCC), are as shown in Table 2-1-1 [1, 2].

Until about 20 years ago, the classification of RCCs was simple. Based on the microscopic appearance of tumor cells, it was either clear cell type, granular cell type, or mixed clear and granular cell type. Because of its poor clinical correlation and the lack of molecular and biochemical evidence, the old classification has been replaced with the current one (Table 2-1-1).

TABLE 2-1-1. Classification of renal epithelial neoplasms

Benign tumors
  Papillary adenoma
  Oncocytoma
  Metanephric adenoma
Malignant tumors
  Clear cell renal cell carcinoma (RCC)
  Multilocular cystic RCC
  Papillary RCC
  Chromophobe RCC
  Carcinoma of collecting ducts of Bellini
  Renal medullary RCC
  Renal carcinoma with XP 11.2 translocation
  Mucinous tubular and spindle cell carcinoma
  Unclassified RCC

Factors significantly affecting the cancer-specific survival are the histologic type in addition to nuclear grade, pathologic stage, presence of necrosis, and sarcomatoid differentiation.

Fuhrman Grading of Renal Cell Carcinomas

We must emphasize that Fuhrman grading of RCCs [3] (Table 2-1-2) has been widely used in the United States because of its simplicity and clinical relevance, being based on the size and shape of nuclei. It is useful for predicting clinical behavior. Fuhrman grading is most useful for grading clear cell RCC, but its application to any other RCC types is controversial. Based on the Fuhrman histologic criteria, grade 1 carcinoma (Fig. 2-1-1) is composed of cells with round nuclei, approximately 10 μm in diameter, with inconspicuous or absent nucleoli. Grade 2 carcinoma (Fig. 2-1-2) consists of cells with larger nuclei, approximately 15 mm with an irregular nuclear shape and small nucleoli that are recognizable only under a high power (×400) examination. Grade 3 carcinoma (Fig. 2-1-3) consists of cells with even larger

TABLE 2-1-2. Fuhrman grading system

Fuhrman grade	Nuclear size (μm)	Nuclear shape	Nucleoli	Nucleoli recognizable
1	10	Small round	Inconspicuous	No
2	15	Larger, irregular	Small	400×
3	20	Larger, irregular	Large	100×
4	30	Pleomorphic	Large	100×

nuclei, approximately 20 mm. Nucleoli are discernible under a medium power examination (100×). Grade 4 carcinoma (Fig. 2-1-4) consists of cells whose nuclei are pleomorphic and are frequently multinucleated and show a high mitotic frequency.

Factors Affecting Survival of Renal Cell Carcinoma Patients

Several recent publications have discussed survival after RCC (Table 2-1-3). Factors significantly affecting the cancer-specific (and overall) survival are the pathologic stage (TNM staging revised in 1997) [4–6], nuclear grade [4–7], the presence of tumor necrosis [4–6], the histologic tumor type [4–7], and the presence of sarcomatoid differentiation [5, 6, 8]. Clear cell carcinoma more frequently presents at advanced stages (pT3 and pT4, $P < 0.0001$) [6] and with high grades (grades 3 and 4, $P = 0.0001$) [6] than the papillary type. This fact is contributory to the unfavorable prognosis associated with clear cell carcinoma. However, even when a comparison is made among tumors at stages pT1 and pT2, the clear cell type carries a worse prognosis than does either papillary or chromophobe cell carcinoma ($P < 0.0001$) [5].

The nuclear grading used by these investigators is different, either three-tiered [6, 9] or four-tiered [4, 7, 8]. Furthermore, even among studies using a four-tiered system, grading criteria are slightly different. They are summarized in Table 2-1-4. Some of the grade 2 tumors by Fuhrman grading may be classified as grade 1 by the Mayo criteria. Despite minor differences among these classification schemes, it

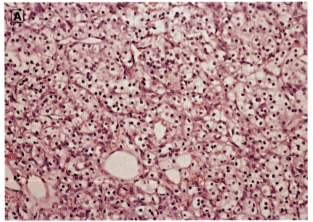
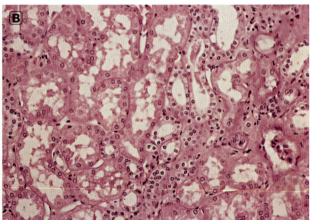

FIG. 2-1-1. **A** Clear cell renal cell carcinoma, Fuhrman grade 1. In this case, clear cells are arranged in compact nests surrounded by an interconnecting vascular stroma. Tumor cells have clear cytoplasm and a small round nucleus. The nuclei are smaller than those in normal tubules (**B**) (×200)

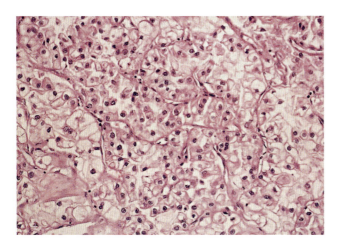

FIG. 2-1-2. Clear cell renal cell carcinoma, Fuhrman grade 2. Clear cells are arranged in a tubular structure. Nuclei are larger than those in Fig. 2-1-1A and are irregular in shape, but nucleoli are not readily discernible at this magnification (×200)

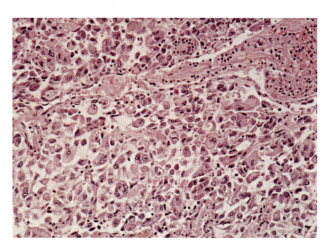

FIG. 2-1-3. Clear cell renal cell carcinoma, Fuhrman grade 3. Tumor cells have opaque cytoplasm and larger and more pleomorphic nuclei than do grade 2 carcinoma cells. Nucleoli can be recognized at this power (×200)

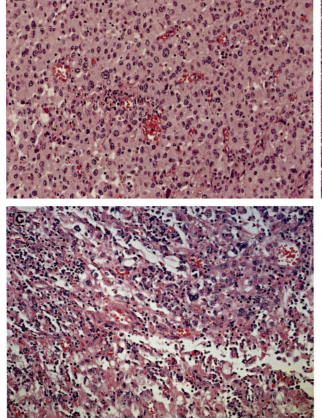

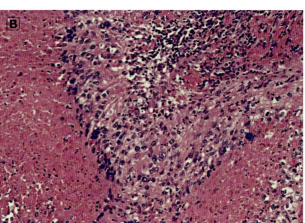

FIG. 2-1-4. **A** Clear cell renal cell carcinoma, Fuhrman grade 4. Eosinophilic carcinoma cells grow in sheets with an abundant vascular supply. The nuclei are more pleomorphic than in grade 3 tumors and have a coarse chromatin pattern. **B, C** Tumor cells are more pleomorphic and assume a spindle shape. Extensive necrosis, another sign of grave prognosis, is noted (×200)

TABLE 2-1-3. Outcome and prognostic features by histologic subtypes of renal cell carcinoma as reported by the Henry Ford Hospital and the Mayo Clinic

	Clear cell RCC		Papillary RCC		Chromophobe RCC		Unclassified RCC		Notes	
	Amin	Cheville	Amin	Cheville	Amin	Cheville	Amin	Cheville	Amin	Cheville
Year reported	2002	2003							Histologic type ($P = 0.002$); Fuhrman's nuclear grade ($P = 0.001$); TNM stage ($P = 0.001$); vascular invasion ($P = 0.001$) and necrosis ($P = 0.001$); significantly associated with disease-specific survival	Collecting duct carcinomas 5 (0.3%) Patients with clear cell RCCs have a worse prognosis than patients with papillary and chromophobe RCCs ($P < 0.001$) No difference in cancer-specific survival between patients with papillary and chromophobe RCC Presence of a sarcomatoid component, nuclear grade; tumor necrosis significantly associated with death from clear cell and chromophobe RCCs
Total cases	255 (67%)	1985 (83.2%)	75 (19.9%)	270 (11.3%)	24 (6.3%)	102 (4.3%)	23 (6.1%)	—		
Nuclear grade (%)										
1	6[a]	9.6[a]	1.4	1.9	0	2	0			
2	21.6	42.6	10.9	60	20.8	64.7	6.7			
3	53.2	39	78.1	35.9	70.8	24.5	48			
4	19.6	8.8	9.6	2.2	9.6	8.8	53.3			
Sarcomatoid change (%)	5.5	5.2	5.4	1.9	4.2	8.8	26			
1997 TNM tumor stage (%)										
I	51.9	44.3	60.6	61.1	50	36.3	11.1			
II	10.8	20.7	18.3	22.6	37.5	48	5.6			
III	25.3	33.9	15.5	15.9	12.5	12.7	27.8			
IV	12	1.1	5.6	0.4	0	2.9	55.5			
Metastasis (%) Regional node Distant	27.4[b]	5.2 15.8	12[b]	7 4.1	4.2[b]	2.9 4.9	69.6[b]			
Cancer-specific survival (%)										
5 Years	76	68.9	86	87.4	100	86.7	24			
10 Years	70	60.3	82	81.9	90	83.3	12			

RCC, renal cell carcinoma.

[a] Fuhrman grade used by The Henry Ford Hospital (Amin group) [4]. Grading in the Cheville study by Mayo criteria (see Table 2-1-4) [7]. Copied with permission of publisher.

[b] Sites of metastasis not stated.

TABLE 2-1-4. Histologic criteria for tumor grading of renal cell carcinomas

Grade	Fuhrman (1982)	Mayo (Cheville) (2002)	UICC/AJCC (Thoenes and Storkel)
I	Round nuclei, about 10 μm, inconspicuous to absent nucleoli	Small round nuclei, inconspicuous nucleoli visible at 400× only	Round, about the size of normal tubule cell, normal tubule nucleoli, mitosis practically absent
II	Irregular nuclear outline, about 15 μm, nucleoli visible at 400×	Round to slightly irregular nuclei, nucleoli mildly enlarged visible at 200×	Round nuclei or roundness lost, 1–2 distinctly enlarged nucleoli, multinucleated cells may be present, mitoses infrequent
III	Irregular nuclear outline, about 20 μm, nucleoli visible at 100×	Round to irregular nuclei, prominent nucleoli visible at 100×	Markedly enlarged polymorphic nuclei, multinucleated cells frequent, nucleoli 1 or multiple, mitoses often atypical and increased
IV	Grade III features plus bizarre often multilobed nuclei, spindle-shaped	Enlarged pleomorphic nuclei, giant cells	
Nuclear grade assignment	By the highest grade even if focal	By the highest grade occupying at least 1 high-power field (400×)	Not stated

appears that grade 1 and 2 tumors by the four-tiered system may be lumped together. When done so, they are comparable with grade 1 tumors by the three-tiered system. Therefore, a three-tiered grading system may be appropriate for classifying renal cell carcinoma [5, 10, 11]. There was no significant difference in the outcome between grade 1 and grade 2 carcinomas so classified by the four-tiered system [5].

We describe the pathologic features of these tumors under Questions 2–6. Readers who wish to know more details are referred to the excellent articles by Amin et al. [4], Moch et al. [6], and Frank et al. [12].

References

1. WHO classification of tumours of the kidney (2004). In: Eble JN, Sauter G, Epstein JI, Sesterhenn IA (eds) Tumours of the urinary system and male genital organs. IARC Press, Lyon, p 10.
2. Storkel S, Eble JN, Adlakha K, Amin M, Blute ML, Bostwick DG, Darson M, Delahunt B, Iczkowski K (1997) Classification of renal cell carcinoma; Workgroup No. 1 (1997) Union Internationale Centre Cancer (UICC) and the American Joint Committee on Cancer (AJCC). Cancer 80:987–989.
3. Fuhrman SA, Lasky LC, Limas C (1982) Prognostic significance of morphologic parameters in renal cell carcinoma. Am J Surg Pathol 6:655–663.
4. Amin MaB, Amin MiB, Tamboli P, Javidan J, Stricker H, De-Peralta Ventrina M, Deshpande A, Menon M (2002) Prognostic impact of histologic subtyping of adult renal epithelial neoplasms. An experience of 405 cases. Am J Surg Pathol 26:281–291.
5. Lohse CM, Blute ML, Zincke H, Weaver AL, Cheville JC (2002) Comparison of standardized and nonstandardized nuclear grade of renal cell carcinoma to predict outcome among 2,042 patients. Am J Clin Pathol 118:877–886.
6. Moch H, Gasser T, Amin MB, Torhorst J, Sauter G, Mihatsch MJ (2000) Prognostic utility of the recently recommended histologic classificaion and revised TNM staging system of renal cell carcinoma. A Swiss experience with 588 tumors. Cancer 89:604–614.
7. Cheville JC, Lohse CM, Zincke H, Weaver AL, Blute ML (2003) Comparisons of outcome and prognostic features among histologic subtypes of renal cell carcinoma. Am J Surg Pathol 27:612–624.
8. Cheville JC, Lohse CM, Zincke H, Weaver AL, Leibovich BC, Frank I, Blute ML (2004) Sarcomatoid renal cell carcinoma. An examination of underlying histologic subtype and an analysis of association with patient outcome. Am J Surg Pathol 28:435–441.
9. Thoenes W, Storkel S, Rumpelt HJ (1986) Histopathology and classification of renal cell tumors (adenomas, oncocytomas and carcinomas). The basic cytological and histological elements and their use for diagnostics. Pathol Res Pract 181:125–143.
10. Storkel S, Thoenes W, Jacobi GH, Lippold R (1989) Prognostic parameters in renal cell carcinoma: A new approach. Eur Urol 16:416–422.
11. Delahunt B, Nacey JN (1987) Renal cell carcinoma, II: histological indicators of prognosis. Pathology 19:258–263.
12. Frank I, Blute ML, Cheville JC, Lohse CM, Weaver AL, Leibovich BC, Zincke H (2003) A multifactorial postoperative surveillance model for patients with surgically treated clear cell renal cell carcinoma. J Urol 170:2225–2232.

Question 2

Does granular cell type renal cell carcinoma exist? What are the features of clear cell renal cell carcinoma? What are the pathologic characteristics and the clinical implication of multilocular cystic renal cell carcinoma?

Answer

The diagnosis of "granular cell-type renal cell carcinoma (RCC)" should be avoided because it does not represent a true subtype of RCC. So-called granular RCC may actually include several subtypes of RCC or even benign oncocytoma, which may require very different therapy. Clear cell (conventional) RCC is not only the most common type but also is responsible for most of the morbidity and mortality of renal neoplasms. Clear cell RCC, particularly of high grade, can display granular cytoplasm. Multilocular cystic RCC, a new entity in the WHO classification system, represents a low-grade clear cell type RCC with a multilocular cyst.

Comments

Although the term "granular cell' type RCC is not a recognized subtype in any of the current renal tumor classification systems, it is being used in the literature and in clinical practice. With advances in molecular biology and immunohistochemistry study, it has become clear that "granular cell" type RCC is not an independent histologic type but a morphologic manifestation of many types of RCC as well as oncocytoma. The granular appearance of tumor cells, typically eosinophilic, can be due to any of the following or their combination: (1) increase in mitochondria or lysosomes; (2) presence of neuroendocrine granules; (3) cytofilaments, or (4) smooth endoplasmic reticulum [1]. Typically, low-grade clear cell RCCs (grades 1 and 2) tend to have clear cytoplasm due high lipid and glycogen content and fewer organelles than high-grade (grades 3 and 4) clear cell RCCs. As the nuclear grade increases, the cytoplasm becomes more eosinophilic and granular. In the past, these tumors were classified as a granular cell type or a mixed granular cell and clear cell type. Cytogenetic analysis has established that these two types of cell share similar genetic characteristics of clear cell carcinoma as is detailed under Question 7.

Studies by us and other investigators have shown that papillary RCC, chromophobe RCC, and oncocytoma all have been mistakenly diagnosed as "granular cell" RCC. Even renal angiomyolipoma and paraganglioma have been misdiagnosed as "granular cell" RCC owing to their granular eosinophilic appearance.

It is important to point out that the diagnosis of "granular cell' RCC should not be used because it does not provide any clinical guidance in terms of the tumors' biologic behaviors. Anyone receiving a diagnosis of "granular cell" RCC should seek a second opinion regarding the nature of the renal tumor.

Clear Cell Renal Cell Carcinoma

Clear cell RCC is the most common type, accounting for approximately 50%–70% of all RCCs.

Gross Appearance

The clear cell RCC may be described as follows.

- A solid well-circumscribed mass with a bulging golden yellow to orange-colored cut surface is characteristic because of a high content of lipid (Fig. 2-2-1).
- Central necrosis, hemorrhage, and cystic changes are common.
- Multifocal development is rare (2%–7%) [2, 3] except in patients with von Hippel Lindau (VHL) disease in which multifocal occurrence approaches 100% (Fig. 2-2-2).

Microscopic Appearance

Several features are characteristic of clear cell RCC.

- Strikingly clear cells (cytoplasmic lipids and glycogen washed out during tissue processing) are arranged in cords and nests (Fig. 2-1-1A) and are bounded by delicate vascular septa. They may form tubules (Fig. 2-1-2).
- The tumor is replete with a well-formed vascular network (Fig. 2-2-3). Vascular endothelial growth factor (VEGF) [4, 5] and basic fibroblast factor [6] secreted by tumor cells are implicated in the high vascularity.

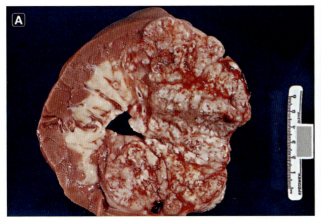
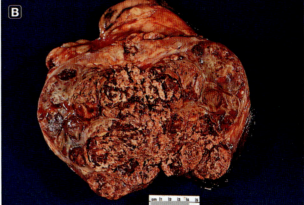

FIG. 2-2-1. **A** Bulging yellow mass of clear cell renal cell carcinoma. **B** Another bulky clear cell renal cell carcinoma with foci of hemorrhage and necrosis. The tumor mass is divided into nodules by septa

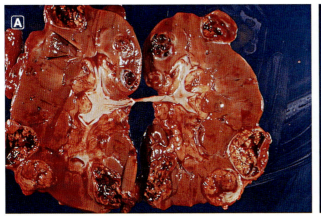
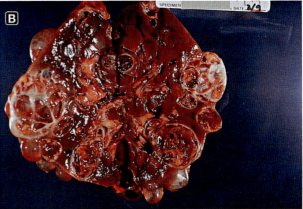

FIG. 2-2-2. **A, B.** Multiple clear cell renal cell carcinomas. These two kidneys are from two young brothers of a von Hippel-Lindau disease family. Both kidneys exhibit multiple tumor nodules of varying size. Many nodules have a delicate fibrous capsule. Some nodules are multiloculated (**B**)

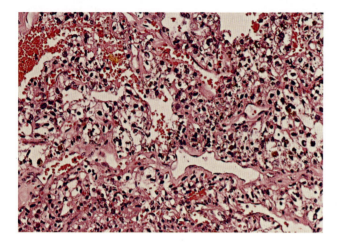

FIG. 2-2-3. Clear cell renal cell carcinoma with a rich vascular supply

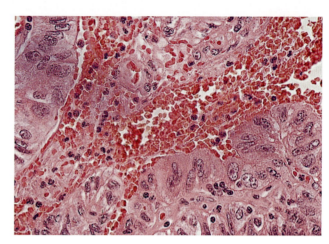

FIG. 2-2-4. Clear cell renal cell carcinoma. This high-grade carcinoma consists of granular cells. Only faint clear cell appearance is suggested

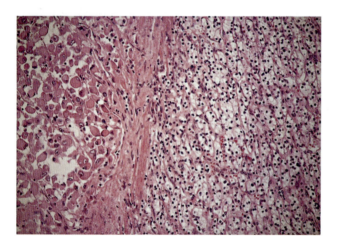

FIG. 2-2-5. Clear cell renal cell carcinoma of two nuclear grades. The right half is composed of grade 1 carcinoma with clear cells, whereas the left half shows a Fuhrman grade 3 carcinoma with granular cytoplasm. If tumor sampling had been limited, an area of a high-grade tumor might not have been detected

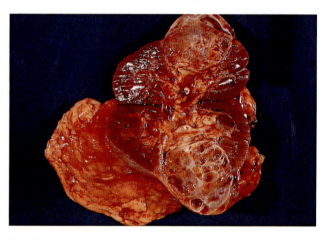

FIG. 2-2-6. Multilocular cystic renal cell carcinoma (clear cell type). It is a low-grade carcinoma (Fuhrman grade 1) and has a favorable prognosis

- Areas of tumor cells with eosinophilic and granular cytoplasm can be seen, particularly in high-grade clear cell RCC (Fuhrman nuclear grade 3/4) (Fig. 2-1-4 A,C; Figs. 2-2-4, 2-2-5).

Multilocular Cystic Renal Cell Carcinoma

Multilocular cystic RCC is recognized as a separate entity in the current (2004) WHO classification system. The tumor is characterized by an encapsulated cystic mass that is divided into multiple locules by septa (Figs. 2-2-6, 2-2-7, 2-2-8), similar to (benign) cystic nephroma (multilocular cyst). However, in contrast to benign cystic nephroma, clusters of clear cells can be identified in the septa (Figs. 2-2-7, 2-2-8). It carries a much better prognosis than the conventional clear cell RCC [7]. It may be considered as a variant of clear cell RCC as *VHL* gene mutations which are characteristic of clear cell RCC, are likewise detected in multilocular cystic RCC [8].

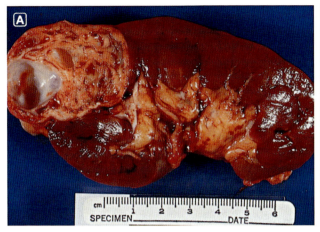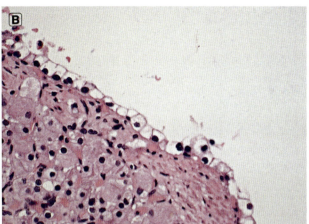

FIG. 2-2-7. **A** Another multilocular cystic renal cell carcinoma. **B** Cysts are lined by a single layer of clear cells of low nuclear grade (Fuhrman grade 1). Underneath the surface epithelial layer are clusters of carcinoma cells

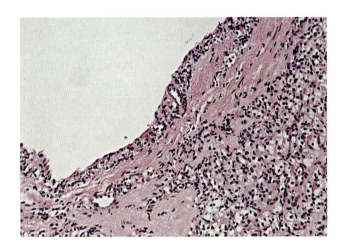

FIG. 2-2-8. Another multilocular cystic renal cell carcinoma. Cysts are lined by multilayered small clear cells of Fuhrman grade 1. Note the nests of clear cells outside the cyst

References

1. Oyasu R (1998) Renal cancer: histologic classification update. Int J Clin Oncol 3:125–133.
2. Amin MaB, Amin MiB, Tamboli P, Javidan J, Stricker H, De-Peralta Ventrina M, Deshpande A, Menon M (2002) Prognostic impact of histologic subtyping of adult renal epithelial neoplasms: an experience of 405 cases. Am J Surg Pathol 26:281–291.
3. Cheville JC, Lohse CM, Zincke H, Weaver AL, Blute ML (2003) Comparisons of outcome and prognostic features among histologic subtypes of renal cell carcinoma. Am J Surg Pathol 27:612–624.
4. Wezigmann-Voos S, Breier G, Risau W, Plate K (1995) Up-regulation of vascular endothelial growth factor and its receptor in von Hippel-Lindau disease-associated and sporadic hemangioblastomas. Cancer Res 55: 1358–1364.
5. Takahashi A, Sasaki K, Kim SJ, Tobisu K, Kakizoe T, Tsukamoto T, Kumamoto Y, Sugimura T, Terada, M (1994) Marked increased amounts of messenger RNAs for vascular endothelial factor and placenta growth factor in renal cell carcinoma associated with angiogenesis. Cancer Res 54:4233–4237.
6. Fujimoto K, Ichimori Y, Yamaguchi H, Arai K, Futami T, Ozono S, Hirao Y, Kakizoe T, Terada M, Okajima E (1995) Basic fibroblast growth factor as a candidate tumor marker for renal cell carcinoma. Jpn J Cancer Res 86:182–186.
7. Murad T, Komaiko W, Oyasu R, Bauer K (1991) Multilocular cystic renal cell carcinoma. Am J Clin Pathol 95:633–637.
8. Grignon DJ, Bismar TA, Bianco F, Sakr WA, Pontes JE, Sarkar F, Che M (2004) VHL gene mutations in multilocular cystic renal cell carcinoma: evidence in support of its classification as a type of clear cell renal cell carcinoma. Mod Pathol: 17(Suppl 1)154A.

Question 3

What is the definition of papillary adenoma? What is the relationship of papillary renal cell carcinoma? Do we need to divide papillary renal cell carcinoma into two subtypes?

Answer

Papillary adenoma is defined as a papillary epithelial tumor with papillary structures <5 mm in size. A renal tumor with similar histologic features but ≥5 mm is considered papillary renal cell carcinoma (RCC). Although the size criterion is arbitrary, a renal papillary tumor <5 mm has no metastatic potential. In reality, a papillary adenoma may grow in size and then satisfy the criteria for papillary RCC. Papillary RCC can be divided into type 1 (scant to basophilic cytoplasm, abundant macrophages, and often low nuclear grade) and type 2 (abundant eosinophilic cytoplasm and often high nuclear grade). However, dividing papillary RCCs by nuclear grade may be more practical and biologically relevant.

Comments

Papillary Adenoma

A minute papillary lesion <1 mm, which is typically not recognizable grossly, is termed papillary hyperplasia. Microscopically, papillary hyperplasia, papillary adenoma (<5 mm) [1], and papillary RCC of low grade share an almost identical histology with low nuclear grade and papillary architecture. The distinction between papillary adenoma and papillary carcinoma in the kidney has been evolving. In the past, the cutoff at 2–3 cm was used for defining renal adenomas. With advances in imaging technology, more and more small renal tumors are incidentally identified on radiographic examination while looking for other lesions. Surgical resection remains the treatment of choice for a renal mass. It is important to point out that the size criterion does not apply to clear cell tumors because a small clear cell epithelial neoplasm can metastasize.

Determination of a neoplasm based on size is obviously not scientific but practical. A papillary tumor <5 mm has no metastatic potential, and a papillary tumor of 5–30 mm has very low metastatic potential. As a papillary tumor increases in size, its genetic alterations are also accumulating; and the potential of invasion and metastasis may be elevated as well. Based on our recent studies on renal papillary lesions, we believe papillary hyperplasia, papillary adenoma, and papillary RCC represent a spectrum of the same process. Papillary adenomas may evolve into papillary RCC over time [2].

Papillary (Chromophile) Renal Cell Carcinoma

Papillary RCC, comprising approximately 10%–15% of RCCs, is the second most common type of renal cancer. Mancilla-Jimenez et al. [3] in 1976 were the first to show that tumors with this histology had a better survival rate than the clear cell type. As with the clear cell RCCs, the hereditary form of papillary RCC exists; and all patients in this group had multiple bilateral lesions ranging from <0.6 cm to 11.0 cm [4].

Gross Appearance

The papillary RCC may be described as follows.

- It is a well-circumscribed solid mass (Figs. 2-3-1, Fig. 2-3-2) that is tan to yellow depending on the content of lipid-laden macrophages in the stroma. In large tumors, a distinct fibrous capsule may be present.
- Papillary RCCs in sporadic cases are frequently multifocal (22.5%) and bilateral (4%) [5].
- Some small nodules considered to be papillary adenomas often coexist.

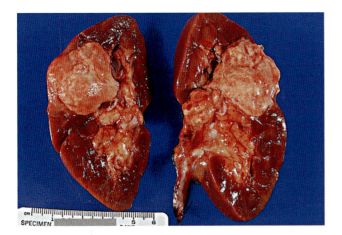

FIG. 2-3-1. Papillary renal cell carcinoma. It shows a solid yellow-tan cut surface. The differential diagnosis based on the gross appearance includes chromophobe cell, clear cell, and papillary carcinomas

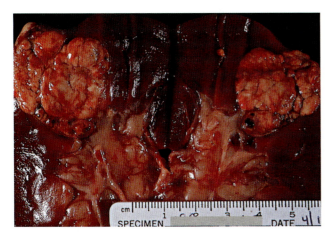

FIG. 2-3-2. Papillary renal cell carcinoma. It is a bulging mass projecting into the perirenal adipose tissue. The cut surface is yellow. The impression on gross examination is that of clear cell renal cell carcinoma

- Massive hemorrhagic necrosis is common in tumors >3 cm in diameter, leading to accumulation of serous and bloody fluid [3, 6].
- Extensive necrosis and hemorrhage can be associated with type 1 (Fig. 2-3-3) or type 2 tumors (see the following section for the definition).

Microscopic Appearance

It predominantly has a papillary architecture supported by a fibrovascular core, although some cases have a mixture of papillary and tubular architecture. Papillary carcinoma can be divided into two subtypes [7, 8] based on the difference in microscopic appearance. The subdivision has been supported by other studies [4, 9, 10] (also refer to Question 7).

- *Type 1*: Papillae (Fig. 2-3-4) and tubules (Fig. 2-3-5) are lined by small cells with a pale cytoplasm and small oval nuclei. Foamy macrophages and psammoma bodies, if found, in papillary cores (Figs. 2-3-6, 2-3-7) are helpful for the diagnosis. Mitotic figures are absent to rare. Expansion of papillary cores by edema fluid is common (73% [7]) leading to a false impression of cysts rather than papillae at a low magnification. If the tumor is extensively cystic, one needs to take numerous sections to verify that it is indeed a papillary carcinoma (Fig. 2-3-8).
- *Type 2*: Papillae are lined by large cells with abundant eosinophilic cytoplasm (Fig. 2-3-9). (Recall that eosinophilic cytoplasm is not the sole property

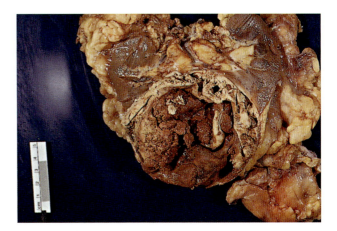

FIG. 2-3-3. Encapsulated cystic papillary renal cell carcinoma showing extensive central necrosis and hemorrhage. Microscopic examination should include sections taken through the capsular portion to ensure that viable neoplastic cells are sampled

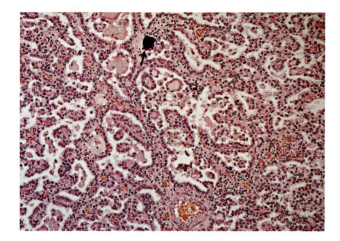

FIG. 2-3-4. Papillary renal cell carcinoma, type 1. The tumor exhibits a typical papillary pattern lined by small pale-stained cuboidal cells. In the lumens are macrophages and a psammoma body (*arrow*)

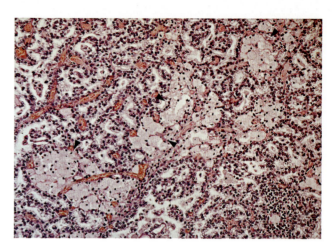

FIG. 2-3-6. Papillary renal cell carcinoma, type 1. Cuboidal pale cells grow in a papillary pattern. Present in the interstitium are collections of macrophages (*arrowheads*), a typical feature of type 1 papillary renal cell carcinoma

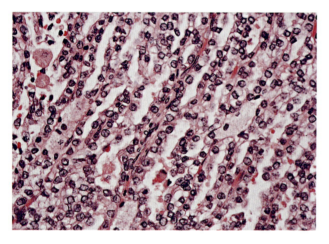

FIG. 2-3-5. Papillary renal cell carcinoma, type 1. Tumor cells grow in a tubular pattern

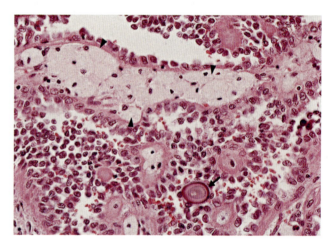

FIG. 2-3-7. Papillary renal cell carcinoma, type 1, with macrophages (*arrowheads*) and a psammoma body (*arrow*). The latter is a common finding in papillary tumors that develop in many organs

of clear cell RCCs). Tumor cells have large spherical nuclei with prominent nucleoli. Psammoma bodies may be found. Foamy macrophages are uncommon [7, 8, 11].

The frequency ratio for type 1/type 2 is about 2:1. Type 2 tumors are larger than type 1 tumors and are more common in patients younger than age 40. Type 1 tumors are of significantly lower Fuhrman grade (P = 0.0001) [7] and are lower TNM stage (P = 0.0001) than type 2 (P = 0.0001) (Delahunt, 1997). Type 2 carcinomas are associated with a higher Fuhrman grade (P < 0.001) and a poor prognosis (P < 0.005) [10]. However, this subclassification could be prob-

lematic because a mixture of type 1 and type 2 cells is seen in up to 30% of cases. Some small type 2 papillary RCCs with low nuclear grade are not expected to behave in an aggressive manner [12]. One of us recently proposed a new classification of papillary RCCs based on molecular analysis. According to this scheme, type 2 papillary RCC is made up of at least two genetically distinct subtypes: Type 2A, of low nuclear-grade, behaves as an indolent tumor, similar to type 1 papillary RCC. Type 2B is an aggressive, metastasizing carcinoma [12].

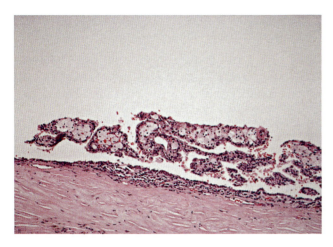

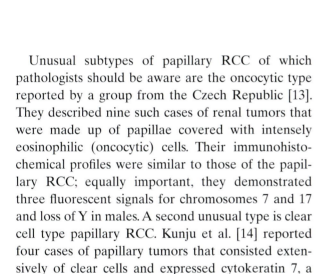

FIG. 2-3-8. Cystic papillary renal cell carcinoma, type 1. Note that the cyst wall is lined by micropapillae of carcinoma cells. The tumor stroma contains macrophages

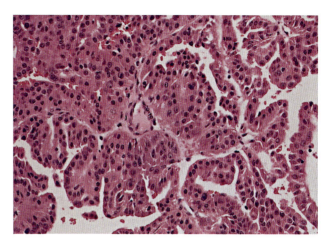

FIG. 2-3-9. Papillary renal cell carcinoma, type 2. Eosinophilic cytoplasm and a higher nuclear grade (than type 1) are characteristic of type 2 carcinoma. Note that nucleoli are visible at this power

Unusual subtypes of papillary RCC of which pathologists should be aware are the oncocytic type reported by a group from the Czech Republic [13]. They described nine such cases of renal tumors that were made up of papillae covered with intensely eosinophilic (oncocytic) cells. Their immunohistochemical profiles were similar to those of the papillary RCC; equally important, they demonstrated three fluorescent signals for chromosomes 7 and 17 and loss of Y in males. A second unusual type is clear cell type papillary RCC. Kunju et al. [14] reported four cases of papillary tumors that consisted extensively of clear cells and expressed cytokeratin 7, a marker for papillary RCC.

In summary, papillary carcinoma, in general, carries a better prognosis because most of them are of type 1, which presents at a low pathologic stage and is more likely to be of a low Fuhrman grade. Occasionally, however, type 2 papillary RCC is small and of a low nuclear grade. It is associated with a good prognosis. The high-grade papillary RCC (type 2B) is associated with a poor prognosis.

References

1. Storkel S, Eble JN, Adlakha K, Amin M, Blute ML, Bostwick DG, Darson M, Delahunt B, Iczkowski K (1997) Classification of renal cell carcinoma; Workgroup No. 1 (1997) Union Internationale Centre Cancer (UICC) and the American Joint Committee on Cancer (AJCC). Cancer 80:987–989.

2. Wang KL, Weinrach DM, Luan C, Han M, Lin F, The BT, Yang XJ (2007) Renal papillary adenoma—a putative precursor of papillary renal cell carcinoma. Hum Pathol 38:239–246.

3. Mancilla-Jimenez R, Stanley RJ, Blath RA (1976) Papillary renal cell carcinoma. Cancer 38:2469–2480.

4. Lubensky IA, Schmidt L, Zhuang Z, Weirich G, Pack S, Zambrano N, Walther MM, Choyke P, Linehan WM, Zbar B (1999) Hereditary and sporadic papillary renal cell carcinomas with *c-met* mutations share a distinct morphological phenotype. Am J Pathol 155: 517–526.

5. Amin MaB, Amin MiB, Tamboli P, Javidan J, Stricker H, De-Peralta Ventrina M, Deshpande A, Menon M (2002) Prognostic impact of histologic subtyping of adult renal epithelial neoplasms: an experience of 405 cases. Am J Surg Pathol 26:281–291.

6. Kovacs G (1989) Papillary renal cell carcinoma: a morphologic and cytogenetic study of 11 cases. Am J Pathol 134:27–34.

7. Delahunt B, Eble JN (1997) Papillary renal cell carcinoma; a clinicopathologic and immunohistochemical study of 105 cases. Mod Pathol 10:537–544.

8. Delahunt B, Eble JN, McCredie MRE, Bethwaite PB, Stewart JH, Bilous AM (2001) Morphologic typing of papillary renal cell carcinoma: comparison of growth kinetics and patient survival in 66 cases. Hum Pathol 32:590–595.

9. Altinok G, Che M, Bismar F, Bianco, F, Sakr W, Pontes JE, Grignon D (2004) Clinicopathologic and immunohistochemical features distinguish type 1 from type 2 sporadic papillary renal cell carcinoma. Mod Pathol 17(suppl 1):136A.

10. Leroy X, Zini L, Leuteurtre E, Zerimech F, Pochet N, Aubert J-P, Gosselin B, Copin M-C (2002) Morphologic subtyping of papillary renal cell carcinoma:

correlation with prognosis and differential expression of MUC1 between the two subtypes. Mod Pathol 15:1126–1130.

11. Renshaw AA, Corless CL (1995) Papillary renal cell carcinoma: histology and immunohistochemistry. Am J Surg Pathol 19:842–849.

12. Yang XJ, Tan MH, Kim HL, Ditlev JA, Betten MW, Png CE, Kort EJ, Futami K, Furge KA, Takahashi M, Kanayama H, Tan PH, Teh BS, Luan C, Wang K, Pins M, Tretiakova M, Anema J, Kahnoski R, Nicol T, Stadler W, Vogelzang NG, Amato R, Seligson D, Figlin R, Belldegrun A, Rogers CG, The BT (2006) A molecular classification of papillary renal cell carcinoma. Cancer Res 65:5628–5637.

13. Hes O, Brunelli M, Michal M, Cossu Rocca P, Chilosi M, Mina M, Menestrina F, Martigoni G (2005) Oncocytic papillary renal cell carcinoma: a clinicopathologic study of 9 cases. Mod Pathol 18(suppl 1):145A.

14. Kunju LP, Bakshi N, Poisson LM, Hafez K, Wojno K, Shah RB (2005) Morphologic subtyping of papillary renal cell carcinoma: clinicopathologic and immunohistochemical analysis. Mod Pathol 18(suppl 1):150A.

Question 4

How is chromophobe renal cell carcinoma diagnosed? How does one distinguish chromophobe renal cell carcinoma from oncocytoma?

Answer

Chromophobe renal cell carcinoma and oncocytoma have certain features in common. (1) Both are considered to derive from the intercalated cells of collecting ducts. (2) The two have a similar gross appearance (discrete mass, light-tan to brown on the cut surface, irregular fibrous bands or scar in the center). Microscopically, however, they are distinctly different. Chromophobe carcinoma cells grow in solid nests and have prominent cell membranes, reticulated or granular cytoplasm, and a perinuclear transluscent zone. Oncocytoma cells, on the other hand, are deeply eosinophilic owing to abundance in mitochondria and are arranged in cords, nests or tubules. However, distinguishing the eosinophilic variant of chromophobe renal cell carcinoma from oncocytoma may be difficult.

Comments

Chromophobe Renal Cell Carcinoma

A subtype termed chromophobe renal cell carcinoma (RCC) was first described and segregated from other types by Thoenes, Storkel, and their colleagues in Germany [1, 2]. This tumor was so named to reflect the perinuclear clearing of cytoplasm in contrast to the complete clearing of the cytoplasm of clear cell RCC. It is an uncommon variant, accounting for 4%–6% of renal epithelial neoplasms [2, 3]. It is less

aggressive than the clear cell type, one reason being that these tumors are at lower stages at diagnosis compared with other RCCs ($P = 0.003$) [4]. The tumor is believed to originate from the intercalated cells of collecting tubules [2], which are also believed to be the source of oncocytoma. As is dealt with later under Question 7, a hybrid tumor of chromophobe and oncocytic features occurs in patients with Birt-Hogg-Dube (BHD) syndrome [5].

Gross Appearance

Chromophobe RCC presents as a sharply circumscribed solid mass with a homogeneously light tan or brown cut surface. Therefore, oncocytoma should be considered in the differential diagnosis (Figs. 2-4-1, 2-4-2). The color is due to a sparse amount of lipid or glycogen. Foci of hemorrhage, necrosis, or cysts are rare. Irregular fibrous bands are common coalesced in the center of the tumor, resembling the central scar of an oncocytoma [3]. In all, 46 of 50 cases were within the renal capsule in the Mayo Clinic series [3].

Microscopic Appearance

The chromophobe RCC appears microscopically as follows.

- The tumor cells are round and are arranged in large sheets separated by delicate fibrovascular septa.
- Two histologic subtypes are recognized, although there is no difference in their behavior. In the first type, tumor cells have a pale finely reticular appearance (partial clearance) (Figs. 2-4-3, 2-4-4). In the second type, tumor cells have a granular eosinophilic appearance (Fig. 2-4-5) that is recognized as the "eosinophilic type" of chromophobe RCC. As a variant of the reticular-type cell, "ballooned" cells may be found in association with granular eosinophilic cells (Fig. 2-4-6).

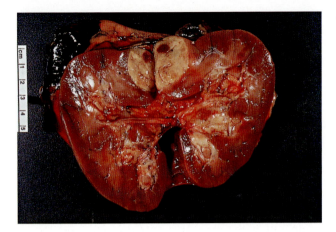

FIG. 2-4-1. Chromophobe renal cell carcinoma. It has a homogeneous yellow to light brown cut surface. Therefore, the differential diagnosis includes clear cell carcinoma and possibly papillary carcinoma

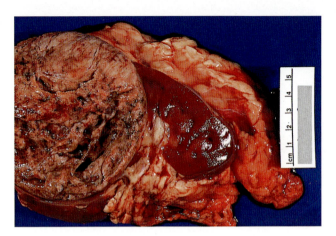

FIG. 2-4-2. Chromophobe renal cell carcinoma. It is a sharply demarcated large mass with a light brown cut surface. Therefore, the differential diagnosis includes clear cell carcinoma and oncocytoma

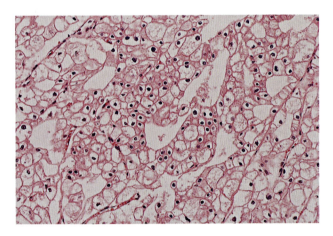

FIG. 2-4-3. Chromophobe renal cell carcinoma with the classic microscopic appearance. Tumor cells are round and have a pale, finely reticulated to opaque cytoplasm. Note that the cytoplasm is condensed against the cell membrane. An ultrastructural study would demonstrate that this appearance is due to accumulation of mitochondria in the peripheral part of the cytoplasm. The perinuclear halo (clearing) is due to accumulation of microvesicles that derive from mitochondria. The perinuclear halo and "thickened cell membrane" are characteristic of chromophobe renal cell carcinoma

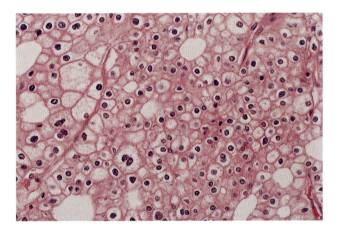

FIG. 2-4-4. Chromophobe renal cell carcinoma. The microscopic appearance is similar to that in Fig. 2-4-3. The nuclei are uniform and small and are Fuhrman grade 2. Binucleated cells are common and should not be construed as evidence of high-grade carcinoma

- A perinuclear translucent zone may be observed in both types of tumor cell, creating a perinuclear halo or fried-egg appearance (Fig. 2-4-4).
- Electron microscopy reveals that the cytoplasm is packed with numerous microvesicles admixed with mitochondria around nuclei, whereas tightly packed mitochondria are distributed in the peripheral zone of individual tumor cells. The microvesicle derives from the outer membrane of a mitochondrion as a saccular dilation [6, 7].
- The number of mitochondria is related to the eosinophilia of tumor cells.

In general, the nuclear grade is Fuhrman grade 2. Binucleated cells, which are often seen, should not be taken as evidence of a high-grade carcinoma (Fig. 2-4-4). The correlation between nuclear grade and biologic behavior is poor. More study with a large number of cases is needed to address this question.

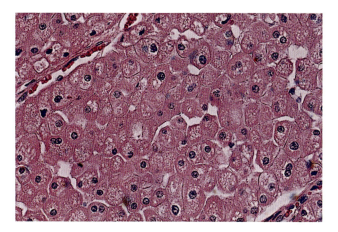

Fig. 2-4-5. Chromophobe renal cell carcinoma. It is composed of eosinophilic granular cells. Nevertheless, note the cytoplasmic condensation against the cell membrane, a feature of chromophobe cell renal cell carcinoma

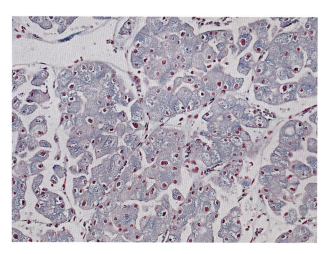

Fig. 2-4-7. Chromophobe renal cell carcinoma. It is positive for colloidal iron stain, a feature with diagnostic utility although not essential for diagnosis. Note the frequent binucleated cells

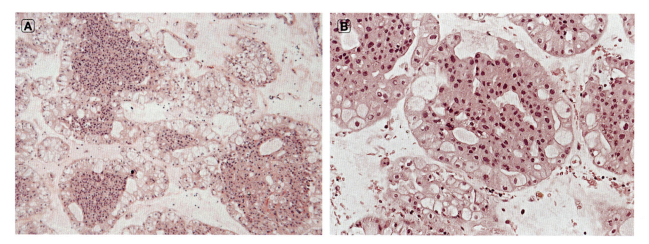

Fig. 2-4-6. **A, B** Chromophobe renal cell carcinoma. A peculiar feature associated with this case is cell nests in loose connective tissue stroma; they are made up of centrally located eosinophilic granular cells and peripherally located large ballooned cells

Chromophobe cells are positive for colloidal iron stain (Fig. 2-4-7). A positive stain is not limited to chromophobe RCC, although a diffuse, strong reticular staining was observed only in cases of chromophobe RCC [8].

Oncocytoma

Oncocytoma is a benign renal epithelial tumor. It is not uncommon and may be mistaken for RCC, especially with chromophobe RCC.

Oncocytoma was first distinguished from RCC as a benign tumor by Klein and Valensi [9] in 1976. It constitutes approximately 6%–7% of renal cortical neoplasms [10, 11]. Ever since, though, controversy has persisted in regard to its absolutely benign nature. The consensus among urologic pathologists is that it is a neoplasm that pursues a benign course if diagnosed correctly, although local invasiveness is demonstrated in rare cases. Occasional metastasis was reported in the early literature. The current prevailing opinion is that "metastasizing" oncocytoma is an incorrectly diagnosed RCC, notably chromophobe RCC. Another possible explanation for the "metastasizing" oncocytoma is that it is due to a coexisting carcinoma of another type in the patient. Oncocytoma not only resembles chromophobe RCC but shares immunohistochemical and molecular features with chromophobe RCC (refer to Question 8).

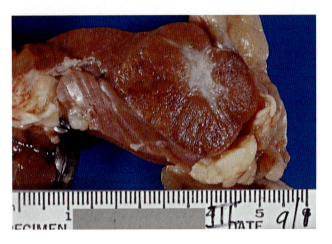

FIG. 2-4-8. Oncocytoma. A discretely outlined mass with a mahogany-colored cut surface and a central scar

Gross Appearance

The typical gross appearance of oncocytoma is that of a well-delineated mass without a capsule. The cut surface is solid and dark brown (mahogany) to dark red, with a central scar recognized in one-third to one-half of cases (Figs. 2-4-8, 2-4-9). The tumor may be large (≥10 cm). Hemorrhage is seen in 20% of cases but no necrosis [10]. The tumor may be multifocal (8%–13%) [10, 12] and bilateral (4%) [10].

Microscopic Appearance

Microscopically, the oncocytoma has the following appearance.

- The characteristic tumor cells are deeply eosinophilic, arranged in cords, nests (Fig. 2-4-9B), or tubules (Fig. 2-4-9C), which may be cystically dilated. The nuclei are small and round (mostly grade 2 by the Fuhrman system) with finely granular chromatin, and they may contain a small nucleolus (Fig. 2-4-9C).

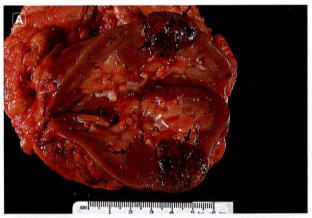

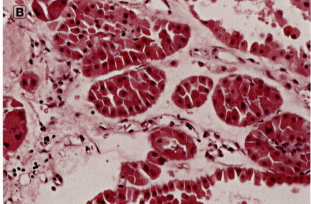

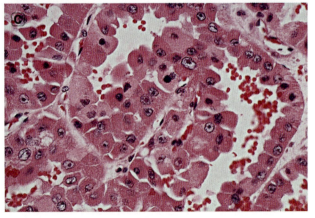

FIG. 2-4-9. **A** Oncocytoma with a dark-brown cut surface. It is difficult to delineate from the normal cortical tissue because of the similar color (*arrows*). **B** Eosinophilic tumor cells in nests are surrounded by a loose fibrovascular stroma. **C** Eosinophilic cells are arranged in tubules in this field

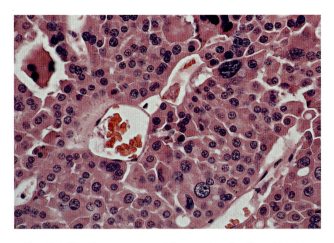

FIG. 2-4-10. Oncocytoma with occasional cells with gigantic nuclei. It does not indicate malignancy

- As variant cells, one may see nucleomegaly, hyperchromasia, and multinucleation. The features of "nuclear atypia" are not signs of aggressive behavior (Fig. 2-4-10).
- Also to be noted is the presence of isolated foci of small tubules and nest of cells with a clear cytoplasm (10% of cases in Perez-Ordonez series [10]). They are found embedded in a hyalinized stroma.
- Mitotic activity may be found (16% of cases [10]), but none of the mitoses is atypical.
- Invasion of perinephric adipose tissue may be seen (20% of cases [10]).
- In the Perez-Ordonez series [10], one case showed invasion of capillary-sized vessels, and two others had invasion of venous-type vessels. One of the latter two cases also had a biopsy-proven metastasis to the liver.

In summary, when the characteristic gross and microscopic appearances are present, the pathologist can make the diagnosis of oncocytoma with reasonable confidence even in the presence of some atypical features. The only time when concern is to be expressed is when there is venous invasion. It may be associated with a progressive behavior.

References

1. Thoenes W, Stoerkel ST, Rumpel HJ (1985) Human chromophobe cell renal carcinoma. Virchows Arch B Cell Pathol 48:207–217.
2. Stoerkel S, Steart PV, Drenckhahn, Thoenes W (1989) The human chromophobe cell renal carcinoma: its probable relation to intercalated cells of the collecting duct. Virchows Arch B Cell Pathol 56:237–245.
3. Crotty TB, Farrow GM, Lieber MM (1995) Chromophobe cell renal carcinoma: clinicopathological features of 50 cases. J Urol 154:964–967.
4. Amin MB, Moch H, Amin M, de Peralta-Venturina M, Stricker H, Tamboli P, Javidan J, Mihatsch M, Menon M (1999) Chromophobe renal cell carcinoma (CH-RCC): study of 65 cases. Mod Pathol 12:88A.
5. Pavlovich CP, Walther MM, Eyler RA, Hewitt SM, Zbar B, Linehan WM, Merino MJ (2002) Renal tumors in the Birt-Hogg-Dube syndrome. Am J Surg Pathol 26:1542–1552.
6. Bonsib SM, Lager DJ (1990) Chromophobe cell carcinoma: analysis of five cases. Am J Surg Pathol 14: 260–267.
7. Akhtar M, Karder H, Linjawi T, McClintock J, Ali MA (1995) Chromophobe cell carcinoma of the kidney: a clinicopathological study of 21 cases. Am J Surg Pathol 19:1245–1256.
8. Tickoo SK, Amin MB, Zarbo RJ (1998) Colloidal iron staining in renal epithelial neoplasms, including chromophobe renal cell carcinoma: emphasis on technique and patterns of staining. Am J Surg Pathol 22:419–424.
9. Klein MJ, Valensi QI (1976) Proximal tubular adenoma of kidney with so-called oncocytic features: a clinicopathologic study of 13 cases of a rarely reported neoplasm. Cancer 38:906–914.
10. Perez-Ordonez B, Hamed G, Campbell S, Erlandson RA, Gaudin PB, Reuter VE (1997) Renal oncocytoma: a clinicopathological study of 70 cases. Am J Surg Pathol 21:871–883.
11. Amin MB, Crotty TB, Tickoo SK, Farrow GM (1997) Renal oncocytoma: a reappraisal of morphologic features with clinicopathologic findings in 80 cases. Am J Surg Pathol 21:1–12.
12. Davis CJ Jr, Sesterhenn IA, Mostofi FK, Ho CK (1991) Renal oncocytoma: clinicopathological study of 166 patients. J Urogenit Pathol 1:41–52.

Question 5

What are the features of collecting duct carcinoma? What is mucinous tubular spindle cell carcinoma?

Answer

What were formerly classified as collecting duct carcinomas consist of four subtypes: (1) classic high-grade collecting duct carcinoma; (2) low-grade (or tubulocystic) collecting duct carcinomas, both of which are believed to derive from the Bellini duct; (3) medullary (high grade) carcinoma currently identified as a malignant tumor closely related to urothelial cell carcinoma; and (4) mucinous tubular spindle cell carcinoma of low malignant potential presumably of the distal tubule or collecting duct origin. Classic collecting duct carcinoma and medullary carcinoma take a highly aggressive clinical course; they demonstrate an infiltrative growth pattern and spread readily to distant sites. Medullary carcinoma is unique in that it affects black young adults and children, predominantly males, with sickle cell trait or hemoglobin SC disease. Tubulocystic carcinoma is characterized by well-differentiated tubules, which in areas are cystically dilated and give rise to the characteristic "bubble-wrap"-like appearance on the cut surface. Mucinous tubular spindle cell carcinoma consists of minimally atypical tumor cells arranged in a vague tubular pattern within myxoid to mucinous stroma.

Comments

Collecting duct carcinoma is the least common type of renal cell carcinoma (RCC), accounting for less than 1% of renal carcinomas. It is believed to derive from the Bellini duct (the inner medullary collecting duct that constitutes the most distal part of the collecting duct opening into the renal pelvis). Storkel [1] divided collecting duct carcinoma into four subtypes: (1) classic type (high grade); (2) collecting duct type of low grade; (3) tubular mucinous type (low grade, now referred to as mucinous tubular spindle cell carcinoma); and (4) medullary renal cell carcinoma (high grade).

High-Grade Collecting Duct Carcinoma, Classic Type

The classic-type high-grade collecting duct carcinoma is one of the most aggressive forms of renal carcinomas and presents as a gray-white firm mass with an irregular infiltrating border located in the medulla (Fig. 2-5-1). These tumors tend to show a connection to the renal pelvis but only rarely extend into it.

Microscopically, unlike the other types of RCC, the tumor shows a destructive intrarenal spread with

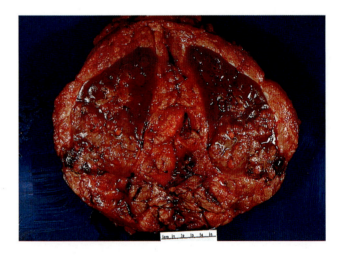

FIG. 2-5-1. Collecting duct carcinoma (classic type). Cross section reveals that almost two-thirds of the cut surface has been replaced by a carcinoma that has invaded the capsule and renal sinuses

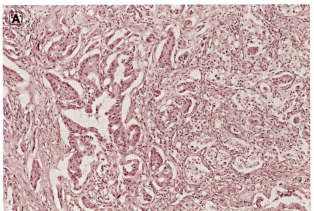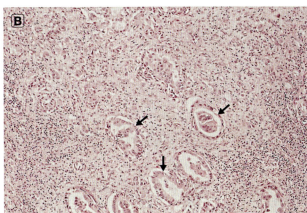

FIG. 2-5-2. Collecting duct carcinoma. **A** Poorly differentiated tumor cells in twisted tubules and cords are surrounded by desmoplastic stroma. **B** Collecting ducts trapped in tumor tissue are replaced by neoplastic cells (*arrows*). (Courtesy of Mareyuki Endoh, MD, Tohoku University Graduate School of Medicine, Sendai)

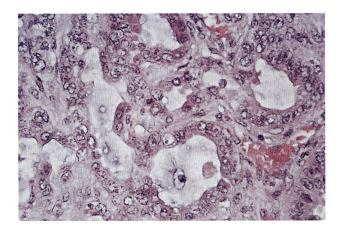

FIG. 2-5-3. Collecting duct carcinoma, classic type (high grade). Large eosinophilic cells are arranged in anastomosing tubules and have nuclei of high grade

a desmoplastic reaction. Foci of necrosis and invasion of intrarenal and hilar veins are common. Large eosinophilic cells are arranged in a microcystic-papillary pattern (Fig. 2-5-2) and, less commonly, in tubular architecture (Fig. 2-5-3) [2–4]. The nuclei are of Fuhrman grades 3 and 4 and have prominent nucleoli. Because of the papillary growth pattern, the differential diagnosis includes papillary RCC. The features in favor of papillary RCC are an absence of desmoplasia, a well-formed papillary structure, circumscribed growth pattern, and frequent multifocality. The features in favor of collecting duct carcinoma are, in addition to the differences described above, the presence of cytologic atypia in the nearby collecting ducts [5] and positive immunohistochemical reac-

tions to high-molecular-weight (HMW) cytokeratin 34βE12 and *Ulex europaeus* lectin. (For more information, refer to Question 8.)

Medullary Renal Cell Carcinoma

Medullary RCC is a recently recognized aggressive form of RCC and involves the medulla and pyramid. It characteristically develops in young adults and children with the sickle cell trait (but not sickle cell anemia) or hemoglobin SC disease [6–8]. The gross appearance is that of a firm, solid invasive mass (Fig. 2-5-4A).

Microscopic features vary and consist of foci of tubular to trabecular (Fig. 2-5-4B), squamoid, yolk sac tumor-like, adenoid cystic differentiations with features in common with the collecting duct carcinoma. Rhabdoid tumor-like foci are reportedly a characteristic feature of this tumor. The tumor is widespread at diagnosis, and most patients die within 14 months [7]. It may be considered a special type of collecting duct carcinoma. Molecular studies have shown that this tumor is more closely related to urothelial carcinoma than to RCC [9], which suggests the possibility of modifying the chemotherapeutic regimens.

Tubulocystic Carcinoma (Low-Grade Collecting Duct Carcinoma)

Tubulocystic carcinoma presents as a discretely circumscribed mass and involves the medulla or cortex. The cut surface reveals a well-circumscribed mass

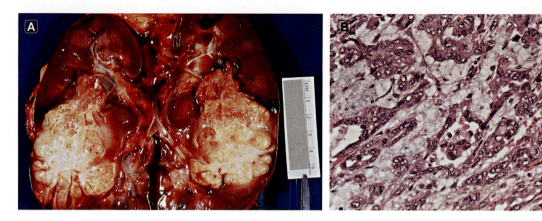

FIG. 2-5-4. Medullary carcinoma (high grade). The patient is a 20 year-old man. **A** Solid mass occupying the medullary region exhibits, on sectioning, a gray-white cut surface. **B** Microscopically, it demonstrates a tubular to a fused tubular pattern in a mucoid background. (Courtesy of Michael Pins, MD, Northwestern University Feinberg School of Medicine, Chicago)

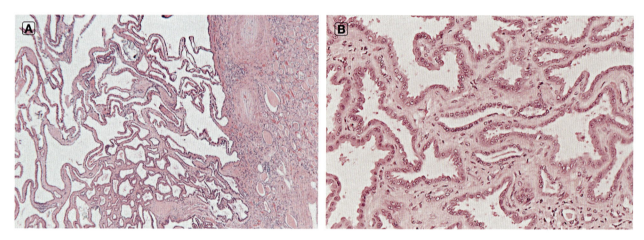

FIG. 2-5-5. **A, B** Tubulocystic carcinoma. It is a sharply demarcated lesion. Cystically dilated tumor glands are lined by low-cuboidal eosinophilic cells with large nuclei and prominent nucleoli. Mitosis is virtually absent. The stroma is relatively oligocellular

composed of multiple cysts [10], described by Amin et al. [11] as a spongy "bubble-wrap"— like appearance created by small cystic structures. The molecular profile and genomic changes, according to a recent study by one of the authors, resemble those of papillary RCC but are still distinct from it (Yang, to be published in Am J Surg Pathol).

Microscopically, it consists of well-differentiated tubules of varying size, which in areas are cystically dilated separated by thin fibrous septa. A desmoplastic reaction is absent. The lining cells are eosinophilic, cuboidal, flattened, or hobnail; and they have uniform nuclei and frequent prominent nucleoli (Fig. 2-5-5). When arranged in well-formed tubules, they have a considerable resemblance to normal renal tubules.

Recently, Amin and his colleagues propose that this low-grade variant be designated tubulocystic carcinoma because of its unique pathologic features and low-grade malignant potential. Immunohistochemical study showed positive reactions to parvalbumin, CK8, CK18, and CK19 (100%); CD10 (85%); P504S (77%); CK7 (62%); and 34β12E (15%). Of 29 cases, 24 were stage pT1, 4 were pT2, and 1 was pT3a. Only two cases showed distant spread.

Mucinous Tubular Spindle Cell Carcinoma

In the past, mucinous tubular spindle cell carcinoma was considered to be a subtype of collecting duct carcinoma based on the immunohistochemical

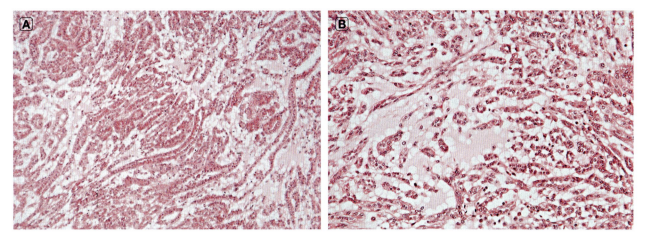

FIG. 2-5-6. **A, B** Mucinous tubular spindle cell carcinoma. This sharply circumscribed mass is from a 34-year-old woman. The tumor cells are uniform, pale-stained, and arranged in twisted slender tubules. Extracellular mucin is a striking feature of this tumor (**B**). (Courtesy of Mareyuki Endoh, MD, Tohoku University Graduate School of Medicine, Sendai)

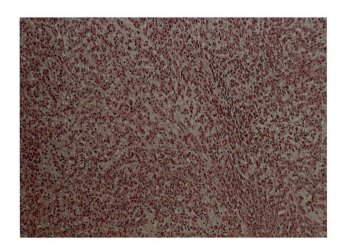

FIG. 2-5-7. Mucinous tubular spindle cell carcinoma. This is another example of mucinous tubular spindle cell carcinoma from an 85 year-old woman. The tumor is a well-circumscribed tan mass localized to the lower pole of the left kidney and measures 5 × 4 × 3 cm. Microscopically it consists of small cells arranged in elongated tubules with a myxoid background. (Courtesy of Michael Pins, MD, Northwestern University Feinberg School of Medicine, Chicago)

expression of site-specific markers but was distinguished from the classic type because of its low malignancy potential [12]. All tumors are sharply circumscribed and show a homogeneous yellow to tan-brown to pinkish cut surface.

Microscopically, "classic" tumors [13] consist of epithelial cells with little intervening myxoid or mucinous stroma. Tumor cells are arranged in a vague tubular pattern, and tubules are lined by cuboidal cells with pale to eosinophilic cytoplasm [12, 14] (Figs. 2-5-6, 2-5-7). Centrally located nuclei are round without significant atypia, and most of them have discernible small to medium-sized nucleoli. Mitoses are rare. The tumor may show areas where cells assume a more spindle shape, although cellular features differ from those of sarcomatoid growth. A striking feature is the presence of abundant, predominantly extracellular mucin (Figs. 2-5-6B, 2-5-7), which is strongly reactive to alcian blue at pH 2.5 but periodic acid-Schiff (PAS)-negative [1]. In the Fine series [13], however, 7 of 17 cases were considered "mucin-poor." Unusual histologic features involving both "classic" and "mucin-poor" types were an accumulation of foamy macrophages, formation of papillary structure, focal clear cells in tubules,, necrosis, and oncocytic tubules.

References

1. Storkel S (2001) Kidney tumors. Workshop presentation at the 18th European Congress of Pathology, Berlin, September 8–13, 2001.
2. Fleming S, Lewi HJE (1986) Collecting duct carcinoma of kidney. Histopathology 10:1131–1141.
3. Rumpelt HJ, Stoerkel S, Moll R, Schaerfe T, Thoenes W (1991) Bellini duct carcinoma: further evidence of this rare variant of renal cell carcinoma. Histopathology 18:115–122.
4. Aizawa S, Kikuchi Y, Suzuki M, Furusato M (1987) Renal cell carcinoma of lower nephron origin. Acta Pathol Jpn 37:567–574.

5. Kennedy SM, Merino MJ, Linehan WM, Roberts JR, Robertson CN, Neumann RD (1990) Collecting duct carcinoma of the kidney. Hum Pathol 21:449–456.

6. Davis CJ, Mostifi FK, Seterhenn IA (1995) Renal medullary carcinoma: the seventh sickle cell nephropathy. Am J Surg Pathol 19:1–11.

7. Abrahams JH, Drachenberg M, Beckwith DS (1998) Medullary renal cell carcinoma (MRC): a report of 28 new cases. Mod Pathol 11:74A.

8. Avery RA, Harris JA, Davis CJ, Borgaonkar DS, Byrd JC, Weiss RB (1996) Renal medullary carcinoma: clinical and therapeutic aspects of a newly described tumor. Cancer 78:128–132.

9. Yang XJ, Sugimura J, Tretiakova MS, Pins M, Teh BT (2004) Molecular profiling of renal medullary carcinoma. Mod Pathol 17(suppl 1):185A.

10. MacLennan GT, Farrow GM, Bostwick DG (1997) Low-grade collecting duct carcinoma of the kidney: report of 13 cases of low-grade mucinous tubulocystic renal carcinoma of possible collecting duct origin. Urology 50:679–684.

11. Amin MB, MacLennan GT, Paraf F, Cheville JC, Viellefond A, Radhakrishnan A, Che M, Srigly JR, Grignon DJ (2004) Tubulocystic carcinoma of the kidney: clinicopathological analysis of 29 cases of a distinctive subtype of renal cell carcinoma (RCC). Mod Pathol 17(suppl1):137A.

12. Rakozy C, Schmahl GE, Bohner S, Storkel S (2001) Low grade tubular-mucinous renal neoplasms: morphologic, immunohistochemical and genetic features. Mod Pathol 15:1162–1171.

13. Fine SW, Argani P, DeMarzo AM, Delahunt B, Sebo TJ, Reuter VE, Epstein JI (2006) Expanding the histologic spectrum of mucinous and spindle cell carcinoma of the kidney. Am J Surg Pathol 30:1554–1560.

14. Parwani AV, Husain AN, Epstein JI, Beckwith JB, Argani P (2001) Low-grade myxoid renal epithelial neoplasms with distal nephron differentiation. Hum Pathol 32:506–512.

Question 6

Why is sarcomatoid renal cell carcinoma not an independent subtype? What is the clinical significance of unclassified renal cell carcinoma?

Answer

The term sarcomatoid carcinoma was coined during the late 1960s by Farrow et al. to describe renal carcinomas in which cells have lost epithelial features and have assumed a sarcomatous, or "sarcomatoid," appearance. The definition was based strictly on the appearance in H&E-stained sections. Thus, it is probable that sarcomatoid components are either sarcoma-like epithelial components or nonepithelial malignant components, such as osteogenic sarcoma or hemangiopericytoma. Strictly defined, it is a carcinoma with sarcoma-like, but epithelial, components as proved by ultrastructural or immunohistochemical studies. Thus, in each case, areas of the usual RCC should be recognized. In practice, however, malignant components could drift away from the epithelial type to the nonepithelial type. Such cases then should be designated carcinosarcoma, mixed carcinoma, or sarcoma. However, because the outcome of such patients is the same as that for patients with tumors having sarcomatoid differentiation, the distinction is more or less academic.

Comments

Sarcomatoid Renal Cell Carcinoma

Sarcomatoid variants of renal cell carcinoma (RCC) [1–3] occurs in approximately 5% of RCCs and can be encountered with any type of RCC. It is associated most frequently, however, with the clear cell type because it is the most common type of RCC. According to de Peralta-Venturina et al. [4], who reported the largest number of sarcomatoid carcinomas (101/952 RCCs), the association frequency was as follows: clear cell type 8%; papillary type 3%; chromophobe type 9%, and collecting duct type 29%. Metastasis was documented at diagnosis in 66% [4] to 77% [5]. Therefore, sarcomatoid RCC represents the very high-grade end of all types of RCC. It is also important to know that sarcomatoid RCCs are more common than true sarcomas in the kidney; the latter typically develop from the renal capsule rather than the renal parenchyma.

Gross Appearance

Sarcomatoid RCC is typically large with accompanying low-malignant components. The sarcomatoid area may be recognized as a hard, gray area in a bulky mass that often exhibits an extracapsular extension (Figs. 2-6-1, 2-6-2A, 2-6-3A). Hemorrhage and necrosis are common. Ro et al. [6] reported that in a good number of cases there was no area grossly identifiable as having sarcomatoid differentiation.

Microscopic Appearance

Microscopically, the sarcomatoid RCC has the following appearance.

- Foci of epithelial differentiation should be found (Figs. 2-6-2B, 2-6-4A). The proportion of the sarcomatoid area varies from case to case—but the more extensive the sarcomatoid component, the worse the prognosis ($P < 0.001$) [6].
- The sarcomatoid component (Figs. 2-6-2C, 2-6-3B, 2-6-4B, 2-6-5) consists of pleomorphic spindle cells that resemble those of fibrous histiocytoma, fibrosarcoma, and others including unclassified sarcoma

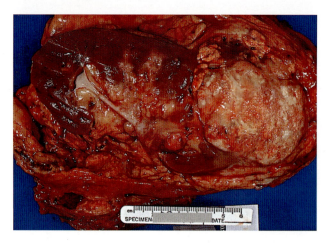

FIG. 2-6-1. Clear cell renal cell carcinoma with a sarcomatoid component extending into the perinephric adipose tissue. On gross examination, it is difficult to identify the sarcomatoid area in this case. Microscopic examination confirmed that it is a clear cell carcinoma with areas of sarcomatoid differentiation

components [1–4, 6–8]. Despite the sarcomatoid appearance, ultrastructural and immunohistochemical studies have confirmed that sarcomatoid cells in most cases exhibit epithelial characteristics [7, 9, 10]. In some cases cells fail to do so, implying that true sarcomatous differentiation has taken place.

• Although most of the epithelial components are of high Fuhrman grades, surprisingly, a fair number of cases were associated with a low-grade carcinoma (6/42 cases) [6] (Fig. 2-6-2B). This is a warning to the pathologist that adequate sampling is essential not to overlook sarcomatoid areas. Even a small fraction of sarcomatoid component affects the prognosis adversely [6].

• Most sarcomatoid RCCs are discovered at advanced stages (Fig. 2-6-1) [4–6], and the prognosis is significantly worse in patients with sarcomatoid RCC and distant metastasis at nephrectomy than in

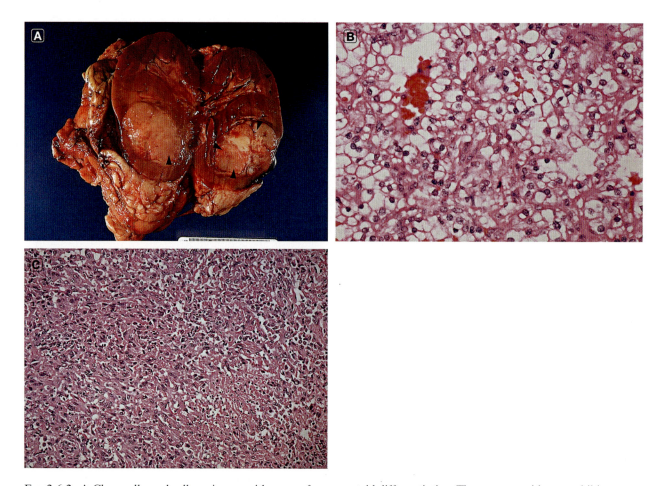

FIG. 2-6-2. **A** Clear cell renal cell carcinoma with areas of sarcomatoid differentiation. The sarcomatoid area exhibits a gray cut surface (*arrowheads*) in contrast to the yellow area of clear cell carcinoma area. **B** Clear cell carcinoma area, Fuhrman grade 2. **C** Sarcomatoid area

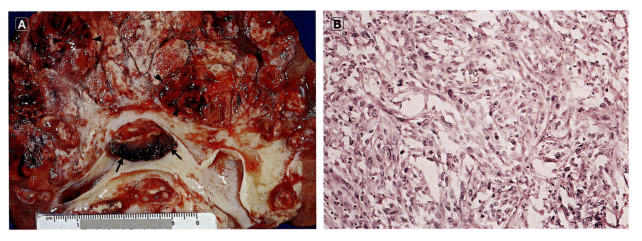

Fig. 2-6-3. **A** Large renal cell carcinoma with sarcomatoid differentiation occupying almost 80% of the kidney. Tumor shows hemorrhagic necrosis and renal vein invasion (*arrows*). **B** The sarcomatoid area is composed of spindle cells. (Case provided by Michael Pins, MD, Northwestern University Feinberg School of Medicine, Chicago)

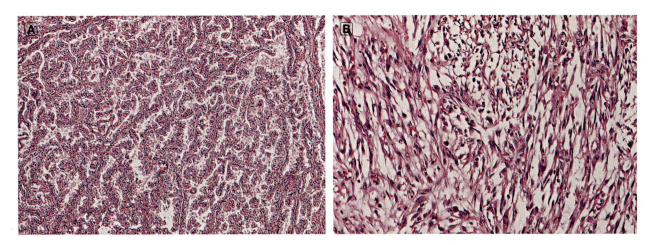

Fig. 2-6-4. Papillary renal cell carcinoma (**A**) with sarcomatoid differentiation (**B**)

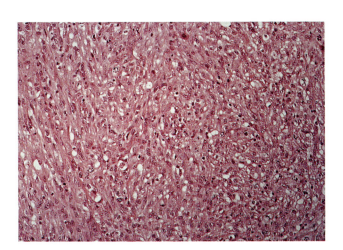

Fig. 2-6-5. Sarcomatoid carcinoma. Epithelial features are faintly suggested

those with sarcomatoid RCC but without evidence of distant metastasis ($P < 0.001$) [11].

- TNM stage (by 1997 and 2003 standards) and tumor necrosis are the only significant variables for predicting outcome among RCCs with a sarcomatoid component [2, 11].

Renal Cell Carcinoma, Unclassified

The diagnostic category "RCC, unclassified" was defined in the 2004 WHO kidney tumor classification system. There is a small number of renal carcinomas that cannot be classified into one of the defined types described above based on their morphologic features. They comprise a group of heterogeneous tumors that are too poorly differentiated to be classified. The tumor cells may include spindle cells and mucin-producing cells, and there may be tubular cribriform growth [12]. These features are of high nuclear grade and high TNM stage. "Renal cell carcinoma, unclassified" may represent a diagnostic term for pathologists to express their uncertainty rather than a true biologic and morphologic entity. Further molecular studies are necessary to elucidate the nature of this group of tumors. Unclassified-type RCCs and collecting duct carcinomas are the most aggressive followed, in descending order of aggressiveness, by clear cell RCC, papillary RCC, and chromophobe RCC.

References

1. Farrow GM, Harrison EG Jr, Utz DC, ReMine WH (1968A) Sarcoma and sarcomatoid and mixed malignant tumors of the kidney in adults. Part I. Cancer 22:545–550.
2. Farrow GM, Harrison EG, Utz DC (1968B) Sarcomas and sarcomatoid and mixed malignant tumors of the kidney in adults. Part II. Cancer 22:551–555.
3. Farrow GM, Harrison EG, Utz DC (1968C) Sarcomas and sarcomatoid and mixed malignant tumors of the kidney in adults. Part III. Cancer 22:556–563.
4. De Peralta-Venturina M, Moch H, Amin M, Tamboli P, Hailemariam S, Mihatsch M, Javidan J, Stricker H, Ro JY, Amin MB (2001) Sarcomatoid differentiation in renal cell carcinoma: a study of 101 cases. Am J Surg Pathol 25:275–284.
5. Mian BM, Bhadakamkar N, Slayton JW, Pisters PWT, Daliani D, Swanson DA, Pisters LL (2002) Prognostic factors and survival of patients with sarcomatoid renal cell carcinoma. J Urol 167:65–70.
6. Ro JY, Ayala AG, Sella A, Samuels ML, Swanson DA (1987) Sarcomatoid renal cell carcinoma: a clinicopathologic study of 42 cases. Cancer 59:516–526.
7. Bonsib SM, Fischer J, Plattner S, Fallon B (1987) Sarcomatoid renal tumors: clinicopathologic correlation of three cases. Cancer 59:527–532.
8. Macke R, Hussain MB, Imray TJ, Wilson RB, Cohen SM (1985) Osteogenic and sarcomatoid differentiation of a renal cell carcinoma. Cancer 56:2452–2457.
9. DeLong W, Grignon DJ, Shum DT, Wyatt JK (1993) Sarcomatoid renal cell carcinoma: an immunohistochemical study of 18 cases. Arch Pathol Lab Med 117;636–640.
10. Akhtar M, Tulbah A, Kardar AH, Ali MA (1997) Sarcomatoid renal cell carcinoma: the chromophobe connection. Am J Surg Pathol 21:1188–1195.
11. Cheville JC, Lohse CM, Zincke H, Weaver AL, Leibovich BC, Frank I, Blute ML (2004) Sarcomatoid renal cell carcinoma: an examination of underlying histologic subtype and an analysis of association with patient outcome. Am J Surg Pathol 28:435–441.
12. Amin MaB, Amin MiB, Tamboli P, Javidan J, Stricker H, De-Peralta Ventrina M, Deshpande A, Menon M (2002) Prognostic impact of histologic subtyping of adult renal epithelial neoplasms: an experience of 405 cases. Am J Surg Pathol 26:281–291.

Question 7

What molecular and genetic changes are characteristic of renal tumors? Based on the new knowledge, is molecular targeting feasible?

Answer

During the past 20 years, consorted efforts of a number of investigator groups have identified several genes that are associated with certain types of renal tumors. To identify the genetic basis of renal tumors, investigators studied the hereditary forms of renal cell carcinoma (RCC) with the hope that gene(s) identified may also be involved in the development of sporadic forms of RCC. The *VHL* gene was identified in association with clear cell RCC. With a similar approach, association of the *C-MET* gene with papillary RCC and the BHD (Birt-Hogg-Dube) gene with chromophobe RCC and oncocytoma was discovered. To date, the *VHL* gene is only one that is significantly associated with the development of clear cell RCC. It is a suppressor gene. Its loss of function either by mutation or loss (physical and functional) leads to the activation of several genes, including the genes for vascular endothelial growth factor (VEGF), platelet-derived growth factor (PDGF), transforming growth factor-α (TGFα), and glucose transporter (GLUT-1), all of which are important for supporting the growth of tumor cells. Thus, these genes are potential targets for suppressing tumor cell growth.

Comments

Those readers interested in this subject are urged to read the excellent review by Linehan et al. [1].

Clear Cell Renal Cell Carcinoma

Inactivation of the VHL Gene by Mutation and Loss

The only gene of known functional significance in clear cell RCCs is the *VHL* (von Hippel-Lindau) gene. Investigation with VHL disease kindred showed that renal tumors that occur in association with this altered gene were uniformly clear cell carcinomas. The tumors develop in 35%–45% of affected individuals and occur as multiple tumors involving both kidneys starting at an early age [1]. In the affected families, there is a constitutional balanced reciprocal translocation of a portion of the short arm of chromosome 3p to chromosome 6, 8, or 11 [2–4]. Thus, the findings suggest that chromosome 3p may harbor a gene involved in the etiology/pathogenesis of the clear cell carcinoma and the translocation breakpoint might disrupt a gene involved in the control of renal cell growth [5]. A subsequent study using the restriction fragment length polymorphism (RFLP) analysis showed that in all 11 cases loss of a segment of chromosome 3 occurred only in tumor tissue and that all showed loss of the same chromosome allele (the wild type—that is, the chromosome derived from the unaffected parent), supporting the notion that there may be an RCC gene in this location [6, 7]. In 1993, *VHL* cDNA was identified on the chromosome 3p25-p26 region as an inactivating mutation in the germline of affected individuals with VHL disease. It is a relatively small gene, composed of three exons with 854 coding nucleotides [5]. It functions as a tumor suppressor gene as evidenced by the following elegant experiment by Gnarra et al. [8]. Clear cell RCC cell lines that are *VHL−/−* (the 2 copies of the *VHL* genes

TABLE 2-7-1. Mechanisms of *VHL* gene inactivation in clear cell RCC

Clear cell RCC type	First copy	Second copy
Familial	Born with a mutated gene derived from an affected parent (germline mutations)[a]	Wild type inactivated mostly by deletion of DNA
Sporadic	Inactivated by mutations[b]	Inactivated by deletion of DNA[c]

[a] Mutations identified in 75% of 144 VHL families [5] and include microdeletion/insertions, deletions, nonsense mutations, or missense mutations involving all three exons. More recently, mutations were identified in 99% of 93 VHL families [9].
[b] Mutations detected in 56%–57% and include missense mutations, deletions, insertions, and nonsense mutations involving all three exons [8, 10].
[c] Loss of one copy in 98% of cases of clear cell carcinomas analyzed [8].

are inactivated) form tumors in nude mice. When a normal (WT) copy of the *VHL* gene was placed in the tumor cell line and the cells were inoculated in the mice, small or no tumors formed. The study provided strong support to the contention that the *VHL* gene acts as a tumor suppressor gene, and loss of function leads to tumor formation.

Thus, in the *VHL*-associated hereditary renal neoplasia, both *VHL* gene copies have lost their function (by different mechanisms) which satisfies the Knudson and Strong's two-hit hypothesis (Table 2-7-1). In the sporadic form of clear cell RCC, 56%–57% of tumors showed (somatic) mutations of one copy; and the second copy is lost at a high frequency.

Recently, another mechanism has been reported in silencing *VHL* gene expression. Herman et al. found in 5 of 27 clear cell carcinomas analyzed that the 5′ region of the VHL gene, which is normally unmethylated, was hypermethylated, whereas no detectable mutations were found in four of the five renal carcinomas studied [11].

Function of the VHL Gene

The *VHL* gene acts as a transcription factor. Based on reported data, *VHL*'s role is summarized in Fig. 2-7-1. In essence, VHL protein (pVHL) plays two major roles: (1) regulation of elongin, which controls the activity of polymerase II; and (2) regulation of hypoxia-inducible factor (*HIF*), which in turn regulates the activities of angiogenesis and cell growth-related genes.

Interaction with Elongin. Elongin controls the transcriptional elongation of RNA by polymerase II. It is a heterotrimer consisting of A, B, and C subunits. Under physiologic conditions, the α domain of VHL protein (pVHL) binds specifically and tightly to the subunits B and C, the regulatory subunits of elongin. The pVHL/elongin C/B complex then binds

to Cul-2 (a member of the multigene cullin family) [12]. This is a ubiquitination (degradation) pathway. The binding of elongin A, the catalytic subunit, to the B/C complex is required for a high level of its transcriptional activity. Mutations of the *VHL* gene result in failure of its binding to elongin, resulting in inhibition of the degradation pathways. As a result, the balance between pVHL/elonginC/B complex and elongin A/B/C complex formation is shifted to the latter and restoration of the polymerase II activity [13–15]. *VHL* mutations thus may involve the failure to regulate some of the target genes such as c-myc family and c-fos, which in turn stimulates cell proliferation.

Interactions with HIF. pVHL, in oxygenated cells, binds directly to HIF through its β domain, thereby targeting HIF for ubiquitination. In this process, a specific domain of the HIF α subunit needs to be hydroxylated (with molecular oxygen) at a proline residue [16, 17]. The pVHL negatively regulates the expression of hypoxia-inducible genes such as VEGF, PDGF, GLUT-1, and erythropoietin [18, 19]. The activity of HIF is induced in hypoxic cells through stabilization and activation of its α subunit. Thus, inactivation of the VHL gene (and hypoxic state) in RCC is associated with activation of the HIF signaling and expression of the hypoxia-inducible genes described above [20]. The biologic significance of the *VHL* gene in this process was demonstrated in an in vitro experiment. Introduction of the wild-type *VHL* gene to renal carcinoma cells lacking the wild-type *VHL* specifically inhibited production of these mRNAs under normoxic conditions [19, 21].

VHL Gene Mutation-Unrelated Clear Cell RCC

The reported mutation rates of the *VHL* gene vary from 56%–57% in sporadic cases to nearly 100% in

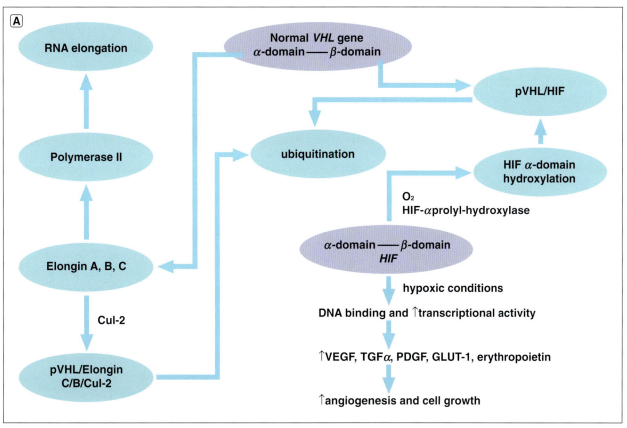

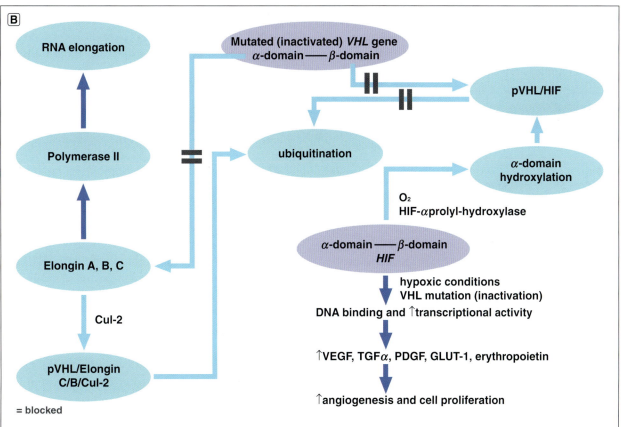

FIG. 2-7-1. **A** Molecular mechanism of wild-type *VHL* and hypoxia-inducible factor (*HIF*) interactions. **B** Molecular mechanism of mutated (inactivated) *VHL* and *HIF* interactions. *Dark arrows* indicate the actiuated steps in consequence of *VHL* gene mutation

familial cases. There is evidence that a sizable number of clear cell RCCs show no mutations of this gene. Existence of pathways leading to clear cell RCC other than mutations of the *VHL* gene has been demonstrated [22, 23]. Chromosomal analysis of clear cell carcinoma during the early 1990s repeatedly suggested the presence of additional genes, which are lost at the breakpoint of chromosome 3p (3p12-14 regions) [4, 24–27]. One such candidate is the fragile histidine triad (*FHIT*), a putative tumor suppressor gene that spans the t(3:8) chromosomal translocation breakpoint identified in a family with RCC [28]. However, subsequent data are conflicting about supporting the hypothesis that *FHIT* is a suppressor gene.

VHL alterations (mutations and hypermethylation) are associated with a better prognosis in patients with stages I–III clear cell carcinoma treated with nephrectomy than in those showing no alterations of *VHL* [29].

Papillary Renal Cell Carcinoma

Cytogenetic studies demonstrated that sporadic papillary RCCs were characterized by trisomy of chromosomes 7, 16, and 17 and in men by loss of the Y chromosome [30–33]. End-stage renal disease patients have an increased risk of renal carcinomas, in particular the papillary type. In one analysis of 14 papillary RCCs, 5 had trisomy of both chromosomes 7 and 17, 3 had either trisomy 7 or trisomy 17 but not both, and 6 had no changes in chromosomes 7 and 17. None had a 3p deletion [33].

Mutation of c-MET Gene

Mutational analysis for papillary RCC was again facilitated by studying the familial form of renal cancer. The responsible gene was found to be located on chromosome 7q31.1-34, and was identified as the *c-MET* gene. Missense mutations were found in its tyrosine kinase domain in the germline of affected members of six of seven hereditary papillary RCC families [34, 35]. C-*MET* mutations also have been identified in tumors of 13% of papillary RCC patients with no family history of renal tumors [36]. To date, 15 different missense mutations have been identified located in a tyrosine kinase domain [37]. They are homologous to those in *c-kit* and *RET*, proto-oncogenes that are targets of naturally occurring mutations. These mutations have been shown to be transforming when transfected into NIH 3T3 cells and cause ligand-independent constitutive phosphorylation of the c-MET protein [36]. The finding suggests that missense mutations lead to activation of the c-MET protein in papillary RCC.

Mutational analysis by Lubensky et al. [37] demonstrated that it is always type 1 lesions that showed c-MET mutations, irrespective of hereditary or sporadic type. Some of small lesions (<0.5 cm) that are classified as papillary adenomas also had *c-MET* mutations. Although all hereditary and sporadic papillary RCCs with *c-MET* mutations showed distinctive type 1 morphology, not all type 1 sporadic cancers had *c-MET* mutations. Study indicates that some other unknown genes are involved in tumorigenesis. What is the significance of chromosome 7 trisomy observed in sporadic and inherited papillary RCC? It is the mutated *c-MET* allele that is duplicated in the tumors [34, 38]. Thus, the trisomy may serve to increase the dosage of the mutant allele [34]. It is to be noted that *c-MET* proto-oncogene is a member of the receptor tyrosine kinase family of proteins. Binding of its ligand, hepatocyte growth factor, to the extracellular portion of *c-MET* triggers autophosphorylation of critical tyrosines in the intracellular tyrosine kinase domain of *MET*, activating a downstream signaling cascade. It must be noted that *MET* has been shown to be overexpressed in a number of other human cancers, including clear cell RCC (Yang, unpublished data).

c-Kit Mutation

Recently a group of investigators from Korea [39] reported a novel point mutation in *c-kit* intron 17 in 17 of 18 papillary RCCs but none in other types, including clear cell and chromophobe RCCs. The significance is unknown. Immunohistochemically, all papillary RCCs demonstrated cytoplasmic staining for c-kit ($n = 18$), while all chromophobe RCCs ($n = 20$) expressed c-kit protein (without mutation) on the cell membranes where c-kit protein is expected to be expressed inasmuch as it is a membrane-associated receptor tyrosine kinase. It has been suggested that diffuse cytoplasmic (not membranous) staining may reflect *c-kit* mutations as is observed in gastrointestinal stromal tumors [40]. The cytoplasmic staining in the papillary RCCs may indicate a functional alteration in c-kit protein [39].

FH (Fumarate Hydratase) Mutations

A familial form of hereditary syndrome designated hereditary leiomyomatosis and renal cancer (HLRCC) syndrome, as well as multiple cutaneous and uterine leiomyomatoses (MCUL), are characterized by germline mutations of fumarase (fumarate hydratase) [41–43]. Fumarase catalyzes the conversion of fumarate to malate as part of the tricarboxylic acid cycle in mitochondria. In the heterozygous mutation/wild-type state, the *FH* gene acts as a tumor suppressor. The renal carcinomas occurring in patients with this syndrome have been described as papillary carcinoma compatible with high Fuhrman nuclear grade [43], although in another report [41] the microscopic appearance was said to be suggestive of collecting duct carcinoma of low grade. It is unknown if FH mutations are involved in the sporadic form of papillary RCC.

Chromophobe Renal Cell Carcinoma

Birt-Hogg-Dube (BHD) syndrome is another familial form of renal tumors associated with benign cutaneous tumors. It is an autosomal dominant dermatosis characterized by the development of small dome-shaped papules on the face, neck, and upper trunk. In addition to these benign hair follicle tumors, the syndrome is associated with the development of pulmonary cysts and renal tumors of a variety of histologic types. The renal tumors are multiple and bilateral. In a study of 130 resected tumors from 30 patients, 44 consisted of chromophobe RCCs (34%), 65 of hybrids of oncocytic tumors that had areas of chromophobe RCC and oncocytoma (50%), and 12 of clear cell RCCs (9%) [44]. Genetic linkage analysis localized the *BHD* gene to chromosome 17p11.2 [45]. It appears to be a suppressor gene. It remains to be determined if the gene is involved in the development of the sporadic form of chromophobe RCC and oncocytoma. The development of at least three types of tumor in patients with this syndrome raises an important question. Is the mutation of the *BHD* gene responsible for the development of these tumors? The clear cell RCCs observed in these patients are indistinguishable morphologically from conventional clear cell RCCs. Molecular analysis of tumors with clear cell morphology indeed showed loss of heterozygosity (LOH) flanking the *VHL* gene on 3p in four of eight tumors, and *VHL* mutations were noted in two of six tumors, both of which also demonstrated 3p LOH. Therefore, they are indeed clear cell RCCs rather than clear cell-rich chromophobe RCCs. We must wait for the identification of the gene, at which time its specific role in tumorigenesis of hybrid oncocytic tumors, chromophobe renal cell carcinomas, and other tumors will be elucidated. Oncocytoma and chromophobe RCCs are thought to originate from the intercalated cells of renal collecting tubules [46], whereas the origin of clear cell renal carcinomas is not clear. Immunohistochemical study suggests the development from an uncommitted cell or a primitive cell rather than any particular portion of the nephron [47]. It is possible that these tumors (oncocytoma, chromophobe and clear cell RCCs) are of the same cell origin.

Unclassifiable Renal Carcinomas and Other Rare Renal Carcinomas

There are tumors that cannot be classified into one the categories described above. Many of them are of high grade and high stage [48] (refer to Question 6). In addition, there are a group of RCCs whose chromosomal abnormality has recently been characterized [49]. They are *PRCC-TFE3* RCC and its related congener *ASPL-TFE3* RCC (Fig. 2-7-2). The former is characterized by t(X;1)(p11.2;q21) and the latter by t(X;17)(p11.2;q25). *TFE3* is a transcription factor gene on Xp11.2. Both types of tumor occur in young persons under age 30. They are characterized by clear to densely granular and eosinophilic cells arranged in a solid nested pattern, alveolar pattern, or papillary architecture, thus resembling the conventional clear cell carcinomas as well as papillary carcinomas. Distinction from the conventional RCC is the immunohistochemical demonstration of TFE3 protein (carboxy-terminal portion) in the nuclei in *PRCC-TFE3* and *ASPL-TFE3* carcinomas and its lack in the former. Furthermore, the conventional clear cell carcinoma is a disease involving adults. Therefore, when a renal tumor with clear cells develops in a young person, the t(X;1) or t(X;17) tumor should be considered in the differential diagnosis, and genetic analysis is warranted.

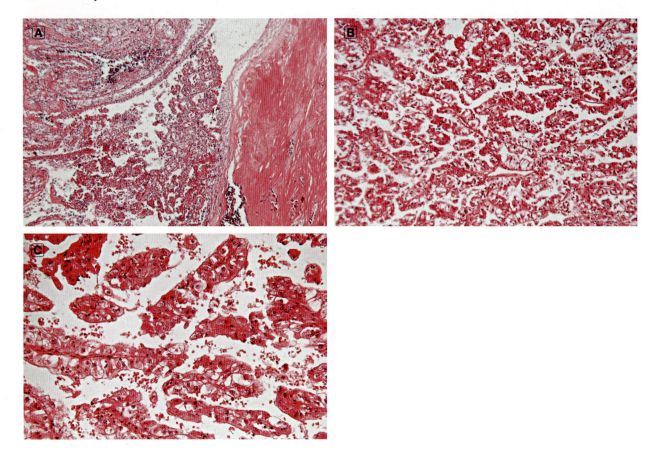

FIG. 2-7-2. PRCC-TFE3 renal carcinoma in a 12-year-old girl. The tumor is sharply demarcated from the degenerated non-neoplastic parenchyma (**A**) and consists of clear and granular cells arranged in either papillary (**B, C**) or alveolar (*right lower corner*) pattern (**C**). Note that some cells are clear and swollen to a balloon shape and have a distinct cell membrane. The tumor cell nuclei are reportedly reactive for TFE3 protein by immunohistochemical reaction. (Courtesy of Mareyuki Endoh, MD, Tohoku University Graduate School of Medicine, Sendai)

References

1. Linehan WM, Waither MM, Zbar B (2003) The genetic basis of cancer of the kidney. J Urol 170:2163–2172.
2. Cohen AJ, Li FP, Berg S, Marchetto DJ, Tsai S, Jacobs SC, Brown RS (1979) Hereditary renal-cell carcinoma associated with a chromosomal translocation. N Engl J Med 301:592–595.
3. Pathak S, Strong LC, Farrel RE, Trindade A (1982) Familial renal cell carcinoma with a 3:11 translocation limited to tumor cells. Science 217:939–941.
4. Kovacs G, Earlandsson R, Boldog F, Ingvarsson S, Mueller-Brechlin R, Klein G, Sumegi J (1988) Consistent chromosome 3p deletion and loss of heterozygosity in renal cell carcinoma. Proc Natl Acad Sci USA 85:1571–1575.
5. Linehan WM, Lerman MI, Zbar B (1995) Identification of the von Hippel-Lindau (VHL) gene: its role in renal cancer. JAMA 273:564–570.
6. Zbar B, Brauch H, Talmadge C, Linehan M (1987) Loss of allele of loci on the shirt arm of chromosome 3 in renal cell carcinoma. Nature 327:721–724.
7. Tory K, Brauch H, Linehan M, Barba D, Oldfield E, Filling-Katz M, Seisinger B, Nakamura Y, White R, Marshal FF, Lerman MI, Zbar B (1989) Specific genetic change in tumors associated with von Hippel-Lindau disease. J Natl Cancer Inst 81:1097–1101.
8. Gnarra JR, Tory K, Weng Y, Schmidt L, Wei MH, Li H, Latif F, Liu S, Chen F, Duh F-M, Lubensky I, Duan DR, Florence C, Pozzatti R, Waether MM, Bander NH, Grossman HB, Brauch H, Pomer S, Brooks ID, Isaacs WB, Lerman MI, Zbar B, Linehan WM (1994) Mutations of the VHL tumor suppressor gene in renal carcinoma. Nat Genet 7:85–90.
9. Stolle C, Glenn G, Zbar B, Humphrey JS, Choyke P, Walther M, Pack S, Hurley K, Andrey C, Klausner R, Linehan WM (1998) Improved detection of germline mutations in the von Hippel-Lindau disease tumor tumor suppressor gene. Hum Mutat 12:417–423.

10. Shuin T, Kondo K, Torigoe S, Kishida T, Kubita Y, Hosokawa Y, Nagashima Y, Kitamura H, Latif F, Zbar B, Lerman MI, Yao M (1994) Frequent somatic mutations and loss of heterozygosity of the von Hippel-Lindau tumor suppressor gene in primary renal cell carcinoma. Cancer Res 54:2852–2855.

11. Herman JG, Latif F, Weng Y, Lerman MI, Zbar B, Liu S, Samid D, Duan D-SR, Gnarr JR, Linehan WM, Baylin SB (1994) Silencing of the VHL tumor suppressor gene by DNA methylation in renal carcinoma. Proc Natl Acad Sci U S A 91:9700–9704.

12. Pause A, Lee S, Worrell RA, Chen DYT, Burgess WH, Linehan WM, Klausner RD (1997) The von Hippel-Lindau tumor-suppressor gene product forms a stable complex with human CUL-2, a member of the Cdc53 family of proteins. Proc Natl Acad Sci USA 94:2156–2161.

13. Krumm A, Groudine M (1995) Tumor suppression and transcription elongation: the dire consequences of changing partners. Science 269:1400–1401.

14. Duan DR, Pause A, Burgers WH, Aso T, Chen DYT, Garret KP, Conaway RC, Conaway JW, Linehan WM, Klausner RD (1995) Inhibition of transcription elongation by VHL tumor suppressor protein. Science 269:1402–1406.

15. Aso T, Lane WS, Conaway JW, Conaway RC (1995) Elongin (SIII): a multisubunit regulator of elongation by RNA polymerase II. Science 269:1439–1443.

16. Jaakkola P, Mole DR, Tian YM, Wilson MI, Gielbert J, Gaskel SJ, von Kriegsheim A, Hebestreit HF, Mukherji M, Schofield CJ, Maxwell PH, Pugh CW, Ratcliff PJ (2001) Targeting of HIF-alpha to the von Hippel-Lindau ubiquitilation complex by O2-regulated prolyl hydroxylation. Science 292:468–472.

17. Ohh M, Park CW, Ivan M, Hoffman MA, Kim TY, Huang LE, Pavletich N, Chau V, Kaelin WG (2000) Ubiquitination of hypoxia-inducible factor requires direct binding to the beta-domain of the von Hippel-Lindau protein. Nat Cell Biol 2:423–427.

18. Gnarra JR, Zhou S, Merrill MJ, Wagner JR, Krumm A, Papavassiliou E, Oldfield EH, Klausner RD, Linehan WM (1996) Post-transcriptional regulation of vascular endothelial growth factor mRNA by the product of the VHL tumor-suppressor gene. Proc Natl Acad Sci U S A 93:10589–10594.

19. Iliopoulos O, Levy AP, Jiang C, Kaelin WG, Goldberg MA (1996) Negative regulation of hypoxia-inducible genes by the von Hippel-Lindau protein. Proc Natl Acad Sci U S A 93:10595–10599.

20. Schofield CJ, Ratcliff PJ (2004) Oxygen sensing by HIF hydroxylases. Nat Rev Mol Cell Biol 5:343–354.

21. Siemeister G, Weindel K, Mohrs K, Barleon B, Martiny-Baron G, Marme D (1996) Reversion of deregulated expression of vascular endothelial growth factor in human renal carcinoma cells by von Hippel-Lindau tumor suppressor protein. Cancer Res 56:2299–2301.

22. Clifford SC, Prowse AH, Affara NA, Buys CH, Maher ER (1998) Inactivation of the von Hippel-Lindau (VHL) tumour suppressor gene and allelic losses at chromosome arm 3p in primary renal cell carcinoma: evidence for a VHL-independent pathway in clear cell renal tumorigenesis. Genes Chromosom Cancer 22:200–209.

23. Martinez A, Fullwood P, Kondo K, Kishida T, Yao M, Maher ER, Latif F (2000) Role of chromosome 3p12-p21 tumor suppressor genes in clear cell renal cell carcinoma: analysis of VHL independent pathways of tumorigenesis. Mol Pathol 53:137–144.

24. Li FP, Decker H-JH, Zbar B, Stanton Jr VP, Lovacs G, Seizinger BR, Aburatani H, Sandberg AA, Berg S, Hosoe S, Brown RS (1993) Clinical and genetic studies of renal cell carcinomas in a family with a constitutional chromosome 3;8 translocation: genetics of familial renal cell, carcinoma. Ann Intern Med 118:106–111.

25. Lubenski J, Hadaczek P, Podolski J, Toloczko A, Sikorski A, McCue P, Gruck T, Huebner K (1994) Common regions of deletion in chromosome regions 3p12 and 3p14.2 in primary clear cell renal carcinoma. Cancer Res 54:3710–3713.

26. Yamakawa K, Morita R, Takahashi E, Hori T, Ishikawa J, Nakamura Y (1991) A detailed deletion mapping of the short arm of chromosome 3 in sporadic renal; cell carcinoma. Cancer Res 51:4707–4711.

27. Wilhelm M, Bugert P, Kenck C, Staehler G, Kovacs G (1995) Terminal deletion of chromosome 3p sequences in nonpapillary renal cell carcinomas: a breakpoint cluster between loci D3S1285 and D2S1603. Cancer Res 55:5383–5385.

28. Ohta M, Inoue H, Cotticelli MG, Kastury K, Baffa R, Palazzo J, Siprashvili Z, Mori M, McCue P, Druck T, Croce CM, Huebner K (1996) The FHIT gene, spanning the chromosome 3p14.2 fragile site and renal carcinoma-associated t(3:8) breakpoint, is abnormal in digestive tract cancer. Cell 84:587–597.

29. Yao M, Yoshida M, Kishida T, Nakaigawa N, Baba M, Kobayashi K, Miura T, Moriyama M, Nagashima Y, Nakatani Y, Kubota Y, Kondo K (2002) VHL tumor suppressor gene alterations associated with good prognosis in sporadic clear cell renal carcinoma. J Natl Cancer Inst 94:1569–1575.

30. Kovacs G (1989) Papillary renal cell carcinoma: a morphologic and cytogenetic study of 11 cases. Am J Pathol 134:27–34.

31. Katter MM, Grignon DJ, Wallis T, Haas GP, Sakr WA, Pontes JE, Visscher DW (1997) Clinicopathologic and interphase cytogenetic analysis of papillary (chromophilic) renal cell carcinoma. Mod Pathol 10:1143–1150.

32. Corless CL, Aburatani H, Fletcher JA, Housman D, Amin MB, Weinberg DS (1996) Papillary renal cell carcinoma: quantitation of chromosome 7 and 17 by FISH analysis of 3p for LOH and DNA ploidy. Diagn Mol Pathol 5:53–64.

33. Hughson MD, Bigler S, Dickman K, Kovacs G (1999) Renal cell carcinoma of end-stage renal disease: an analysis of chromosome 3,7, and 17 abnormalities by microsatellite amplification. Mod Pathol 12:301–309.

34. Schmidt L, Duh F-M, Chen F, Kishida T, Glenn G, Choyke P, Scherer SW, Zhuang Z, Lubensky I, Dean M, Allikmets R, Chidambaram A, Bergerheim UR, Feltis JT, Casadevall C, Zamarron A, Bernues M, Richard S, Lips CJM, Walther MM, Tsui L-C, Geil L, Orcutt ML, Stackhouse T, Lipan J, Slife L, Brauch H, Decker J, Niehans G, Hughson MD, Moch H, Storkel S, Lerman MI, Linehan WM, Zbar B (1997) Germline and somatic mutations in the tyrosine kinase domain of the MET proto-oncogene in papillary renal carcinomas. Nat Genet 16:68–73.

35. Schmidt L, Junker K, Weirich G, Glenn G, Choyke P, Lubensky I, Zhuang Z, Jeffers M, Vande Woude G, Neumann H, Walther M, Linehan WM, Zbar B (1998) Two North American families with hereditary papillary renal carcinoma and identical novel mutations in the MET proto-oncogene. Cancer Res 58:1719–1722.

36. Schmidt L, Junker K, Nakaigawa N, Kinjerski T, Weirich G, Miller M, Lubensky I, Neumann HPH, Brauch H, Decker J, Vocke C, Brown JA, Jenkins R, Richard S, Bergerheim U, Gerrard B, Dean M, Linehan WM, Zbar B (1999) Novel mutations of the MET proto-oncogene in papillary renal carcinomas. Oncogene 18:2343–2350.

37. Lubensky IA, Schmidt L, Zhuang Z, Weirich G, Pack S, Zambrano N, Walther MM, Choyke P, Linehan WM, Zbar B (1999) Hereditary and sporadic papillary renal cell carcinomas with c-met mutations share a distinct morphological phenotype. Am J Pathol 155:517–526.

38. Fisher J, Palmedo G, Bugert P, Prayer-Galeti T, Pagono F, Kovacs G (1998) Duplication and overexpression of the mutant allele of the met proto-oncogene in multiple hereditary renal cell tumors. Oncogene 17:733–739.

39. Lin Z-H, Han EM, Lee ES, Kim CW, Kim HK, Kim I, Kim Y-S (2004) A distinct expression pattern and point mutation of c-kit in papillary renal cell carcinomas. Mod Pathol 17:611–616.

40. Berman J, O'Leary TJ (2001) Gastrointestinal stromal tumor workshop. Hum Pathol 32:578–582.

41. Alam NA, Rowan AJ, Wortham NC, Pollard PJ, Mitchell M, Tyrer JP, Barclay E, Calonje E, Manek S, Adams SJ, Bowers PW, Burrows NP, Charles-Holmes R, Cook LJ, Daly BM, Ford GP, Fuller LC, Hadfield-Jones SE, Hardwick N, Highet AS, Keefe M, MacDonald-Hull SP, Potts EDA, Crone M, Wilkinson S, Camacho-Martinez F, Jablonska S, Ratnavel R, MacDonald A, Mann RJ, Grice K, Guilett G, Lewis-Jones MS, McGrath H, Seukeran DC, Morrison PJ, Fleming S, Rahman S, Kelsell D, Leigh I, Olpin S, Tomlinson IPM (2003) Genetic and functional analysis of FH mutations in multiple cutaneous and uterine leiomyomatosis, hereditary leiomyomatosis and renal cancer, and fumarate hydratase deficiency. Hum Mol Genet 12:1241–1252.

42. Launonen V, Vierimaa O, Kiuru M, Isola J, Roth S, Pukkala E, Sistonen P, Herva R, Aaltonen LA (2001) Inherited susceptibility to uterine leiomyomas and renal cell cancer. Proc Natl Acad Sci USA 98:3387–3392.

43. Kiuru M, Launonen V, Hietala M, Aittomaki K, Vierimaa O, Salovaara R, Arola J, Pukkala E, Sistonen P, Herva R, Aaltonen LA (2001) Familial cutaneous leiomyomatosis is a two-hit condition associated with renal cell cancer of characteristic histopathology. Am J Pathol 159:825–829.

44. Pavlovich CP, Walther MM, Eyler RA, Hewitt SM, Zbar B, Linehan WM, Merino MJ (2002) Renal tumors in the Birt-Hogg-Dube syndrome. Am J Surg Pathol 26:1542–1552.

45. Schmidt LS, Warren MB, Nickeerson ML, Weirich G, Matrosova V, Toro JR, Turner ML, Duray P, Merino M, Hewitt S, Pavlovich CP, Glenn G, Greenberg CR, Linehan WR, Zbar B (2001) Birt-Hogg-Dube syndrome, a genodermatosis associated with spontaneous pneumothorax and kidney neoplasia, maps to chromosome 17p11.2. Am J Hum Genet 69:876–882.

46. Stoerkel S, Steart PV, Drenckhahn, Thoenes W (1989) The human chromophobe cell renal carcinoma: its probable relation to intercalated cells of the collecting duct. Virchows Arch B Cell Pathol 56:237–245.

47. Cohen C, McCue PA, Derose PB (1988) Histogenesis of renal cell carcinoma and renal oncocytoma: an immunohistochemical study. Cancer 62:1946–1951.

48. Amin MaB, Amin MiB, Tamboli P, Javidan J, Stricker H, De-Peralta Ventrina M, Deshpande A, Menon M (2002) Prognostic impact of histologic subtyping of adult renal epithelial neoplasms: an experience of 405 cases. Am J Surg Pathol 26:281–291.

49. Argani P, Antonescu CR, Coutrier J, Fournet J-C, Sciot R, Debiec-Rychter M, Hutchinson B, Reuter VE, Boccon-Gibod L, Timmons C, Hafez N, Ladanyi M (2002) PRCC-TFE3 renal carcinomas: morphologic, immunohistochemical, ultrastructural, and molecular analysis of an entity associated with the t(X;1)(p11.2;q21). Am J Surg Pathol 26:1553–1566.

Question 8

Are there immunohistochemical markers for the differential diagnosis of renal cell neoplasms, especially when tumor cells have an eosinophilic/granular cytoplasm?

Answer

Standard microscopic examination is sufficient for classifying most renal tumors, but there are occasions on which ancillary studies are helpful in reaching the final diagnosis. They are, in order of practical usefulness: immunohistochemistry, chromosomal analysis by fluorescence in situ hybridization (FISH), and molecular analysis. The last method should be considered for renal cell carcinomas arising in children or young adults.

The need for immunohistochemical analysis may arise when tumors are composed almost exclusively of eosinophilic cells or clear cells in a papillary pattern. No markers are available that are specific to a certain type of renal tumor with 100% distinction. In some cases, a combination of markers is advised. For the differential diagnosis between clear cell renal cell carcinoma (RCC) and papillary RCC, three markers are available: a positive reaction to glutathione S-transferase-α (GSTα) and carbonic anhydrase IX (CA IX) favor the diagnosis of clear cell RCC, whereas a positive reaction to α-methylacyl coenzyme A racemase (AMACR) favors a diagnosis of papillary RCC. For the differential diagnosis between papillary RCC and chromophobe RCC/oncocytoma, AMACR is useful. In practice, the differential diagnosis between chromophobe RCC and oncocytoma is the most difficult. The marker that is expressed more strongly and specifically by chromophobe RCCs is the epithelial cell adhesion molecule (EpCAM). E-cadherin may be used for the differential diagnosis because of different staining patterns. Loss of chromosomes 2, 6, 10, and 17, recognized by FISH analysis, is reported to be characteristic of chromophobe RCC, whereas these chromosomes are preserved in oncocytoma.

Comments

Standard light microscopic histopathology is sufficient for classifying most renal tumors. However, as stated under Question 2, tumors with eosinophilic cytoplasm can pose difficulty for the pathologist. With the use of cDNA or tissue microarrays, a number of genes have been identified as potential molecular markers with immunohistochemistry or other techniques. They are RCC, carbonic anhydrase IX, CD10, parvalubumin, KIT, CK7, CK19, E- and N-cadherins, vimentin, AMACR, and most recently EpCAM. Complex expression profiles can be screened to identify a number of differentially expressed genes. Although powerful, as you might imagine, there has been no single gene which is found to be expressed with 100% distinction in a specific tumor type. This fact suggests that all tumors may stem from a primitive cell and may be committed to express to varying degrees either proximal nephron or distal nephron characteristics. A recent study by Shen et al. using a proximal nephron marker RCC and a distal nephron marker Ksp-cadherin [1], indicates that more than 95% of chromophobe RCCs (RCC) and oncocytoma

125

are stained with Ksp-cadherin sharing close genetic characteristics. Although clear cell RCC and papillary RCC express the proximal nephron marker RCC in more than 90% of cases, there are a small number of chromophobe RCCs that are reactive to the antibody to RCC.

Here we discuss selected markers that are useful for differentiating certain renal tumors.

Differential Diagnosis Between Clear Cell Renal Cell Carcinoma and Papillary Renal Cell Carcinoma

In most cases, the pathologist has no problem distinguishing clear cell RCC from papillary RCC in H&E-stained sections. Diagnostic difficulty may arise when a papillary RCC shows nonpapillary growth patterns such as trabecular, tubular, or solid areas, or when it is made up of eosinophilic (oncocytic) or clear cells in a papillary pattern. For a clear cell carcinoma that comprises almost exclusively eosinophilic cells, the differential diagnosis from other types of tumor may be problematic.

Several markers are available, including AMACR, GSTα, and carbonic anhydrase IX.

α-Methylacyl Coenzyme A Racemase (AMACR)

Xu et al. [2] in 2000 first described *AMACR* as a gene uniquely overexpressed in prostate carcinoma cells with the use of cDNA library subtraction and the tissue microarray technique. AMACR showed strong cytoplasmic staining in prostate carcinoma but not in benign prostate cells. It soon became apparent, however, that AMACR protein was detectable in normal tissues such as hepatocytes and renal tubule cells. It was also discovered that a number of neoplasms—colonic adenoma and adenocarcinoma; hepatocellular carcinoma; RCCs; carcinoma of the lung, breast, and ovary; lymphoma; melanoma—were immunohistochemically reactive to AMACR antibody [3, 4]. Thus, its usefulness in evaluating metastatic carcinomas may be limited.

In a normal kidney, AMACR is expressed in the proximal tubules [5]. We first reported elevated AMACR mRNA in papillary RCCs [6]. In the original report by Takahashi et al. [6], we showed, by immunostaining, that all 10 papillary RCCs were AMACR-positive, whereas AMACR was expressed

in only a small number of clear cell RCCs (1/10) and in none of the chromophobe RCCs ($n = 10$) or oncocytomas ($n = 5$). Subsequently, a more detailed study based on a larger number of cases was reported by Tretiakova et al. [5]. We confirmed and extended the previous observation by Takahashi et al. [6] by demonstrating a strong immunohistochemical reaction of AMACR in all cases ($n = 41$) of papillary RCC including six metastases with high sensitivity (reaching 100%). The reaction was only focal or weak in most of the other renal tumors (18/124, 15%) including 13 of 52 clear cell RCCs, 3 of 20 oncocytomas, and 2 of 17 urothelial cell carcinomas. All chromophobe RCCs ($n = 18$) and sarcomatoid components of RCCs ($n = 15$) were negative for AMACR. Weak or focal AMACR immunoreactivity was detected in only 4 of 51 (8%) papillary carcinomas arising in other organs (2/14 thyroid, 2/13 lung, 0/6 breast, 0/6 endometrium, 0/6 ovarian, and 0/6 pancreas tumors).

More recently, Li et al. [7], in an abstract presented in the United States and Canadian Academy of Pathologists meeting (2005) reported that focal/diffuse staining was observed in 94% (53/56) of papillary RCCs as expected but it was also observed in 16% (11/70) of clear cell RCCs, 21% (8/38) of chromophobe RCCs, and 7% (3/43) of oncocytomas. Thus, caution should be exercised when one uses AMACR for the diagnosis of papillary RCC.

Readers may recall that we introduced under Question 3 a report on seven papillary RCCs that were composed of "oncocytic" cells. By chromosomal analysis, most of these cases showed trisomies 7 and 17 and loss of the Y chromosome (in males), features supporting papillary RCC differentiation [8]. All seven cases were positive for AMACR, indicating that a papillary tumor with eosinophilic (oncocytic) cells is a variant papillary RCC.

Glutathione S-transferase-α (GSTα)

Immunohistochemically GSTα is detectable in the proximal convoluted tubules but not in the distal convoluted tubules, glomeruli, or stromal cells [9]. It was expressed in 9 of 10 clear cell RCCs but in none of the other types except in one chromophobe RCC in the Takahashi study. Later we [9] demonstrated strong, diffuse GSTα immunoreactivity in clear cell

RCCs (166/202, 82%) with a mean staining intensity of 2.41. Other tumors had a lower frequency and lower intensity: 11 of 54 papillary carcinomas with a mean intensity of 0.30, 1 of 52 chromophobe RCCs with a mean intensity of 0.02, and 5 of 40 oncocytomas with a mean intensity of 0.20. The elevated staining intensity was correlated with a marked elevation in mRNA of the GSTα gene.

Carbonic Anhydrase IX (CA IX)

In the study presented in an abstract by Tu et al. [10], all 15 clear cell RCCs stained positive for CA IX; 14 of them, including the sarcomatoid areas (two cases), showed more than 10% of tumor cells stained, whereas 5 of 16 papillary RCCs expressed the marker in less than 10% of tumor cells. Chromophobe RCCs ($n = 18$), oncocytomas ($n = 13$), and unclassified type/collecting duct carcinomas ($n = 3$) were negative. Although additional studies are needed to confirm this favorable result, it appears that CA IX is a promising marker with good sensitivity and specificity for clear cell RCC.

Other Markers

Other markers, such as CD10, vimentin, and RCC, can also be detected in most clear cell RCCs. However, they have limited value in the differential diagnosis of papillary and clear cell RCCs as they are also expressed in most papillary RCCs.

In summary, for the positive identification of clear cell RCCs, CA IX and GSTα are good markers with a reasonable sensitivity and specificity, and AMACR is a sensitive marker with a reasonable specificity for papillary RCCs.

Differential Diagnosis Between Clear Cell/Papillary Renal Cell Carcinomas and Chromophobe Renal Cell Carcinoma/Oncocytoma

Several markers are available for distinguishing clear cell/papillary RCCs from chromophobe RCC/oncocytoma. They are CD10, parvalbumin, c- KIT, E- and N-cadherins, AMACR, and CA IX.

CD10

CD 10 is an acute lymphoblastic leukemia antigen (CALLA) and is expressed on the brush border of normal proximal renal tubular epithelial cells [11]. It was expressed in high frequency in clear cell/papillary RCCs (58/62 clear cell RCCs and 13/14 papillary RCCs) and in low frequency in chromophobe RCCs (0/19) and oncocytomas (3/9) [12]. Matrignoni et al. [13] also found that CD10 was expressed in high frequency in clear cell RCCs (75/75) and papillary RCCs (32/57). However, a sizable number of chromophobe RCCs also expressed it (11/42). It is of interest that five of seven chromophobe RCCs that had aggressive features (stages pT3a/pT3b—2002 TNM staging) were positive to CD10. Thus, the study found a statistically significant association between the expression of CD10 and clinicopathologic aggressiveness among chromophobe RCCs ($P < 0.003$, univariate analysis).

It appears that CD10 is a positive marker for clear cell and papillary RCCs, although a fraction of aggressive chromophobe RCCs also expresses CD10.

Parvalbumin

Parvalbumin is a calcium-binding protein expressed in the distal nephron. In the studies reported by Matrignoni et al. [13, 14], it was specifically expressed by chromophobe RCC and oncocytoma. All 42 cases of chromophobe RCC expressed the marker, whereas no "significant" level of expression was noted in 75 clear cell RCCs or 51 papillary RCCs.[1] Young et al. [15] also reported their study on parvalbumin in addition to vimentin and β-defensin-1. All of eight oncocytomas and all of six chromophobe RCCs were positive for parvalbumin. Only 1 of 23 clear cell RCCs was positive for parvalbumin, whereas four of seven papillary RCCs were positive. It appears that parvalbumin is a good marker for differentiating clear cell RCCs from chromophobe cell RCCs and oncocytomas.

c-KIT

The *c-KIT* gene encodes a transmembrane tyrosine kinase growth factor receptor. Its ligand, stem cell

---

[1] In their 2001 report, which includes most of the cases reported in the 2004 paper, 0/75 of clear cell RCCs, 0/17 papillary RCCs, 32/32 chromophobe RCCs, and 11/16 oncocytomas were positive for parvalubumin [14].

factor (SCF), or alternatively known as the mast cell growth factor, is a hematopoietic growth factor that, in conjunction with other hematopoietic factors, supports the proliferation and differentiation of multiple cell lineages from early precursors [16]. Its interaction with the SCF is also essential for development of germ cells [17]. The c-KIT gene has attracted investigators' attention because it belongs to the tyrosine kinase group that includes BCR-ABL, platelet-derived receptor, and ARG. Its protein interaction with ATP is inhibited by a new drug STI571 (imatinib mesylate, or Gleevec) [18]. Gain-of-function mutations in c-KIT result in oncogenic activity in gastrointestinal stromal tumors [19], and Gleevec has been shown to inhibit their growth [20].

Comparative gene expression analysis has identified the c-KIT gene to be upregulated in chromophobe RCCs [21]. In a normal kidney, weak expression of c-KIT is detected in the cytoplasm of renal tubules [21]. In renal neoplasms, the protein is localized to the cell membrane of chromophobe RCC cells, suggesting a possible functional role in the tumor. Investigation by three groups [22–24] showed high rates of immunohistochemical expression in the cell membrane of chromophobe RCCs and oncocytomas and a nearly totally negative reaction in clear cell and papillary RCCs. In the Petit group study [22], the expression frequency was 0 of 21 clear cell RCCs, 0 of 10 papillary RCCs, 22 of 25 chromophobe RCCs, and 10 of 14 oncocytomas (polyclonal antibody A4502, 1:100 dilution). In the series we reported [24], the frequency was 1 of 40 clear cell RCCs, 1 of 21 papillary RCCs, 38 of 49 chromophobe RCCs, and 36 of 41 oncocytomas (monoclonal; Dako). In Pan's series [23], the frequency was 0 of 256 clear cell RCCs, 0 of 25 papillary RCCs, 24 of 29 chromophobe RCCs, and 5 of 7 oncocytomas (polyclonal antibody A4502, Dako, 1:200 dilution).

E-Cadherin, N-Cadherin

Although studies have been limited, cadherins appear to be promising markers. However, further investigation is needed for validation. In the report by Taki et al. [25], E-cadherin was shown to be a positive marker for chromophobe RCCs (19/19) and oncocytomas (3/3) in contrast to a negative reaction in clear cell RCCs (0/19). On the other hand, a positive reaction to N-cadherin was limited to clear cell RCCs (10/19) and was absent in chromophobe RCCs and oncocytomas. Unfortunately, papillary RCCs were not included in this study.

Vimentin

Both clear cell and papillary RCCs exhibit a high rate of positive reaction to vimentin antibody. In the Taki series [25], 13 of 21 clear cell RCCs were positive for vimentin, whereas chromophobe RCCs ($n = 21$) and oncocytomas ($n = 8$) were totally negative. In the Young study [15], 17 of 20 clear cell and 6 of 7 papillary RCCs were positive, whereas none of chromophobe RCCs ($n = 8$) or oncocytomas ($n = 8$) showed a positive reaction.

Differential Diagnosis Between Papillary Renal Cell Carcinoma and Chromophobe Renal Cell Carcinoma/Oncocytoma

AMACR appears to be a useful tool in the differential diagnosis between papillary RCCs and chromophobe RCCs/oncocytomas because, as stated earlier, it is expressed by papillary RCCs (41/41) with high sensitivity, whereas chromophobe RCCs are negative for the marker (0/18) and oncocytomas showed low reactivity (3/20) [5].

Differential Diagnosis Between Chromophobe Renal Cell Carcinoma and Oncocytoma

Chromophobe RCCs and oncocytomas are believed to be derived from the distal tubule/collecting duct [26], which is reflected in the similar immunologic reactions to various of the markers cited above. Because the prognosis of these two neoplasms is different, a marker to distinguish these two categories would be highly desirable. To date, a few markers are proposed to be potentially useful.

EpCAM

EpCAM, a 40-kDa epithelial transmembrane glycoprotein, functions as an epithelial cell-specific Ca^{2+}-independent intercellular adhesion molecule [27]. Went et al. [28] reported their experience with an epithelial cell adhesion molecule designated EpCAM. In large conventional tissue sections, 19 of 21 chromophobe RCCs (90%) showed strong membranous EpCAM expression in more than 90% of cells.

Moreover, 13 of 15 oncocytomas (87%) showed EpCAM expression. Expression was detectable in less than 10% of tumor cells, and staining was less intense ($P < 0.0001$, by χ^2 analysis). Only single cells or small clusters of cells expressed EpCAM. This observation raised the possibility to the authors that some of the positively stained cells, especially in tubules, might represent trapped normal tubules, as distal cortical tubules of the normal kidney stains intensely to the antibody.

Combination of CK7/CK20/CD15

Although CK7 was observed in both chromophobe RCCs and oncocytomas, the CK7 staining pattern in these two tumors are different. We have reported that CK7 mRNA levels in chromophobe RCCs was higher than those of oncocytomas. Furthermore, by immunohistochemistry, 27 of 41 (66%) chromophobe RCCs expressed CK7 diffusely compared to only 3 of 55 oncocytomas (5%) [29].

Magi-Galluzzi et al. [30], from the Cleveland Clinic, at the 2005 USCAP annual meeting proposed a combination of CK7/CK20/CD15 for the differential diagnosis of the two tumors. They advocated that the diagnosis favors chromophobe RCC if (1) the immunohistochemical reaction to CK7 is diffusely positive (>90% of cells stained), or (2) CK7 staining is focal (at least 5% of cells stained) but CK20 and CD15 are negative. In contrast, the diagnosis of oncocytoma is favored if (1) CK7 is negative, (2) CK7 and CK20 are focally positive, or (3) CK7 and CD15 are focally positive.

E-Cadherin

Berbescu and Lager [31] proposed that the pattern of E-cadherin expression is useful for distinguishing chromophobe RCCs from oncocytomas. All chromophobe RCCs ($n = 58$) were positive for E-cadherin with a pure membranous staining pattern including six eosinophilic variants. On the other hand, all oncocytomas ($n = 54$) were positive for E-cadherin but with a mixed granular cytoplasmic and partially membranous staining pattern.

S100A1

The Martignoni group recently introduced utility of immunohistochemical expression of S100A1 protein in differentiating chromphobe RCC from oncocytoma; it was expressed in 93% (37 of 40 cases) of oncocytomas whereas 94% (48 of 51) were negative for S100A1 (p < 0.001) [32].

Fluorescence In Situ Hybridization Analysis for Chromosomes 1, 2, 6, 10, and 17

Recently, Brunelli et al. [33] has described differential losses of chromosomes 1, 2, 6, 10, and 17 by the fluorescence in situ hybridization (FISH) technique. Losses of chromosomes 1, 2, 6, 10, and 17 are frequent in chromophobe RCCs (both granular and classic types). In contrast, there were no oncocytomas that showed loss of chromosomes 2, 6, 10, or 17, although loss of chromosome 1 occurred occasionally.

Differential Diagnosis Among Collecting Duct Carcinoma, Papillary Renal Cell Carcinoma, and Urothelial Carcinoma

Marker studies on collecting duct carcinoma have been limited because of its rarity and the poor definition of this tumor. Collecting duct carcinoma is distinct from other renal cell carcinomas by its more aggressive clinical behavior. Morphologically, it is characterized by the presence of cuboidal cells forming tubules similar to collecting ducts. The differential diagnosis from papillary RCC needs to be considered. However, distinction from high-grade papillary RCC may be impossible. Furthermore, there are tumors with morphologic features of both collecting duct carcinoma and high-grade papillary RCC.

The features in favor of collecting duct carcinoma are higher nuclear grade, destructive invasion of surrounding normal tissue, desmoplasia, and cytologic atypia in the nearby collecting ducts. By immunohistochemistry, positive UEA (*Ulex europaeus*) [35], negative CD10, and negative AMACR [5] are supportive of collecting duct carcinoma. However, the UEA antibody is often difficult to work with. Urothelial carcinoma of the renal pelvis, in particular with a papillary pattern, could be a challenging lesion because it may share some morphologic and antigenic properties with the collecting duct carcinoma [35]. A positive reaction to UEA is the only realistic marker to favor the diagnosis of collecting duct carcinoma (Table 2-8-1). The utility of various markers in the differential diagnosis is summarized in Table 2-8-2. Because none of the markers is exclusive to a certain type of tumor, a combination of more than one marker is preferred.

TABLE 2-8-1. Useful markers in the differential diagnosis among various types of renal epithelial neoplasms

Clear cell carcinoma GST-α ↑ Carbonic anhydrease↑	vs.	Papillary carcinoma AMACR ↑
Clear cell/papillary carcinoma CD10 ↑[a] N-Cadherin↑[c] Vimentin↑	vs.	Chromophobe cell carcinoma/oncocytoma Parvalbumin ↑[b] KIT↑ E-cadherin ↑[c]
Papillary carcinoma	vs.	Chromophobe cell carcinoma/oncocytoma AMACR ↑
Chromophobe cell carcinoma EpCAM ↑ CK7 ↑ E-cadherin (pure membranous stain) Chromosomes 2,6,10, and 17 frequently lost (FISH analysis)	vs.	Oncocytoma E-cadherin (granular cytoplasmic and partial membranous stain) S100A1 ↑ Chromosomes 2, 6, 10, and 17 preserved (FISH analysis)

GSTα, glutathione-S-transferase-α; FISH, fluorescence in situ hybridization; AMACR, α-methylacyl CoA racemase.
[a] Most of CD10 positive cases have aggressive clinical/pathologic features (Martignoni, 2004)
[b] Useful for differentiating chromophobe cell carcinoma/oncocytoma from clear cell carcinoma.
[c] Papillary carcinoma cases not studied.

TABLE 2-8-2. Expression of immunohistochemical markers by renal neoplasms

Renal neoplasms	AE 1/3	Cam 5.2	34 β E12	EMA	Vimentin	CD10	RCC	AMACR	CK7	Kit	Parvalbumin	CK20	UEA
RCC, clear cell	+[1]	+[2,5]	−[2]	+[1,2]	+[1,2,10]	+[2,7]	+[2]	−/+[6,18]	−[1]	−[11,12,14]	−[10,13]		
RCC, papillary	+[2]		−[2]		+/−[10]	+[7]	+[2]	+[6]	+[2] (type 1 > 2)	−[10–12,14]	+[2,10]−[13]		
RCC, chromophobe	+[5]	+[5]	−[2,5]	+[2]	−[2,10]	−[7]/+[13]	+/−[2]	−[6]	+[2,8,9]	+[11,12,14,15]	+[10,13]	−[9]	−[5]
Collecting duct Ca	+[5]	+[5]	+[2,17]	+[2,16]	−[5]/+[16]	−[17]	−[2]	−[6]	+[2]	−[12]			+[5,17]
Oncocytoma	+[2]		+[2]	+[2]	+[2]	−/+[7]	−[2]	−/+[6]	+/−[2,9]−[8]	+[11,14]	+[2,10,13]	+[2]−[9]	−[5]
Urothelial Ca	+[5]	+[5]	+[4,5]					−[6]	+[14]	−[12]		−/+[3]+[4]	−[5]

−/+, a small fraction positive; +/−, a large fraction positive; RCC, renal cell carcinoma marker; UEA, *Ulex europaeus*.
[1]Taki et al.; [2]Murphy et al. (AFIP); [3]Genega et al.; [4]Parker et al.; [5]Orsola et al.; [6]Tretiakova et al.; [7]Avery et al.; [8]Adley et al.; [9]Wu et al.; [10]Young et al.; [11]Petit et al.; [12]Pan et al.; [13]Martignoni et al. (2004); [14]Huo et al.; [15]Yamazaki et al.; [16]Paraf et al.; [17]Srigley et al. (WHO); [18]Li et al.

References

1. Shen SS, Chirala M, Krishnan B, Amato R, Liu YL, Zhai J, Truong LD (2005) Renal cell neoplasm with dual differentiation of proximal and distal nephron: an immunohistochemical study. Mod Pathol 18(suppl 1):164A.
2. Xu J, Stolk JA, Zhang X, Silva SJ, Houghton RL, Matsumura M, Vedvick TS, Leslie KS, Badaro R, Reed SG (2000) Identification of differentially expressed genes in human prostate cancer using subtraction and microarray. Cancer Res 60:1677–1682.
3. Jiang Z, Fanger G, Woda B, Banner BF, Algate P, Dresser K, Xu J, Chu PG (2003) Expression of alpha-methylacyl-CoA racemase (P504S) in various malignant neoplasms and normal tissue: a study of 761 cases. Hum Pathol 34:792–796.
4. Zhou M, Chinnaiyan AM, Kleer GC, Lucas PC, Rubin MA (2002) Alpha-methylacyl-CoA racemase: a novel tumor marker over-expressed in several human cancers and their precursor lesions. Am J Surg Pathol 26:926–931.
5. Tretiakova MS, Sahoo S, Takahashi M, Turkyilmaz M, Vogelzang NJ, Lin F, Krausz T, The BT, Yang XJ (2004) Expression of alpha-methyl-CoA racemase in papillary renal cell carcinoma. Am J Surg Pathol 28:69–76.
6. Takahashi M, Yang XJ, Sugimura J, Backdahl J, Tretiakova M, Quian C-N, Gray SG, Knapp R, Anema J, Kahnoski R, Nicol D, Vogelzang NJ, Furge KA, Kanayama H, Kagawa S (2003) Molecular subclassification of kidney tumors and discovery of new diagnostic markers. Oncogene 22:6810–6818.
7. Li C, Jiang J, Banner B, Wu C-L (2005) Expression of alpha-methylacyl-CoA racemase (AMACR)/P504S in renal neoplasms. Mod Pathol 18(suppl 1):152A.

8. Hes O, Brunelli M, Michal M, Cossu Rocca P, Chilosi M, Mina M, Menestrina F, Martigoni G (2005) Oncocytic papillary renal cell carcinoma: a clinicopathologic study of 9 cases. Mod Pathol 18(suppl 1):145A.

9. Chuang ST, Chu P, Sugimura J, Tretiakova M, Papavero V, Wang K, Tan M, Lin F, The BT, Yang XJ (2005) Overexpression of glutathione S-transferase alpha in clear cell renal cell carcinoma. Am J Clin Pathol 123:421–429.

10. Tu JJ, Chen Y-T, Hyjek E, Tickoo SK (2005) Carbonic anhydrase IX as a highly sensitive and specific marker of clear cell renal cell carcinoma: a comprehensive immunohistochemical study using a panel of commonly utilized antibodies in the differential diagnosis of renal cell tumors. Mod Pathol 18(suppl 1):169A.

11. McIntosh GG, Lodge AJ, Watson P, Hall AG, Wood K, Anderson JJ, August B, Horne CW, Milton ID (2003) NCL-CD10-270: a new monoclonal antibody recognizing CD10 in paraffin-embedded tissue. Am J Pathol 154:77–82.

12. Avery AK, Beckstead J, Renshaw AA, Corless CL (2000) Use of antibodies to RCC and CD10 of renal neoplasms. Am J Surg Pathol 24:203–210.

13. Matrignoni G, Pea M, Brunelli M, Chilosi M, Zamo A, Bertaso M, Cossu-Rocca P, Eble JN, Mikuz G, Puppa G, Badoual C, Ficarra V, Novella G, Bonetti F (2004) CD10 is expressed in a subset of chromophobe renal cell carcinomas. Mod Pathol 17:1455–1463.

14. Matrignoni G, Pea M, Chilosi M, Brunelli M, Scarpa A, Colato C, Tardanico R, Zamboni G, Bonetti F (2001) Parvalbumin is constantly expressed in chromophobe renal carcinoma. Mod Pathol 14:760–767.

15. Young AN, de Oliveira Salles PG, Lim SD, Cohen C, Petros JA, Marshall FF, Neish AS, Amin MB (2003) Beta defensin-1, parvalbumin, and vimentin: a panel of diagnostic immunohistochemical markers for renal tumors derived from gene expression profiling studies using cDNA microarray. Am J Surg Pathol 27:199–205.

16. Krystal GW, Hines SJ, Organ CP (1996) Autocrine growth of small cell lung cancer mediated by coexpression of c-kit and stem cell factor. Caner Res 56:370–376.

17. Mauduit C, Hamamah S, Behnamed M (1999) Stem cell factor/c-kit system in spermatogenesis. Hum Reprod Update 5:535–545.

18. Schindler T, Bornmann W, Pellicena P, Miller WT, Clarkson B, Kuriyan J (2000) Structural mechanism for STI-571 inhibition of Abelson tyrosine kinase. Science 289:1938–1942.

19. Hirota S, Isozaki K, Moriyama Y, Hashimoto K, Nishida T, Ishiguro S, Kawano K, Hanada M, Kurata A, Takeda M, Tunio GM, Matsuzawa Y, Kanakura Y, Shinomura Y, Kitamura Y (1998) Gain-of-function mutations in c-kit in human gastrointestinal stromal tumors. Science 279:577–580.

20. Joensuu H, Roberts PJ, Sarlomo-Rikala M, Andersson LC, Tervahartiala P, Tuveson D, Silberman SL, Capedeville R, Dimitrijevic S, Druker B, Demetri G (2001) Effect of the tyrosine kinase inhibitor STI571 in a patient with a metastatic gastrointestinal stromal tumor. N Engl J Med 344:1052–1056.

21. Yamazaki K, Sakamoto M, Ohta T, Kanai Y, Ohki M, Hirohashi S (2003) Overexpression of KIT in chromophobe renal cell carcinoma. Oncogene 22:847–852.

22. Petit A, Castillo M, Santos M, Mellado B, Alcover JB, Mallofre C (2004) KIT expression in chromophobe renal cell carcinoma: comparative immunohistochemical analysis of KIT expression in different renal cell neoplasms. Am J Surg Pathol 28:676–678.

23. Pan C-C, Chen PC-H, Chiang H (2004) Overexpression of KIT (CD117) in chromophobe renal cell carcinoma and renal oncocytoma. Am J Clin Pathol 121:878–883.

24. Huo L, Patton KT, Adley BP, Gupta R, Papavero V, Laskin WB, Yeldandi A, Yang XJ (2004) Analysis of c-kit expression in 171 renal neoplasms. Mod Pathol 17(suppl 1):150A.

25. Taki A, Nakatani Y, Misugi K, Yao M (1999) Chromophobe renal cell carcinoma: an immunohistochemical study of 21 Japanese cases. Mod Pathol 12:310–317.

26. Storkel S, Eble JN, Adlakha K, Amin MB, Blute ML, Bostwick DG, Darson M, Delahunt B, Iczkowski K (1997) Classification of renal cell carcinoma: workshop no. 1—Union Internationale Contre le Cancer (UICC) and American Joint Committee on Cancer (AJCC). Cancer 80:987–989.

27. Litvinov SV, Bakker HA, Gourevitch MM, Velders MP, Warnaar SO (1994) Evidence for a role of the epithelial glycoprotein 40 (EP-CAM) in epithelial cell-cell adhesion. Cell Adhes Commun 2:417–428.

28. Went P, Dirnhofer S, Salvisberg T, Amin MB, Lim SD, Diener P-A, Moch H (2005) Expression of epithelial cell adhesion molecule (EpCam) in renal epithelial tumors. Am J Surg Pathol 29:83–88.

29. Adley BP, Teh BT, Yang XJ (2006) Diagnostic value of cytokeratin 7 and parvalbumin in differentiating chromophobe renal cell carcinoma from renal oncocytoma. Anal Quant Cytol Histol 28:228–236.

30. Magi-Galluzzi C, Levin HS, Willis-Epinger G, Hood L, Zhou M (2005) CK7, CK20, and CD15 can reliably differentiate renal oncocytoma from chromophobe renal cell carcinoma. Mod Pathol 18(suppl 1):154A.

31. Berbescu EA, Lager DJ (2005) E-cadherin pattern of expression differentiates chromophobe renal cell carcinoma from oncocytoma: An immunohistochemical study of 137 renal neoplasms. Mod Pathol 18(suppl 1):129A.

32. Rocca PC, Brunelli M, Gobbo S, Eccher A, Bragantini E, Mina MM, Ficarra V, Zattoni F, Zamò A, Pea M, Scarpa A, Chilosi M, Menestrina F, Bonetti F, Eble JN, Martignoni G (2007) Diagnostc utility of S100A1 expression in renal cell neoplasms: an immunohistochemical and quantitative RT-PCR study. Mod Pathol 20:722–728.

33. Brunelli M, Eble JN, Zhang S, Martignoni G, Delahunt B, Cheng L (2005) Eosinophilic and classic chromophobe renal cell carcinomas have similar frequent losses of multiple chromosomes from among chromosomes 1, 2, 6, 10, and 17, and this pattern of genetic

abnormality is not present in renal oncocytoma. Mod Pathol 18:161–169.

34. Paraf F, Viellefond A, Bouvier R, Droz D, Toublanc M, Dupuytren CHRU (1999) Collecting duct carcinoma of the kidney: study of 29 cases. Mod Pathol 12(suppl):103A.

35. Orsola A, Trias I, Raventos CX, Espanol I, Cecchini L, Orsola I (2005) Renal collecting (Bellini) duct carcinoma displays similar characteristics to upper tract urothelial cell carcinoma. Urology 65:49–54.

36. Srigley JR, Moch H (2004) Carcinoma of the collecting ducts of Bellini. In: Eble JN, Sauyer G, Epstein JI, Sesterhenn IA (eds) World Health Organization classification of tumours. IARC Press, Lyon, pp 33–38.

37. Murphy WM, Beckwith JB, Farrow GM (1994) Tumors of the kidney, bladder, and related urinary structures. Atlas of Tumor Pathology. Armed Forces Institute of Pathology, Bethesda, pp 92–145.

38. Genega EM, Hutchinson B, Reuter VE, Gaudin PB (1999) Immunophenotype of intermediate and high grade prostatic and urothelial carcinoma. Mod Pathol 12 (suppl 1): 87A.

39. Parker DC, Folpe AL, Bell J, Oliva E, Young RH, Cohen C, Amin MB (2003) Potential utility of uroplakin III, thrombomodulin, high molecular weight cytokeratin, and cytokeratin 20 in noninvasiv, invasive, and metastatic urothelial (transitional cell) carcinomas. Am J Surg Pathol 27:1–10.

40. Wu SL, Kathari P, Wheeler TM, Reese T, Connelly JH (2002) Cytokeratins 7 and 20 immunoreactivity in chromophobe renal cell carcinomas and renal oncocytomas. Mod Pathol 15:712–717.

Question 9

How does adrenal gland involvement by renal cell carcinoma affect the prognosis, if any? Should a tumor directly infiltrating the ipsilateral adrenal gland be kept as a pT3a tumor?

Answer

There have been several reliable reports that recommended cases of adrenal involvement by renal cell carcinoma (RCC) by direct invasion be removed from the pT3a category and moved to pT4 because of their grave prognosis, which is comparable to that of pT4 carcinoma.

Comments

The current (2002) TNM classification defines T3a tumors as tumors that directly invade the ipsilateral adrenal gland or perinephric tissue (including sinus invasion) but do not go beyond Gerota's fascia (Table 2-9-1) [1]. There are two ways by which RCC invades the adrenal gland. The first is by way of direct invasion of a renal cancer, a mode of spread that is rare. The frequency is reported to be 1.2%–10.0% in a large series [2–7]. The second method of spread is discontinuously either by a hematogenous route or by an unknown mechanism.

Our discussion focuses on the significance of ipsilateral adrenal gland involvement by direct invasion. In a recent retrospective study, Han et al. [2] noted that patients with pT3a tumors with direct invasion of the adrenal gland have an unfavorable prognosis that is comparable to that of patients with pT4 tumors.

Of 1087 patients who underwent nephrectomy, 27 were identified with direct invasion of the adrenal gland (pT3a, adrenal), and 187 were found to show perinephric fat or sinus involvement (pT3a, perinephric fat). The median survival of patients with pT3a (perinephric fat) was 36 months with a 36% five-year cancer-specific survival rate. In contrast, patients with pT3a (adrenal involved) had a significantly worse survival rate at a median of 12.5 months and 0% five-year cancer-specific survival rate ($P < 0.001$). The rate was similar to the median survival of those with stage pT4 tumor (11 months). They therefore recommended moving cases showing direct adrenal invasion to the pT4 category. Although the number of cases is small, Sandock et al. [4] also observed that direct extension of tumor into the ipsilateral adrenal resulted in progression to disseminated disease.

Recently, there came another article from the Mayo Clinic group reporting a significant association of direct adrenal gland invasion with an increased risk of cancer-specific mortality comparable to that of pT4 tumors [5]. Cancer-specific survival for 22 patients with pT3a or pT3b tumors that directly invaded the ipsilateral adrenal gland was significantly worse than that of patients with pT3a ($P < 0.001$) or pT3b ($P = 0.011$) disease that did not invade the adrenal gland. Even among the subset of pT3a and pT3b patients with pNx/pN0 pM0 status, direct adrenal gland invasion was still significantly associated with death from renal cancer ($P = 0.011$). Furthermore, there was no significant difference in the 5-year cancer-specific survival between patients with pT3a or pT3b disease accompanied by direct adrenal invasion and patients with pT4 tumors.

After removing cases with direct adrenal involvement, T3a would then comprise only tumors with perirenal fat infiltration including sinus invasion. Siemer et al. [8] then questioned if T3a can remain

TABLE 2-9-1. TNM staging of renal cell carcinoma (2002)

Classification	2002
T1	Tumor 7 cm or less, limited to kidney
T1a	Tumor 4 cm or less
T1b	Tumor more than 4 cm but not more than 7 cm
T2	Tumor more than 7 cm, limited to kidney
T3	Tumor extends into major veins or directly invades adrenal gland or perinephric tissues but not beyond Gerota's fascia
T3a	Tumor directly invades adrenal gland or perinephric tissues[a] but not beyond Gerota's fascia
T3b	Tumor grossly extends into renal vein(s)[b] or vena cava below diaphragm
T3c	Tumor grossly extends into vena cava above diaphragm
T4	Tumor invades beyond Gerota's fascia

[a] Includes renal sinus (peripelvic) fat.
[b] Includes segmental (muscle-containing) branches.

TABLE 2-9-2. Effect of tumor size on survival rates in stages pT1, pT2, and PT3a cases with pN_{all} and cM0

Stage	No.	P
pT1 vs. pT2		<0.001
pT1	744	
pT2	256	
pT3a < 7 cm vs. > 7 cm		
<7 cm	100	<0.04
>7 cm	93	
pT1 vs. pT3a < 7 cm		NS
pT1	744	
pT3a < 7 cm	100	
pT2 vs. pT3a > 7 cm		NS
pT2	256	
pT3a > 7 cm	93	
pT1, modified vs. pT2, modified		<0.001
pT1, modified	895	
pT2, modified[l]	419	
pT3b+c vs. pT2, modified		<0.001
pT3b+c	453	
pT2, modified	419	
pT3b+c vs. pT4, modified		<0.001
pT3b+c	453	
pT4, modified	27	

Data are from Siemer et al. [8].
pT1, modified includes pT1 + pT3a ≤ 7 cm; pT2, modified includes pT2 + pT3a > 7 cm; pT4, modified includes pT4 and pT3a with direct adrenal invasion; pT3b+c, tumor thrombus extending into vena cava, either below or above diaphragm.

as a useful category in kidney cancer staging. Because direct invasion of the ipsilateral adrenal gland [2] and distant metastasis regardless of TNM staging are unfavorable signs, these cases were excluded from their T3a case analysis (but cases with adrenal involvement by the indirect route were included because they represent "perirenal fat infiltration"[1]). Then, in an attempt to obtain the best cutoff point, the tumor size and tumor-specific survival were analyzed by receiver operating characteristics (ROC) curves. It was found that the tumor-specific survival rate in patients with pT3a tumors <7 cm was significantly better than in patients with pT3a tumors >7 cm (P < 0.04). Of considerable interest were the additional findings shown in Table 2-9-2.

Although it is no surprise that pT1 (by definition <7 cm in size) had a better survival rate than pT2 (by definition >7 cm), among the pT3a group, tumor size (divided into two subgroups by size 7 cm) likewise demonstrated a significant influence on the prognosis. In other words, in their opinion, perirenal invasion per se does not affect the prognosis overtly; thus, when all cases of tumors <7 cm were combined as a modified pT1 and compared with the cases >7 cm as a modified pT2 group, the former had a better sur-

vival rate than the latter (P < 0.001). Thus, the category pT3a, when cases with direct invasion into the adrenal gland were excluded, does not serve a useful purpose. The Siemer group correctly pointed out that infiltration of perirenal fat tissues is usually diagnosed postoperatively by the pathologist, and it has no impact on clinical decision making; therefore, they concluded it should not be used for assigning the T category.

References

1. Greene FL, Page DL, Fleming ID, Fritz A, Balch CM, Heller DG, Morrow M (2002) AJCC cancer staging manual. Springer-Verlag, New York, pp 323–328.
2. Han KR, Bui MHT, Pantuck AJ, Freitas DG, Leibovich BC, Dorey FJ, Zisman A, Janzen NK, Mukouyama H, Figlin RA, Belldegrun AS (2003) TNM T3a renal cell carcinoma: adrenal gland involvement is not the same as renal fat invasion. J Urol 169:899–904.
3. Sagalowsky AJ, Kadesky KT, Ewalt DM, Kennedy TJ (1994) Factors influencing adrenal metastasis in renal cell carcinoma. J Urol 151:1181–1184.

[1] Although this in not justifiable without reasonable explanation, they [9] have data to suggest that solitary metastasis to the adrenal gland has a reasonably favorable cancer-specific survival rate.

4. Sandock DS, Seftel AD, Resnick MI (1997) Adrenal metastases from renal cell carcinoma: role of ipsilateral adrenalectomy and definition of stage. Urology 49: 28–31.
5. Thompson RH, Leibovich BC, Cheville JC, Lohse CM, Frank I, Kwon ED, Zincke H, Blute ML (2005) Should direct ipsilateral adrenal invasion from renal cell carcinoma be classified as pT3a? J Urol 173:918–921.
6. Angervall L, Wahlqvist L (1978) Follow-up and prognosis of renal cell carcinoma in a series operated by perifascial nephrectomy combined with adrenalectomy and retroperitoneal lymphadenectomy. Eur Urol 4:13–17.
7. Kobayashi T, Nakamura E, Yamamoto S, Kamoto T, Okuno H, Terai A, Kakehi Y, Terachi T, Fujikawa K, Fukuzawa S, Takeuchi H, Ogawa O (2003) Low incidence of ipsilateral adrenal involvement and recurrences in patients with renal cell carcinoma undergoing radical nephrectomy: a retrospective analysis of 393 patients. Urology 62:40–45.
8. Siemer S, Lehmann J, Loch L, Becker F, Stein U, Schneider G, Ziegler M, Stoeckle M (2005) Current TNM classification of renal cell carcinoma evaluated: revising stage T3a. J Urol 173:33–37.
9. Siemer S, Lehmann J, Kamradt J, Loch T, Remberger K, Humke U, Ziegler M, Stoeckle M (2004) Adrenal metastases in 1,635 patients with renal cell carcinoma: outcome and indication for adrenalectomy. J Urol 171: 2155–2159.

Question 10

How does the tumor thrombus in the renal vein or inferior vena cava and its level of extension affect the prognosis of renal cancer?

Answer

Tumor extension into the renal vein or the inferior vena cava signifies an unfavorable prognosis because it is frequently associated with other adverse prognostic factors including large tumor size, perirenal invasion, regional lymph node involvement (N), and distant metastasis (M). After adjusting for N and M status, the level of thrombus extension in the inferior vena cava is negatively associated with the prognosis. The Mayo group proposed a new classification scheme for the T3 category by combining the level of thrombus and perirenal extension of the renal cell carcinoma.

Comments

Renal cell carcinoma (RCC) invades the venous system in 4%–9% of newly diagnosed patients [1–4]. The prognostic significance of tumor extension into the renal vein (RV) or inferior vena cava (IVC) has been debated for a long time. Some investigators claim that the prognosis is worsened not only by tumor extension into the RV/IVC but also by the level of extension of the thrombus. On the other hand, others have claimed that venous extension, when the tumor is removed surgically, does not affect the prognosis significantly.

After having reviewed a number of articles on this subject, we conclude that the evaluation should be based on recent publications because the early litera-ture cannot be reliably cited due to inadequacy in both clinical (including intraoperative) and pathologic assessment of disease extent and inadequacy of the statistical analyses.

Vascular invasion generally indicates an unfavorable outcome for patients with a malignant neoplasm. Controversy remains, however, about the prognostic significance of RV/IVC invasion in patients with RCC. In the TNM/AJCC staging system published in 1997 and 2002 [5], T3b is defined as a tumor with extension into the RV or IVC or its wall below the diaphragm and T3c as a tumor with extension into the IVC or its wall above the diaphragm. No consideration is given to the status of local pericapsular invasion. The prognostic significance of RV/IVC extension should be evaluated with consideration of other concurrent adverse pathologic factors. Thus, T3b/c comprises a heterogeneous group of tumor status. Data accumulated over the past 20 years have clearly established that T2b/c tumors in most cases are frequently associated concurrently with other adverse factors such as perinephric tumor extension, regional lymph node involvement, distant metastasis, and large tumor size. The last three items are known to be independent adverse factors [6–9] and their presence dictates the prognosis adversely in patients with tumor thrombus in the RV/IVC. According to Ficarra et al. [6], the frequency of these adverse factors was as follows: Among 118 patients in whom tumor thrombus was limited to the RV, perirenal invasion, lymph node metastasis, and distant metastasis were observed, respectively, in 20%, 11%, and 25%. Among 24 patients with tumor extending into the ICV, the frequency was, respectively, 33%, 4%, and 25%. When the 118 patients with RV involvement only were divided into those with ($n = 66$) and without ($n = 52$) the concurrent adverse prognostic factors described above, the cause-specific survival was significantly worse in the former group (log rank $P < 0.0001$) (Table 2-10-1). In 52 of 114 patients with

TABLE 2-10-1. Effects of concurrent presence of adverse prognostic factors on cause-specific survival of RCC patients with renal vein and inferior vena cava tumor thrombus

Pathologic features	No.	5-Year survival	10-Year survival	P*
Tumor in renal vein				
No other factors[a]	52	83%	71%	<0.0001
Adverse factors[a]	66	30%	14%	
Tumor extends into IVC				
No other factors[a]	7	69%		0.008
Adverse factors[a]	17	10%		

Data from Ficarra et al. [6].
[a] Perirenal invasion, metastasis to regional node(s) and distant site(s).
*Log-rank test.

tumor involving the RV but without concurrent adverse factors, the cancer-specific survival was 83% after 5 years and 71% after 10 years. These are excellent numbers for RCC. Similarly, among the 24 patients with IVC extension, the cause-specific survival of 7 patients with no concurrent adverse factors had a significantly better survival rate than those with concurrent adverse factors ($P = 0.008$, log rank) and showed no difference from T2N0M0 patients ($P = 0.191$).

Most recently, cancer-specific survival data for pT3b cancer patients were presented by the Mayo Clinic group [10]. The strength of this study is that they controlled perirenal fat invasion, node metastasis (pN), and distant spread (M) status for evaluating RV/IVC thrombus formation. Their data are as comprehensive as they should be but are somewhat complex. First, perirenal fat invasion including pericapsular extension and sinus fat invasion were considered in the analysis. Second, the level of thrombus extension was divided into four groups; level 0, thrombus limited to the RV; level I, thrombus extending ≤2cm above the RV; level II, thrombus extending >2cm above the RV but below the confluence of the hepatic veins; level III, thrombus at the level of or above the hepatic veins but below the diaphragm; and level IV, thrombus extending above the diaphragm. Cancer-specific survival at 5 years after nephrectomy was calculated by the 2002 RCC classification. For a total of 675 patients with pT3 (after excluding 22 cases with evidence of direct adrenal invasion for the reason cited under Question 9), the rates were 54.7%, 45.9%, 34.4%, and 18.1% for patients with pT3a, pT3b, pT3c, and pT4 cancer, respectively. By univariate analysis using pT3a as the reference, the staging designations for pT3b, pT3c, and pT4 were all significantly different but with a low

c index[1] of 0.548. Although the c index increased to 0.704 after accounting for regional node involvement (pN) and distant metastasis (M) at nephrectomy, the 2002 tumor classification was no longer statistically significantly associated with the outcome. Among the 422 patients with pT3b tumors, patients with level I, II, or III tumor thrombus were significantly more likely to die of renal carcinoma than patients with level 0 thrombus ($P < 0.001$). The risk persisted even after adjusting for pN and M status ($P < 0.001$). Similarly, patients with perinephric or renal sinus fat invasion were almost twice as likely to die of renal carcinoma than patients without fat invasion by univariate analysis ($P < 0.001$). The risk persisted even after adjusting for pN and M status at nephrectomy. With these data they reclassified pT3 renal carcinomas into four groups by combining perirenal fat invasion and the level of thrombus extension. They are as follows (Fig. 2-10-1): group 1, thrombus level 0 without fat invasion; group 2, fat invasion only; group 3, thrombus level 0 with fat invasion or thrombus levels I, II, or III without fat invasion; and group 4, thrombus level I, II, or III with fat invasion. Also added for comparison were 28 patients whose tumors extended beyond Gerota's fascia (proposed group 5). Cancer-specific survivals for these five groups are shown in Fig. 2-10-1. The estimated cancer-specific survival rates for these five groups at 5 years after nephrectomy were 63.5%, 54.7%, 42.4%, 25.5%, and 18.1%, respectively; and the associations of this proposed classification with death from renal carcinoma were highly significant not only by univariate analysis but after adjustment for pN and M status (group 1

---

[1] This is a statistical measure to assess the reliability of the proposed model. The higher the c index, the better is the model.

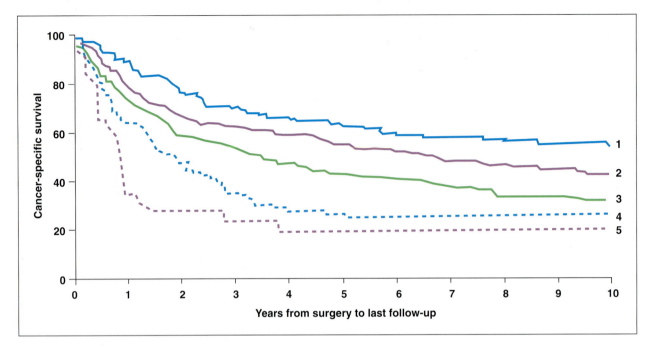

FIG. 2-10-1. Cancer-specific survival by proposed primary tumor classification for 675 patients with pT3 and pT4 renal cell carcinoma. From Leibovich et al. [10], with permission. Group 1: thrombus level 0 without fat invasion; group 2: fat invasion only; group 3: thrombus level 0 with fat invasion or thrombus levels I, II, or III with fat invasion; group 4: thrombus level I, II, or III with fat invasion, or thrombus level IV; and group 5: tumor extension beyond Gerota's fascia.

vs. group 2, $P = 0.262$; group 1 vs. groups 3, 4, and 5, $P < 0.001$ for each comparison).

In summary, tumor thrombus extension (which indicates the likelihood of distant metastasis) into the RV or IVC is frequently associated with adverse factors and is therefore associated with a worse prognosis. After adjusting for pN and M status, perirenal fat invasion is associated with a higher risk of dying of renal cancer. Likewise, the level of tumor extension into the IVC is negatively associated with the prognosis. The Mayo group proposed a new classification scheme for T3 category by combining the level of thrombus extension and perirenal extension of renal cell carcinoma.

References

1. Pagano F, Bianco M, Artibani W, Pappagallo G, Prayer Galetti T (1992) Renal cell carcinoma with extension into the inferior vena cava: problems in diagnosis, staging and treatment. Eur Urol 22:200–203.
2. Casanova GA, Zingg EJ (1991) Inferior vena caval tumor extension in renal cell carcinoma. Urol Int 47:216–218.
3. Hatcher PA, Anderson EE, Paulson DF, Carson CC, Robertson JE (1991) Surgical management and prognosis of renal cell carcinoma invading the vena cava. J Urol 145:20–24.
4. Hoehn W, Hermanek P (1983) Invasion of veins in renal cell carcinoma: frequency, correlation and prognosis. Eur Urol 9:276–280.
5. Greene FL, Page DL, Fleming ID, Fritz A, Balch CM, Heller DG, Morrow M (2002) AJCC cancer staging manual. Springer-Verlag, New York, pp 323–328.
6. Ficarra V, Righetti R, D'Amico A, Rubilotta E, Novella G, Malossini G, Mobilio G (2001) Renal vein and vena cava involvement does not affect prognosis in patients with renal cell carcinoma. Oncology 61:10–15.
7. Kuczyk MA, Bokemeyer C, Koehn G, Stief CG, Machtens M, Truss M, Hoefner K, Jonas U (1997) Prognostic relevance of intracaval neoplastic extension for patients with renal cell cancer. Br J Urol 80:18–24.
8. Rabbani F, Halimian P, Reuter VE, Simmons R, Russo P (2004) Renal vein or inferior vena cava extension in patients with renal cortical tumors: impact of tumor histology. J Urol 171:1057–1061.
9. Golimbu M, Tessler A, Joshi P, Al-Askari S, Sperber S, Morales P (1986) Renal cell carcinoma: survival and prognostic factors. Urology 27:291–301.
10. Leibovich BC, Cheville JC, Lohse CM, Zincke H, Kwon ED, Frank I, Thompson RH, Blute ML (2005) Cancer specific survival for patients with pT3 renal cell carcinoma: can the 2002 primary tumor classification be improved? J Urol 173:716–719.

Question 11

How does the renal sinus involvement in renal cell carcinoma affect the prognosis?

Answer

In the 2002 TNM/AJCC formulation, sinus involvement was recognized for the first time as an anatomic site of perirenal invasion. Thus, as you can imagine, there has been hardly any quality study addressing the importance of sinus invasion on the prognosis. Sinus invasion can take place in two ways. The first is direct extension of a renal tumor located primarily in the column of Bertin; and the second is extravascular extension of tumor thrombus in small veins coming off the renal parenchyma and subsequent extravascular extension into the sinus fat. A comprehensive study reported recently by the Mayo Clinic group indicates that the presence of extrarenal extension (perinephric fat invasion including renal sinus invasion), compared with its absence, is twice as likely to result in patients' death from renal cell carcinoma.

Comments

The renal sinus is the cavity that opens on the medial border of the kidney and contains fatty tissue, the renal pelvis and its calices, branches of the renal artery and veins, lymphatics, nerves, and a small amount of adipose tissue [1] (Fig. 2-11-1A).

It was the 2002 TNM/AJCC formulation [2] in which renal sinus invasion was recognized for the first time as a specific anatomic structure for invasion and was classified under T3a (Fig. 2-11-1B). Articles that specifically address the invasion of the sinus were virtually nonexistent until two reports came from Bonsib and his associates [3, 4]. Whereas the renal cortex is separated from the veins and lymphatics of the perinephric fat by the renal capsule, there is no fibrous capsule separating the renal cortex of the columns of Bertin from the renal sinus. Thus, a tumor involving a column of Bertin may have easy access to the renal sinus, which is rich in blood vessels and lymphatics.

The Bonsib study consisted of 100 renal cell carcinomas (RCCs). Most of the nephrectomy specimens were handled by Bonsib himself. In the first 50 cases the entire interface between the renal sinus and the tumor was totally embedded, but in the second 50 cases sampling was more selective. Five blocks of the renal sinus interface with tumor were submitted. Sections of the peripheral capsule were also submitted from the most suspicious area for capsular invasion. Using the 2002 TNM staging formulation, 49 cases were T1, 5 were T2, and 46 were T3 or T4. A total of 74 cases were clear cell type, 16 papillary type, 7 chromophobe type, and 3 unclassified type. The results are summarized in Table 2-11-1. No tumor invaded the capsule without invading the sinus. There were two ways by which the sinus was invaded. The first was by tumor thrombi formed in small veins, which was discernible on careful gross inspection (personal communication), and, second, by direct extension of the tumor into the sinus's fat tissue. More often than not, sinus fat invasion was secondary to initially involved sinus veins rather than direct extension from the main cortical tumor. In 9 of 46 sinus-invasive tumors, venous invasion was identified only without sinus soft tissue invasion. Extension to the renal vein was observed 21 of 38 cases. The sinus invasion correlated with Fuhrman grade ($P < 0.001$), tumor type, and tumor size. It was seen in 16% cases of stage T1a (<4 cm) carcinomas. The frequency of sinus invasion abruptly increased with tumors >4 cm

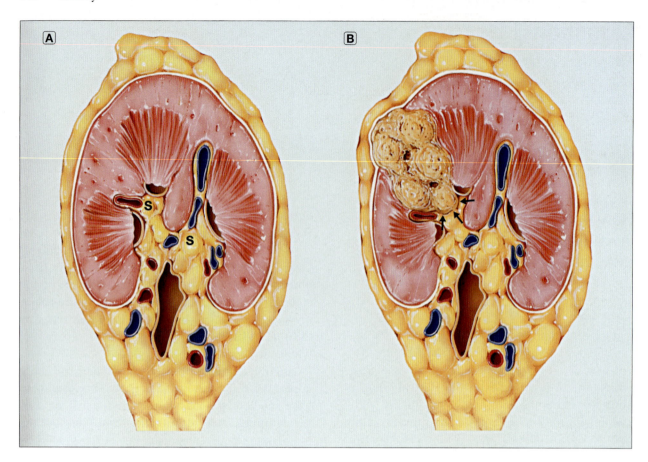

FIG. 2-11-1. **A** Bisected kidney to demonstrate the anatomic relation of renal parenchyma to renal sinus. The renal sinus (*S*) contains lymphatics (not shown), veins (*blue*), and arteries (*red*). **B** Renal cell carcinoma invading the renal sinus (*arrows*)

TABLE 2-11-1. Relation between sinus invasion and capsular invasion

Renal carcinoma	Sinus negative (no.)		Sinus positive (no.)	
	Negative capsule	Positive capsule	Negative capsule	Positive capsule
Clear cell/unclassified	33	0	17	27
Papillary	15	0	0	1
Chromophobe	6	0	1	0
Total	54	1	18	28

From Bonsib [4], with permission.

($P < 0.001$). As the consequence of careful study of sinus invasion, 28% of cases were up-staged from T1 or T2 to T3.

The Bonsib studies have several important messages: (1) The pathologist must pay more attention to the possibility of sinus invasion when examining nephrectomy specimens. As a result, more cases may be classified as T3 instead of T2. (2) If one excludes the less common and less aggressive renal carcinomas (papillary and chromophobe cell types), the number of T1b and T2 clear cell RCCs by the 2002 TNM

staging formulation may diminish. Most tumors >4 cm are likely to have invaded the sinus and are classified as T3 tumors. Bonsib and colleagues justifiably argued that stage T1b and T2 categories need to be redefined to remain as meaningful staging categories. Their preliminary data suggest that sinus invasion is associated with an unfavorable prognosis. Three of the four cases that involved the lumens of the sinus veins but not the main renal vein developed metastasis [3].

As we noted under Question 10, the Mayo Clinic group evaluated the effect of renal sinus fat invasion

[5]. Of 206 pT3a cases (excluding cases with direct adrenal gland invasion), prerinephric fat invasion, renal sinus invasion, and both were observed, respectively, in 166 (80.6%), 13 (6.3%), and 27 (13.1%) cases. The presence of extrarenal extension versus their absence was twice as likely to result in the death of the patient with renal carcinoma ($P < 0.001$ by univariate analysis). Note that, compared with the Bonsib data, there is a big difference in the frequency of renal sinus invasion and pericapsular extension.

The Bonsib study should stimulate other pathologists to study sinus invasion and its effects on prognosis. In any future study, sinus invasion should be divided into two categories: extension of tumor by way of vein invasion only (T3b) and extension into the sinus fat (T3a).

References

1. Schaeffer JP (1951) Morris' human anatomy: a complete systemic treatise. Blackstone, Toronto, pp 1427.
2. Greene FL, Page DL, Fleming ID, Fritz A, Balch CM, Heller DG, Morrow M (2002) AJCC cancer staging manual. Springer-Verlag, New York, pp 323–328.
3. Bonsib SM, Gibson D, Mhoon M, Greene GF (2000) Renal sinus involvement in renal cell carcinoma. Am J Surg Pathol 24:451–458.
4. Bonsib SM (2004) The renal sinus is the principal invasive pathway: a retrospective study of 100 renal cell carcinomas. Am J Surg Pathol 28:1594–1600.
5. Leibovich BC, Cheville JC, Lohse CM, Zincke H, Kwon ED, Frank I, Thompson RH, Blute ML (2005) Cancer specific survival for patients with pT3 renal cell carcinoma: can the 2002 primary tumor classification be improved? J Urol 173:716–719.

Question 12

What is the significance of microvascular tumor invasion observed in a renal cell carcinoma?

Answer

The possible prognostic significance of intratumoral microvascular invasion by tumor cells has been mentioned sporadically over the past decade. All reports have determined that it is an adverse factor that negatively affects tumor recurrence or cancer-specific death. Its frequency is closely related to tumor size, Fuhrman nuclear grade, and pathologic stage. The presence of microvascular invasion may be more meaningful in predicting the prognosis in a low-stage, low nuclear grade tumor. For the pathologist, the presence (or absence) of tumor thrombus in a renal cancer mass should be stated in the pathology report. The ability to invade an intratumoral vessel must be a manifestation of aggressive biologic potential even for a tumor that is removed at an early stage of growth that is presumed to carry a favorable prognosis.

Comments

Despite the favorable outcome anticipated for patients with favorable pathology findings (low stage, low grade, no evidence of cancer spreading outside the kidney, negative lymph nodes, no distant metastasis), it is clear that a sizable number of patients succumb to cancer-specific death. This fact has directed the attention of investigators to look for additional factors. One of them, renal sinus invasion, has been discussed already. A second was the signifi-

cance of intratumoral microscopic tumor vascular invasion in regard to the prognosis. We cite here five articles that are acceptable in terms of case selection and data analyses (Table 2-12-1). All of these studies concluded that microscopic tumor vascular invasion is a potent prognostic factor, and some of them concluded that microscopic tumor vascular invasion is either one of several independent risk factors or the only significant independent factor affecting tumor recurrence or cancer-specific death [1–5].

Several interesting findings can be recognized in these studies. First, the frequency of microscopic tumor vascular invasion rises with tumor size, nuclear grade (by Fuhrman et al. [6]), and stage [2, 3]. According to Goncalves et al. [2], the frequency of microscopic tumor vascular invasion was 10 of 66 tumors <7 cm (15%), whereas it rose to 14 of 29 (48%) tumors >7 cm ($P < 0.001$). According to Van Poppel et al. [1], the frequency of microscopic tumor vascular invasion by pT stage was 0 of 14 for pT1 (<2.5 cm, 1987 TNM formulation), 31 of 128 pT2 (24%), 19 of 36 pT3 (53%), and 1 of 1 pT4 ($P = 0.0005, \chi^2$). The frequency of microscopic tumor vascular invasion by Fuhrman grade was 0 of 19 grade 1, 25 of 96 grade 2 (26%), 17 of 49 grade 3 (35%), and 9 of 15 grade 4 tumors (60%) ($P = 0.001$).

Second, a pertinent question is whether a relation exists between microscopic tumor vascular invasion and tumor thrombus formation in the renal vein (RV) or inferior vena cava (IVC). There are only two studies that have addressed this question. Samma et al. [3] found microscopic tumor vascular invasion in seven of eight cases of RV/IVC thrombus formation, whereas microscopic tumor vascular invasion alone was seen in only 7 of 60 patients ($P < 0.01$). Similarly, in the study by Goncalves et al. [2], 9 of 10 patients with macroscopic tumor vascular invasion also had microscopic tumor vascular invasion. Moreover, in the Goncalves study, macrovascular tumor involve-

TABLE 2-12-1. Effects of microscopic intratumoral microvascular invasion on cancer-specific survival or recurrence

Study	No. of cases	No. of paraffin blocks examined	Follow-up period	MV+	MV−	Effects on outcome	Comments
Samma [3], 1991	68	2–3/tumor	Not stated	14	54	Cancer-specific survival, $P < 0.025$ (univariate analysis)	Report is faulted in the lymph node metastasis is not stated, analysis includes cases not surgically treated, and cases of all stages (T1-T4) are included.
Mrstik [4], 1992	58 (M+, LN+ excluded)	Mean 5 (4–10)	Median 37 mos.	14	44	5-Year disease-free survival, $P < 0.0001$	MV+ has significant impact on disease-free survival irrespective of Fuhrman grade or pT stage.
Kinouchi [5], 1999	204 (TNM T1 and T2, 1997 only)	Not stated	Mean 5.4 years	11	193	Cancer-specific survival, $P = 0.0125$ (univariate analysis), $P = 0.0068$ (multivariate analysis)	Tumor size and MV+ invasion are independent factors of cancer-specific survival.
Van Poppel [1], 1997	180 (M+, LN+, renal vein/ inferior vena cava-positive cases excluded)	One or more block per cm tumor diameter	Mean 52 mos.	57	129	Disease-free survival, $P < 0.00001$ (univariate analysis)	MV+ is the single most important risk factor by multivariate analysis for disease-free survival.
Goncalves [2], 2004	95 (T1/T2 Nx M0)	Not stated	Median 45 mos.	24	71	Disease-free survival, $P < 0.001$ (univariate analysis)	MV invasion significantly correlated with tumor >7 cm, perirenal invasion, macrovascular involvement, Fuhrman grade, lymph node metastasis, and presence of sarcomatoid component (all comparisons $P < 0.001$). MV invasion and perirenal invasion are independent factors of cancer-specific survival by multivariate analysis.

MV, microvascular invasion.

ment has the same unfavorable predictive value as microscopic tumor vascular invasion ($P < 0.001$, univariate analysis). However, by multivariate analysis, only microscopic tumor vascular invasion was a significant prognostic factor, indicating that RV/IVC involvement is a phenomenon occurring together with other, more potent adverse factors (refer to Question 10).

In summary, we have identified a number of prognostically important pathologic parameters. Most of them are closely interrelated.

During the process of neoplasia, initially a tumor emerges as a tiny mass. Its progression rate is dictated by its inherent biologic potential of aggressiveness, such as nuclear grade, growth rate, and ability to invade the surrounding normal tissues including intratumoral vessels. One such biologic potential could be IMP3, a recently reported RNA-binding protein that has been shown to be closely associated with the metastatic potential of RCCs. Compared with nonmetastatic RCCs, IMP expression was greatly increased not only in metastatic tumors but also in a subset of primary tumors that were likely subsequently to develop metastasis [7].

Because macrovascular involvement should occur only after invasion of small vessels in the tumor has been established, it is reasonable to suggest that microvascular tumor vascular invasion is probably a determining factor for a worse outcome [2].

To date, it is unusual for the pathologist to mention the presence (or absence) of microvascular invasion in the report to the urologist. Based on the reports cited above, it is clear that this information may be useful for predicting outcome, especially in those with low stage and perhaps low-grade clear cell carcinoma. Although data regarding RCCs other than the clear cell type are absent, microscopic tumor vascular invasion, if found, should be similarly meaningful in predicting the outcome.

References

1. Van Poppel H, Vandendriessche H, Boel K, Mertens V, Goethuys H, Haustermans K, Van Damme B, Baert L (1997) Microscopic vascular invasion is the most relevant prognosticator after radical nephrectomy for clinically nonmetastatic renal cell carcinoma. J Urol 158:45–49.
2. Goncalves PD, Srougi M, Dall'Oglio F, Leite MKR, Ortiz V, Hering F (2004) Low clinical stage renal cell carcinoma: relevance of microvascular tumor invasion as a prognostic parameter. J Urol 172:470–474.
3. Samma S, Yoshida K, Ozono S, Ohara S, Hayashi Y, Tabata S, Uemura H, Iwai A, Hirayama A, Hirao Y, Okajima E (1991) Tumor thrombus and microvascular invasion as prognostic factors in renal cell carcinoma. Jpn J Clin Oncol 21:340–345.
4. Mrstik C, Salamon J, Weber R, Stögermayer F (1992) Microscopic venous infiltration as predictor of relapse in renal cell carcinoma. J Urol 148:271–274.
5. Kinouchi T, Saiki S, Meguro N, Maeda O, Kuroda M, Usami M, Kotake T (1999) Impact of tumor size on the clinical outcomes of patients with Robson stage I renal cell carcinoma. Cancer 85:689–695.
6. Fuhrman SA, Lasky LC, Limas C (1982) Prognostic significance of morphologic parameters in renal cell carcinoma. Am J Surg Pathol 6:655–663.
7. Jiang Z, Chu PG, Woda BA, Rock KL, Liu Q, Hsieh C-C, Li C, Chen W, Duan HQ, McDougal S, Wu C-L (2006) Analysis of RNA-binding protein IMP3 to predict metastasis and progression of renal-cell carcinoma: retrospective study. Lancet Oncol 7:556–564.

Question 13

How does one distinguish benign from malignant renal cysts clinically? Which renal neoplasms are characterized by cyst formation?

Answer

Renal cysts are common. According to a recent ultrasonographic study, they are seen in 14% of men and 8% of women in the general population. Clinically important disease categories include multilocular cystic renal cell carcinoma, cystic nephroma (multilocular cyst), mixed epithelial and stromal tumor, cystic partially differentiated nephroblastoma, and renal cell carcinomas (RCCs) arising in dialysis-associated acquired renal cystic disease. Among these disease entities, partially differentiated nephroblastoma is a disease of the pediatric population under the age of 24 months and is curative after complete resection. Cystic nephroma and mixed epithelial and stromal tumors are benign, affect predominantly women, and are exceptional before the age of 30. There has been controversy whether these two are a single entity with different histologic manifestations. Studies by several groups have indicated that this is indeed the case.

Multilocular cystic RCC is a newly defined RCC subtype that has an excellent prognosis after complete resection. Nevertheless, its distinction from cystic nephroma is important, as these two entities exhibit a similar radiologic picture. There is a distinct difference in the microscopic appearance between the two. Ultimately, the final diagnosis rests on pathology study of the resected specimen.

Renal cell carcinomas developing in acquired renal cystic disease kidneys are predominantly of the papillary type, although clear cell and chromophobe cell carcinomas may arise. Imaging studies such as computed tomography (CT), ultrasonography (US), and magnetic resonance imaging (MRI) are useful tools for evaluating a cystic lesion. The Bosniak classification is useful for clinical decision-making, but correlation with the pathologic findings is moderate.

Comments

Renal cysts are common. With the increasing use of abdominal CT scans, they are frequently discovered as an incidental finding. Several important benign and malignant entities in the kidney present as a cystic mass, including multilocular cystic RCC, cystic nephroma (multilocular renal cyst), mixed epithelial and stromal tumor, cystic partially differentiated nephroblastoma, and carcinomas arising in dialysis-associated acquired renal cystic disease.

Bosniak Classification

The Bosniak classification of renal cysts, introduced in 1986, has been used to evaluate cystic renal masses and for the decision-making of clinical management [1]. Based on the complexity of the cystic lesions on CT images, the Bosniak classification divides cystic renal lesions into four categories.

- Category I lesions are benign simple cysts with hairline-thin walls. These cysts contain no septa, calcification, or solid components.
- Category II masses are benign cystic lesions that may contain hairline-thin septa. Fine calcification may be present in the wall or septa. Category IIF lesions (the F indicates a need for follow-up

imaging) are more complex cystic lesions that cannot be classified as category II or III. These cysts may contain an increased number of hairline-thin septa or have minimal but smooth thickening of the wall or septa. The wall or septa may contain calcifications.

- Category III lesions are intermediate masses, and it cannot be determined at imaging whether they are benign or malignant. They have thickened, irregular walls or septa in which enhancement can be demonstrated.
- Category IV lesions are malignant cystic masses. They may have findings similar to those seen in category III masses, but they also have enhancing soft tissue components adjacent to, but independent of, the wall or septa.

Thus, categories III and IV lesions would be the important ones that require a correlative study between CT findings and pathology studies. The Bosniak group claims that addition of MRI helps, in some cases, in depicting additional septa and upgrading the Bosniak cyst classification [1].

A correlative study between Bosniak lesions and pathologic findings has been reported by Picken et al. [2]. Four, seven, and eight patients of Bosniak II, III, and IV lesions, respectively, underwent surgery. By pathology examination, the correlative findings are tabulated in Table 2-13-1.

Although the Bosniak classification is useful for distinguishing benign cystic lesions from malignant ones, the correlation is only moderate. A benign lesion such as mixed epithelial and stromal tumor with complex structures mimics a malignant lesion on CT and MRI. By US (which is inferior to CT or MRI for detecting cystic disease), Terada et al. [3] found renal cysts in 15% of men and 8% of women in the general population. In their follow-up of these men and women, the cysts increased in size and number more rapidly in the younger generation. Although most of the cases were simple cysts, 6 of 45 were described as "multilocular" cysts, and they grew more rapidly than simple cysts ($P < 0.001$). The histologic nature of "multilocular" cysts is unknown. A possible correlation with cystic nephromas (multilocular cysts) is of interest.

Multilocular Cystic Renal Cell Carcinoma

Multilocular cystic RCC was a newly defined entity in the 2004 WHO classification system [4]. Although it may be an early phase of clear cell renal cell RCC, it is associated with an excellent prognosis [5]. This entity has been discussed in detail under Question 2. Multilocular cystic RCC is different from clear cell RCC with its cystic changes in which solid areas of clear cell tumor are present. Although cysts are common in clear RCCs, only rarely is the tumor composed entirely of cysts (Fig. 2-13-1A).

The multiloculated cysts vary in size and contain fluid that ranges from clear to hemorrhagic. Calcification is present in the septa in more than 20% of tumors [6]. Microscopically, the cysts are, for the most part, lined by a single layer of epithelial cells that characteristically have clear cytoplasm and a small, uniform-sized nucleus (Fuhrman nuclear grade 1) [7] (Fig. 2-13-1B). Sometimes, however, the lining is multilayered. The stroma is loosely to densely collagenous but characteristically contains nests of clear carcinoma cells (Fig. 2-13-1C). The latter finding is a feature that supports the diagnosis of multilocular cystic RCC and not of cystic nephroma, an important differential diagnosis.

Cystic Nephroma (Multilocular Cyst)

Cystic nephroma is a benign cystic neoplasm of adults that occurs predominantly in women (9:1) [8]. Most patients are asymptomatic, and the tumor is discovered incidentally. It forms an expansile mass limited by a pseudocapsule. On sectioning, it is divided into multiple locules that, by definition, do not communicate among themselves (Figs. 2-13-2A, 2-13-3A). In 5% of cases, the lesion involves both kidneys [9].

Microscopically the tumor is composed entirely of numerous cysts of varying size (Fig. 2-13-2B). The cysts are lined by a single layer of low cuboidal to flat, inconspicuous epithelial cells (Figs. 2-13-2B, 2-13-

TABLE 2-13-1. Pathologic correlation of Bosniak II, III, and IV lesions

Bosniak category	No.	Pathologic findings	
		Benign	Malignant
II	4	2 CN	2 CPRCC
III	7	1 CN	6 (3 CRCC, 2 PRCC, 1 ChRCC)
IV	8	3 MEST	5 (1 CCRCC, 4 PRCC)

From Picken et al. [2].
CN, cystic nephroma; RCC, renal cell carcinoma; CPRCC, cystic papillary renal cell carcinoma; CRCC, clear cell RCC; PRCC, papillary RCC; ChRCC, chromophobe RCC; MEST, mixed epithelial and stromal tumor; CCRCC, cystic clear cell RCC.

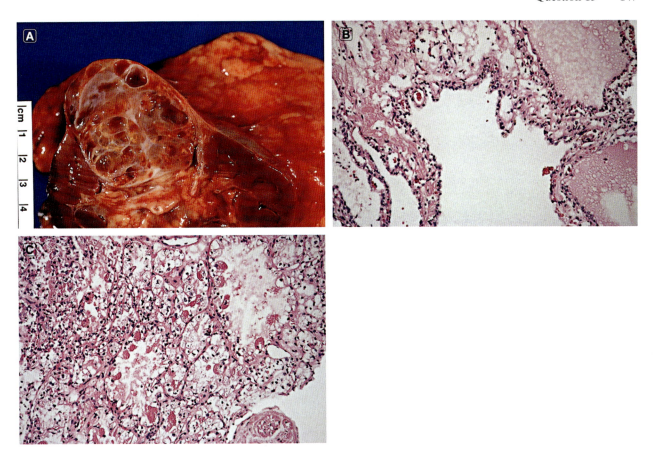

FIG. 2-13-1. **A** Multilocular cystic renal cell carcinoma. Cross section reveals a sharply demarcated cystic mass divided into multiple locules separated by thin fibrous septa. On gross examination alone, this case would be difficult, if not impossible, to distinguish from cystic nephroma. (This is the same case presented in Fig. 2-2-7 under Question 2.) **B, C** Microscopic examination revealed that the thin septa are lined by a single layer of cuboidal clear cells with small, round nuclei. In other areas, however, the interseptal tissue contains nests of clear cells characteristic of clear cell renal cell carcinoma. The presence of clear cell nests is against the diagnosis of multilocular cysts (cystic nephroma)

3B). The low cuboidal cells have eosinophilic cytoplasm and small hyperchromatic nuclei that may be pushed toward the lumen of the cyst, producing a hobnail appearance (Fig. 2-13-2C). The cells lining the cysts may have clear cytoplasm (Figs. 2-13-2C,D, 2-13-3B) [10], but this feature alone is insufficient to consider the diagnosis of multicystic renal cell carcinoma [11]. The stroma consists of dense fibrous connective tissue containing spindle cells. In areas and in some cases, the stroma is densely cellular and resembles ovarian stroma (Fig. 2-13-3B). The presence of ovarian-type stroma is a unique feature of cystic nephroma. It was detected in 7 of 10 cases according to Mukhopadhay et al. [8]. The cells were reactive to antibody to estrogen receptors in 4 of 10 and to progesterone receptors in 6 of 10 cases, whereas the stromal cells of "nonovarian" areas were negative to these markers. Despite the similarities between normal ovarian stroma and the ovarian-like stroma of cystic nephroma (both types of cells positive for vimentin and progesterone receptors), there was a difference in the reaction to other markers: The ovarian-like stroma of cystic nephroma was positive for smooth muscle actin (SMA) and desmin, whereas ovarian stroma was negative for both markers. Cyst epithelial cells showed consistent positive reactions for markers of distal tubule/collecting duct markers (CK19, AE1/3, epithelial membrane antigen) and variable reactivity for proximal tubule markers (α_1-antitrypsin, lysozyme, CD15, and CD10).

The differential diagnosis from multilocular cystic RCC is important. The features favoring cystic nephroma are flattened to eosinophilic cells, often with a hobnail appearance, and loose to myxoid stroma. The presence of ovarian-type stroma is distinctly in favor of a cystic nephroma diagnosis. Clear

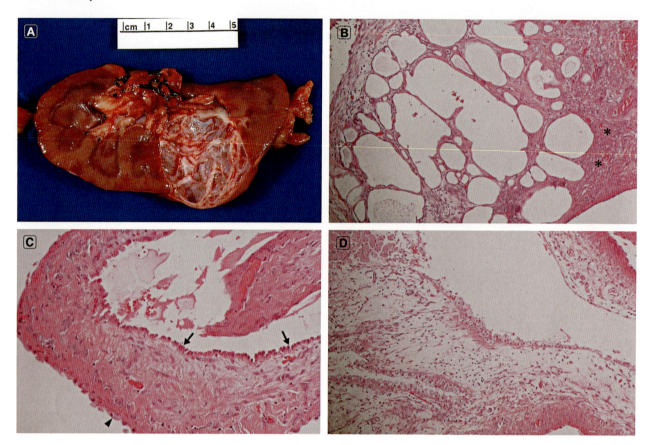

FIG. 2-13-2. **A** Cystic nephroma from a 52-year-old woman. Note that the sharply demarcated cystic mass is divided into multiple locules that have a smooth inner lining. **B** Cysts vary in size; here they are microcysts with inconspicuous lining epithelial cells. The tissue outside the cysts is cellular and resembles ovarian stroma (*). **C** In this portion of the tumor, the cysts are lined by eosinophilic cuboidal cells with a hobnail appearance (*arrows*), whereas in another area, the lining cells have amphophilic cytoplasm (*arrowhead*). **D** In another area, the cyst is lined by a single layer of cuboidal cells with clear cells. (Case provided by Michael Pins, MD, Northwestern University Feinberg School of Medicine, Chicago)

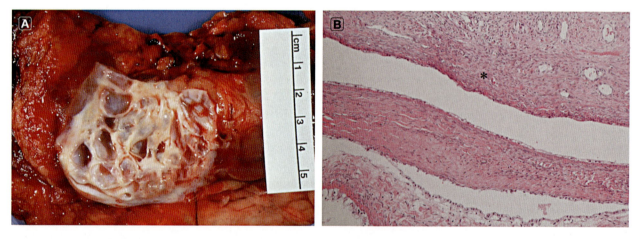

FIG. 2-13-3. **A** Cystic nephroma from a 55-year-old woman. **B** In this portion of the tumor the cysts are lined by a single layer of cuboidal clear cells, which may resemble the cells of multilocular cystic renal cell carcinoma. However, there are no clear cell nests underneath the cyst lining, and the stroma consists of cellular connective tissue that resembles ovarian stroma (*). These features support the diagnosis of cystic nephroma. (Case provided by Michael Pins, MD, Northwestern University Feinberg School of Medicine, Chicago)

cells may line the cyst wall; but if accompanied by ovarian-like stroma, the diagnosis of multilocular cystic RCC is untenable. Features that support the diagnosis of multiocular cystic RCC are clear cells lining all cyst surfaces and frequent aggregates of the same type of cells below the cyst lining (refer to Fig. 2-2-7 and Fig. 2-2-8).

Mixed Epithelial and Stromal Tumor

Mixed epithelial and stromal tumor is a recently described benign adult renal tumor that is composed of a mixture of epithelial and stromal cells. Whether they represent a single or two entities has been debated because of overlapping clinical and pathologic features. Three correlative studies were reported at the 2005 United States–Canadian Academy of Pathology annual meeting that discussed the similarities and dissimilarities of the two entities [12–14]. The consensus was that they represent a spectrum of one entity. It is based on the predominance of both entities in middle-aged women, variably cystic architecture, eosinophilic cells, hobnail cells, and ovarian-type stroma [15]. In the stromal component, estrogen receptor and progesterone receptor staining was 62% and 85% in mixed epithelial and stromal tumors and 19% and 40% in cystic nephromas [15].

If cases are made up "entirely" of thin fibrous-walled cysts, the diagnosis would be cystic nephroma, whereas if the lesion is a mixture of cystic and solid (fibrous) areas, the diagnosis would be mixed epithelial and stromal tumor. Note that in all cases diagnosed as mixed epithelial stromal tumor by Jevremovic et al. [13], there were areas of cystic nephroma. It is probable that most cases fall in the middle and have combined features. Note also that in the Antic study [14], mixed epithelial and stromal tumor occurred exclusively in women 40–80 years old: Five of the seven women were on long-term estrogen therapy, and two were obese. Turbiner et al. has proposed that the name "renal epithelial and stromal tumor" encompasses the cystic nephroma and mixed epithelial and stromal tumors [15].

The tumors are grossly composed of multiple cysts and solid areas. The solid areas may be extensive. Microscopically, the mass consists of large cysts, microcysts, and tubules lined by columnar and cuboidal cells. These epithelial components are scattered in the stroma with variable cellularity ranging from scar-like areas to spindle cells arranged in fascicles

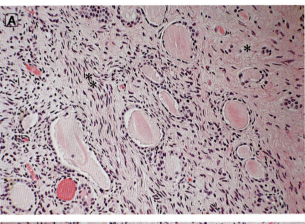
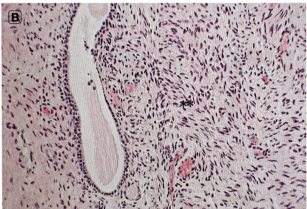

FIG. 2-13-4. **A, B** Mixed epithelial and stromal tumor in an 80 year-old woman. There are small cysts scattered in variably cellular stroma ranging from a scar-like area (*) to spindle cells showing smooth muscle cell differentiation (**). (Case provided by Michael Pins, M. D., Northwestern University Feinberg School of Medicine, Chicago)

(Fig. 2-13-4). Immunohistochemistry shows that the spindle cells are reactive with smooth muscle cell markers [16].

Cystic Partially Differentiated Nephroblastoma

The cystic partially differentiated nephroblastoma is related to Wilms' tumor because it contains blastema and other immature elements. It is a disease of infants, usually occurring within the first 24 months of life and with a 2:1 male predominance [11]. It is, however, benign [17], and complete resection is curative. Cysts are common in Wilms' tumors but are a minor component. Rarely, however, is there a type of lesion that presents as a totally cystic mass indistinguishable from cystic nephroma on gross examination. What distinguishes partially differentiated nephroblastoma from cystic nephroma is the presence of blastema and immature stromal and immature epithelial elements. The lining of the cysts is similar to that of cystic nephroma, with flattened, cuboidal, or hobnail cells.

Carcinoma Arising in Acquired Renal Cystic Disease

It has been well established that hemodialysis applied to patients with end-stage renal disease induces acquired renal cystic disease [18]. Acquired renal cystic disease is characterized by the development of multiple cysts in the kidneys of patients with end-stage renal disease in the absence of congenital cystic disease [19]. Acquired renal cystic disease is more prevalent in males than females ($P < 0.001$, Fisher's exact test) [20] and increases with the years on dialysis ($P < 0.001$, multivariate analysis) [20]. It occurs in 20% of patients who have been on dialysis for 1–3 years and rises to 90% when they have been on dialysis for 5–10 years [19]. There is a high incidence of RCCs in patients with end-stage renal disease, and most of them occurred in the setting of acquired renal cystic disease (91%, 10/11 cases) [20]. According to Denton et al. [20], among 260 nephrectomy cases undergoing renal transplantation, acquired renal cystic disease, adenoma (all papillary type), RCC, and oncocytoma were found in 33%, 14%, 4.2%, and 0.6% of cases, respectively. These incidences are based on pathology examinations of removed kidneys which were sliced at 0.5-cm intervals. RCCs were detected in 4.2% (11/260); six (55%) were clear cell type with cystic changes in three cases. Four of the remaining cases, including one case that also had a coexisting clear cell RCC, were papillary type (three type 1, two type 2); and the remaining case was chromophobe RCC. In general, however, RCCs associated with end-stage renal disease (Fig. 2-13-5), are predominantly the papillary type, accounting for 42%–86% of cancers [21, 22].

Generally, patients with preexisting solid organ malignancies are deferred from renal transplantation for at least 2 years after treatment of the malignancy. However, data from the Cincinnati Tumor Registry reveals that an incidentally detected RCC with no capsular invasion is at very low risk for recurrence after transplantation, and no waiting period is recommended in this selected group of patients [23, 24].

What seems to be the mechanism involved in cancer development in patients with acquired renal cystic disease? Histologic examination of kidneys reveals three types of cysts: those lined by flat, cuboi-

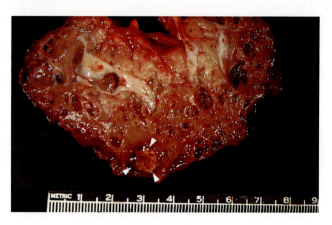

Fig. 2-13-5. Acquired cystic renal disease after hemodialysis. There are many cysts in this atrophic kidney. Note a small renal cell carcinoma (*arrowheads*). (Case provided by Michael Pins, MD, Northwestern University Feinberg School of Medicine, Chicago)

dal, or hyperplastic epithelium, progressing to micropapillary hyperplasia [21, 25]. Increased proliferative activity has been demonstrated in hyperplastic cysts [26]. Expression of hepatocyte growth factor (HGF) and its receptor oncogene MET is demonstrated in the hyperplastic epithelia by immunohistochemistry and reverse transcription–polymerase chain reaction (RT-PCR) [25]. Expression of these proto-oncogenes is not specific to end-stage cystic disease-associated cancer as they are also expressed in sporadic RCCs of various types [27, 28], including the hereditary form of papillary RCC in which germline mutation is found in the MET gene [29].

Trisomies of chromosomes 7 and 17 are observed in most of the sporadic papillary RCCs. Houghson et al. [21] analyzed chromosomes 7 and 17 in papillary carcinomas in end-stage renal disease kidneys. Trisomies of these chromosomes, both or either, were found in 8 of 14 cases studied; no changes were demonstrated in the remaining 6. These findings suggest that a different genetic mechanism, in addition to the conventional mechanism, may underlie the development of many papillary carcinomas developing in end-stage renal disease-associated kidneys.

References

1. Israel GM, Hindman N, Bosniak MA (2004) Evaluation of cystic renal masses: comparison of CT and MR by using the Bosniak classification system. Radiology 231:365–371.
2. Picken MM, Antic T, Jahoda A, Damos T, Campbell SC (2005) Cystic adult renal lesions: radiologic and

pathologic correlations. Mod Pathol 18(suppl 1): 158A.

3. Terada N, Ichioka K, Matsuta Y, Okubo K, Yoshimura K, Arai Y (2002) The natural history of simple renal cysts. J Urol 167:21–23.

4. WHO (2004) WHO classification of tumours of the kidney. In: Eble JN, Sauter G, Epstein JI, Sesterhenn IA (eds) Tumours of the urinary system and male genital organs. IARC Press, Lyon, p 10.

5. Murad T, Komaiko W, Oyasu R, Bauer K (1991) Multilocular cystic renal cell carcinoma. Am J Clin Pathol 95:633–637.

6. Eble JN (2005) Cystic tumors of the kidney. In: 2005 Companion Meeting Syllabus, United States and Canadian Academy of Pathology Annual Meeting, San Antonio.

7. Fuhrman SA, Lasky LC, Limas C (1982) Prognostic significance of morphologic parameters in renal cell carcinoma. Am J Surg Pathol 6:655–663.

8. Mukhopadhay S, Valente AL, de la Roza G (2004) Cystic nephroma: a histologic and immunohistochemical study of 10 cases. Arch Pathol Lab Med 128: 1404–1411.

9. Castillo OA, Boyle Jr ET, Kramer SA (1991) Multilocular cysts of kidney: a study of 29 patients and review of literature. Urology 37:156–162.

10. Davila RM, Kissane JM, Crouch EC (1992) Multilocular cyst: immunohistochemical and lectin-binding study. Am J Surg Pathol 16:508–514.

11. Murphy WM, Grignon DJ, Perlman EJ (2004) Tumors of the kidney, bladder, and related urinary structures. In: AFIP atlas of tumor pathology, Series 4. American Registry of Pathology. Washington, DC, pp 53–55.

12. Turbiner J, Amin MB, Radhakrishnan A, Humphrey PA, Srigley JR, De Leval L, Oliva E (2005) Cystic nephroma (CN) and mixed epithelial and stromal tumor (MEST) of the kidney: are they one and the same entity? Mod Pathol 18(suppl 1):169A.

13. Jevremovic D, Lager DJ, Lewin ML (2005) Cystic nephroma and mixer epithelial and stromal tumor of the kidney: a spectrum of the same entity? Mod Pathol 18(suppl l):148A.

14. Antic T, Fresco R, Pins MR, Picken MM (2005) Mixed epithelial and stromal tumor of the kidney vs adult cystic nephroma: one or two entities? Reappraisal of 14 lesions. Mod Pathol 18(suppl 1):127A.

15. Turbiner J, Amin, MB, Humphrey PA, Srigley JR, de Val L, Radhakrishnan A, Oliva E (2007) Cystic nephroma and mixed epithelial and stromal tumor of kidney: a detailed clinicopathologic analysis of 34 cases and proposal for renal epithelial and stromal tumor (REST) as a unifying term. Am J Surg Pathol 31: 489–500.

16. Adsay NV, Eble JN, Srigley JR, Jones EC, Grignon DJ (2000) Mixed epithelial and stromal tumor of the kidney. Am J Surg Pathol 24:958–970.

17. Joshi VV, Banerjee AK, Yadav K, Pathak IC (1997) Cystic partially differentiated nephroblastoma: a clinicopathologic entity in the spectrum of infantile renal neoplasia. Cancer 40:789–795.

18. Truong LD, Bhuvaneswari K, Cao JTH, Barrios R, Suki WN (1995) Renal neoplasm in acquired cystic kidney disease. Am J Kidney Dis 26:1–12.

19. Matson MA, Cohen EP (1990) Acquired cystic kidney disease: occurrence, prevalence, and renal cancers. Medicine (Baltimore) 69:217–226.

20. Denton MD, Magee CC, Ovuworie C, Mayiyyedi S, Pascual M, Colvin RB, Cosimi AB, Tolkoff-Rubin N (2002) Prevalence of renal cell carcinoma in patients with ESRD pre-transplantation: a pathologic analysis. Kidney Int 61:2201–2209.

21. Hughson MD, Bigler S, Dickman K, Kovacs G (1999) Renal cell carcinoma of end-stage renal disease: analysis of chromosomes 3, 7, and 17 abnormalities by microsatellite amplification. Mod Pathol 12:301–309.

22. Chudek J, Herbers J, Wilhelm M, Bugert P, Ritz E, Waldman F, Kovacs G (1998) The genetics of renal tumors in end-stage renal failures differs from those occurring in the general population. J Am Soc Nephrol 9:1045–1051.

23. Gulanikar AC, Daily PP, Kilambi NK, Hamrick-Turner JE, Butkus DE (1998) Prospective pretransplant ultrasound screening in 206 patients for acquired renal cysts and renal cell carcinoma. Transplantation 66:1669–1672.

24. Goldbarb DA, Neumann HPH, Penn I, Novick AC (1997) Results of renal transplantation in patients with renal cell carcinoma and von Hippel-Lindau disease. Transplantation 64:1726–1729.

25. Konda R, Sato H, Hatafuku F, Nozawa T, Ioritani N, Fujioka T (2004) Expression of hepatocyte growth factor and its receptor c-met in acquired renal cystic disease associated with renal cell carcinoma. J Urol 171:2166–2170.

26. Nadasdy T, Laszik Z, Lajoie G, Blick KE, Wheeler DE, Silva FG (1995) Proliferative activity of cyst epithelium in human renal cystic disease. J Am Soc Nephrol 5:1462–1468.

27. Horie S, Aruga S, Kawamata H, Okui N, Kakizoe T, Kitamura T (1999) Biological role of HGF/MET in renal cell carcinoma. J Urol 161:990–997.

28. Pisters L, El-Nagger AK, Luo W, Malpica A, Lin S-Hm (1997) C-*met* proto-oncogene expression in benign and malignant renal tissues. J Urol 158:724–728.

29. Schmidt L, Duh F-M, Chen F, Kishida T, Glenn G, Choyke P, Scherer SW, Zhuang Z, Lubensky I, Dean M, Allikmets R, Chidambaram A, Bergerheim UR, Feltis JT, Casadevall C, Zamarron A, Bernues M, Richard S, Lips CJM, Walther MM, Tsui L-C, Geil L, Orcutt ML, StackhouseT, Lipan J, Slife L, Brauch H, Decker J, Niehans G, Hughson MD, Moch H, Storkel S, Lerman MI, Linehan WM, Zbar B (1997) Germline and somatic mutations in the tyrosine kinase domain of the *met* proto-oncogene in papillary renal carcinomas. Nat Genet 16:68–73.

Question 14

Is angiomyolipoma a neoplasm or a hamartoma? Does cytologic atypia seen in angiomyolipomas denote aggressive behavior? Does an angiomyolipoma need treatment if it is benign? What is the indication for surgical intervention if it is required?

role in the preoperative diagnosis, but the role may be limited because of the difficulty of finding HMB45-positive cells in the tumor. Hemorrhage, as one of the major clinical complications, is seen more commonly in patients with tumors >4 cm. Therefore, for a renal tumor that is a possible angiomyolipoma, surgical treatment should be considered.

Answer

Renal angiomyolipoma is a benign neoplasm, not a hamartoma. Angiomyolipoma may be included in a group of tumors of perivascular epithelioid cells (PEComas). Renal angiomyolipoma occurs as either a sporadic form or a hereditary form as a part of syndrome of tuberous sclerosis.

Although cytologic atypia can be seen in this tumor, it is usually not associated with aggressive biologic behavior. True malignant angiomyolipoma is extremely rare, with only a few case reports in the literature. However, a subset of epithelioid variants of angiomyolipoma may exhibit aggressive behavior. Nevertheless, the diagnosis of malignant angiomyolipoma should be restricted to a case with obvious malignant features, such as metastasis, in addition to significant cytologic atypia.

The preoperative diagnosis of renal angiomyolipoma is difficult and not reliable. Radiographic findings may suggest the diagnosis of an angiomyolipoma only if fat tissue is observed by CT or MRI. However, many angiomyolipomas have a limited lipomatous component, which makes radiographic diagnosis impossible. Fine-needle biopsy and needle core biopsy may also have a

Comments

Angiomyolipoma (AML) is one of a few common benign renal tumors that we encounter in our practice. The other benign tumors are adenoma and oncocytoma, which have been discussed under Questions 1 and 4. AML occurs in two forms: as a sporadic disease and as part of tuberous sclerosis. It may arise in association with several histologically related tumors under the umbrella of PEComa.

Concept of PEComa

Bonetti et al. [1] in 1992 proposed that a group of tumors have a common origin in the perivascular epithelioid cells (PECs). The hypothesis was based on the observation that a group of vessel-rich spindle cell/clear cell tumors have one thing in common; that is, they are all reactive to the melanogenesis marker antibody HMB45. To date, the normal counterpart of the PEC has not been identified [1]. This family of tumors shows a spectrum of cells from epithelioid to spindle cells with clear to eosinophilic cytoplasm, many of which are arranged in a perivascular distribution [2]. It is not conclusive from molecular studies that these PEComas are actually related, although they share some morphologic and immunohistochemical features.

Ultrastructurally, these tumors characteristically show premelanosomes [3, 4]. In common with all tumors of this family is the cytoplasmic staining reaction to HMB45, a melanoma-specific monoclonal antibody and a variable staining reaction to the antibodies for smooth muscle actin and negative reactivity for epithelial markers and vimentin [2]. Several histologic subtypes exist. They are angiomyolipoma, lymphangiomyoma (Fig. 2-14-1), the clear cell "sugar" tumor (Fig. 2-14-2), and others, so-called PEComas, not otherwise specified. As stated already, the seemingly morphologically different tumors have one thing in common—a positive reaction to HMB45.

Angiomyolipoma is the prototype of PEComas and the most common one. It characteristically consists of three types of cell: smooth muscle cells, fat cells, and vessels. The smooth muscle cells are typically not mature-looking as one would expect in a hamartoma. Recently, it was shown that all cell types are clonal [5, 6], which indicates that AML is a neoplasm rather than a hamartoma.

Bonetti et al. [1] hypothesized that PECs have the potential to differentiate into three morphologic cell types: spindle cells (smooth muscle cell type), adipocytes, and epithelioid round clear-to-eosinophilic cells (Fig. 2-14-3). AML occurs most commonly in the kidney but also has been observed at other sites including the liver [7–9], retroperitoneum [10], retroperitoneal lymph nodes [11], lung [12], cardiac atrium [13], spleen [14], and colon [15]. Its modified form, generally referred to as PEComa, is found at various sites, including the falciform ligament and ligamentum teres of the liver [16], pancreas [17], prostate [18], bladder [19], uterus [20], rectum [4], ileum [4], vulva [4], heart [4], bile duct [2], skull base [21], and soft tissue [16, 22, 23].

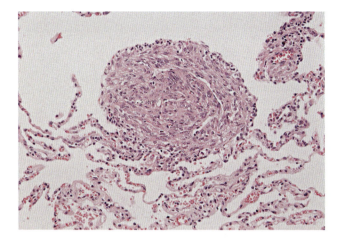

FIG. 2-14-1. Lymphangiomyoma of lung. The patient, a woman in her thirties, developed progressive dyspnea on exertion. Chest computed tomography (CT) scan demonstrated multiple minute nodules present throughout both lung fields. An open biopsy revealed subpleural nodules composed of smooth muscle cells in alveolar septa. The cells were positive to HMB45 (not shown). Subsequently, she was found to have an abnormal brain CT scan suggestive of tuberous sclerosis lesions. (Case provided by Yukinori Inadome, MD, Tsukuba Medical Center Hospital, Tsukuba, Japan)

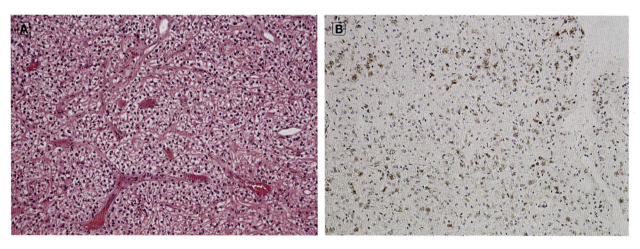

FIG. 2-14-2. "Sugar tumor" of the lung. The patient, a 43-year-old man who had had one testis removed for seminoma 9 years previously, was found to have a pulmonary coin lesion on a routine checkup. An open biopsy revealed a small discrete nodule. **A** The tumor is vascular and consists of clear cells in a lobular architecture. The cells are positive to PAS stain but negative after diastase digestion, proving that the PAS-positive material is glycogen. **B** Scattered tumor cells are positive to HMB45. The patient has no renal mass that suggests renal cell carcinoma

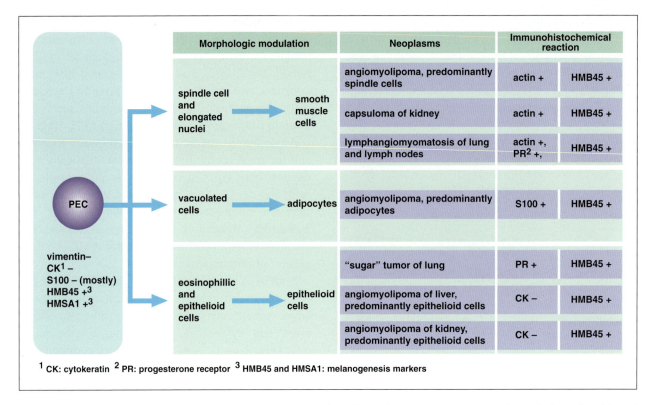

	Morphologic modulation		Neoplasms	Immunohistochemical reaction	
PEC	spindle cell and elongated nuclei	smooth muscle cells	angiomyolipoma, predominantly spindle cells	actin +	HMB45 +
			capsuloma of kidney	actin +	HMB45 +
			lymphangiomyomatosis of lung and lymph nodes	actin +, PR[2] +,	HMB45 +
	vacuolated cells	adipocytes	angiomyolipoma, predominantly adipocytes	S100 +	HMB45 +
	eosinophillic and epithelioid cells	epithelioid cells	"sugar" tumor of lung	PR +	HMB45 +
			angiomyolipoma of liver, predominantly epithelioid cells	CK −	HMB45 +
			angiomyolipoma of kidney, predominantly epithelioid cells	CK −	HMB45 +

vimentin−
CK[1] −
S100 − (mostly)
HMB45 +[3]
HMSA1 +[3]

[1] CK: cytokeratin [2] PR: progesterone receptor [3] HMB45 and HMSA1: melanogenesis markers

Fig. 2-14-3. Histogenetic mechanism of perivascular epithelioid cell neoplasms *(PEComas)*. The figure is formulated based on the proposal by Bonetti et al. [1]

The PEComas that occur in the lung are lymphangiomyoma and "sugar" tumor. The names are still commonly being used because they were assigned before the concept of PEComa was proposed. "Sugar" tumor reportedly occurs at extrapulmonary sites as well [4, 17, 24]. It is to be noted that "sugar" tumor has features overlapping with PEComas. Most PEComas, particularly AML, are benign, although rare cases behave as malignant tumors. It is also to be noted that AML and some other forms of PEComas, such as lymphangiomyoma, may occur in lymph nodes, but it does not indicate metastasis.

Molecular Mechanism Involving Tuberous Sclerosis Cluster *(TSC)* Genes 1 and 2

Tuberous sclerosis (TS) is an autosomal dominant disorder characterized by seizures, mental retardation, and a number of lesions typical of TS, including cerebral cortical tumors and subependymal giant cell astrocytomas, rhabdomyomas in the heart, angiofibromas of the skin and periungal fibromas, and angiomyolipoma of the kidney [25, 26]. Genetically, disease-determining genes for TS have been posi-

tioned on chromosomes 9 [27] and 16 [28]. In 1993, the gene on chromosome 16 was identified and characterized by the European Chromosome 16 Tuberous Sclerosis Consortium [29]. Discovery of the loss of heterozygosity (LOH) in the *TSC1* and *TSC2* genomic regions in TS lesions suggested that the *TSC* genes act as tumor suppressor genes [30–34]. Approximately one-half of TS families demonstrate linkage to *TSC1* and another half to *TSC2*. Hamartin, the product of the *TSC1* gene, is strongly expressed in various normal tissues including the proximal and distal tubules of the kidney. The expression pattern of tuberin, a product of the *TSC2* gene, is almost identical to that of hamartin, consistent with the recent finding that tuberin and hamartin interact directly. In *TSC*-linked AMLs, two types of immunoreactivity were observed as the manifestation of gene mutation: tumors lacking the expression of either hamartin or tuberin [35]. This suggests that tuberin and hamartin function in the same molecular pathway, leading to the nearly indistinguishable clinical phenotypes of the *TSC1*- and *TSC2*-linked disease [35]. The gene mutations are observed in both sporadic and *TSC*-linked lesions at varying frequency. In the TS patients, the allelic loss rates vary; LOH was observed in 56% of renal AMLs but in only 4% of brain lesions (cortical tuber and subependymal giant cell astrocytoma) [34].

Pathologic Features of AML

Angiomyolipoma most commonly occurs in the renal parenchyma. It may arise in the renal cortex and medulla or occasionally from stromal nodules associated with the renal capsule [36]. Grossly, typical AMLs range from yellow (abundant fat cells) to pink-tan (abundant smooth muscle cells), depending on the relative proportion of smooth muscle and fat cells. They are well demarcated from the surrounding renal parenchyma (Fig. 2-14-4). When multiple AMLs are present and coalesce, the gross appearance may resemble infiltration by renal cell carcinoma [36]. Multiple tumors and bilateral involvement should alert the pathologist to the possibility of TSC. Infrequently, renal AML invades the intrarenal venous system, the renal vein/inferior vena cava (RV/IVC) and even the right atrium of the heart [37]. Multifocality and vascular invasion should not be interpreted as evidence of malignancy; the prognosis is invariably favorable following nephrectomy and removal of tumor thrombi [36, 38].

A typical AML consists of a mixture of smooth muscle cells of variable maturity, fat, and abnormal blood vessels (Fig. 2-14-5). Fat cells are of mature (adult) type, but lipoblasts may be found [39]. Smooth muscle cells are arranged in fascicles. However, some AMLs consist almost entirely of relatively normal-appearing smooth muscle and mimic leiomyoma or leiomyosarcoma [40, 41], whereas some with extensive lipid accumulation may resemble lipomas or well-differentiated liposarcomas [42, 43].

Several types of morphologically different vessels are observed in AML. The most typical are thick-walled collagenized vessels that resemble arteries and are a neoplastic component of AML. These vessels are deficient in the elastic layers (Fig. 2-14-5B) and are believed to be responsible for rupture, leading to bleeding that requires an emergency nephrectomy.

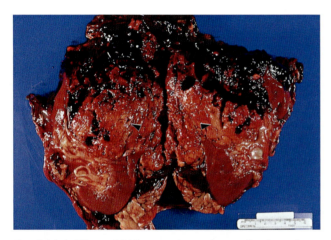

Fig. 2-14-4. Bisected kidney to show a hemorrhagic angiomyolipoma (*arrowheads*). This woman came in with a sudden onset of abdominal pain and hypovolemic shock. At operation a massive hemorrhage from the tumor was discovered

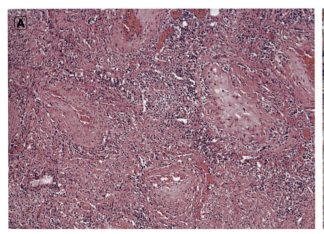
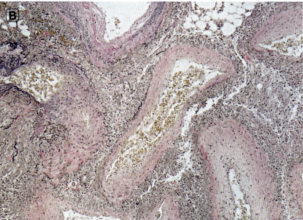

Fig. 2-14-5. Angiomyolipoma of the kidney. **A** In this field several partly collagenized thick-walled vessels are distributed in a smooth muscle background. **B** Elastica-Van Gieson-stained section reveals these vessels to be only partly decorated by an elastic layer

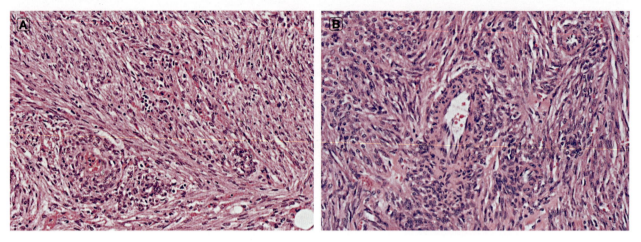

FIG. 2-14-6. **A, B** Angiomyolipoma. In these fields, smooth muscle cells are arranged in whorls and streams around vessels. Note that the smooth muscle cells form a cuff around vessels, a feature of perivascular arrangement of cells supporting the PEComa concept

The smooth muscle cells are typically spindle cells; their nuclei are small and regular and lack mitotic activity. Often, smooth muscle cells form a cuff around these vessels, merging in the surrounding smooth muscle cells (Fig. 2-14-6), and giving the appearance of spinning around vessels. This is a typical feature of PEComa cells, arranged in a perivascular distribution [2]. It is not unusual to see smooth muscle cells with enlarged, irregular atypical nuclei with enlarged nucleoli [36]. Mitotic figures may be present in these cells. Although alarming, the presence of cytologic atypia in AMLs does not alter their benign behavior.

A malignant form of AML, though rare, has been reported in the world literature. More recently, AML with foci composed of epithelioid cells has been reported. Instead of a spindle shape, smooth muscle cells become round to polygonal and have either clear (Fig. 2-14-7) or eosinophilic (Fig. 2-14-8), cytoplasm, resembling RCCs. Epithelioid cells may be separated by hyaline cords and accompanied by foamy macrophages (Figs. 2-14-8, 2-14-9) [44]. Only a subset of epithelioid AMLs take an aggressive clinical course.

Biologic Features of AML and Management Considerations

The AMLs occur in about 50%–70% of patients with tuberous sclerosis [45, 46], although it accounts for only a small number of AMLs encountered in daily practice. In contrast to the sporadic form of AML,

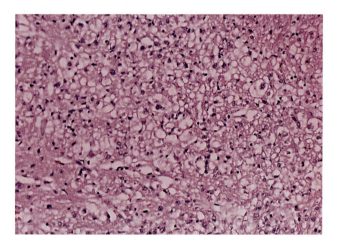

FIG. 2-14-7. Epithelioid angiomyolipoma. The patient is a 54-year-old woman. In this field, polygonal epithelioid cells in sheets make up the lesion

familial AMLs are typically multiple, bilateral, and involve younger patients. Most AMLs behave in a benign fashion and are asymptomatic. The only well-known complication is massive bleeding, which leads to hypovolemic shock [47] (Fig. 2-14-4). The defect or lack in the elastic layers in the walls of vessels is believed to be responsible for the bleeding (Fig. 2-14-5). The risk of hemorrhage is minor in tumors <4 cm in diameter but rises to more than 50% for tumors any larger than that [48].

In a small fraction of AMLs, the smooth muscle cells show an "epithelioid" appearance (Figs. 2-14-7, 2-14-8), and it is not uncommon for these cells to

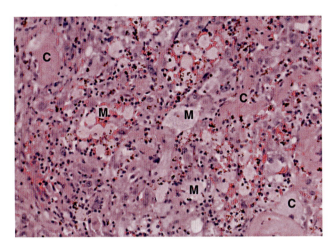

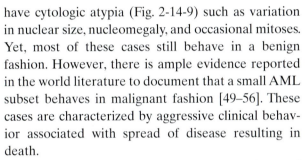

FIG. 2-14-8. Epithelioid angiomyolipoma. The patient is a 54-year-old woman. She had multiple angiomyolipomas but no tuberous sclerosis. In this field, the tumor cells are eosinophilic and epithelioid and are accompanied by foamy macrophages (*M*) and collagenous islands (*C*)

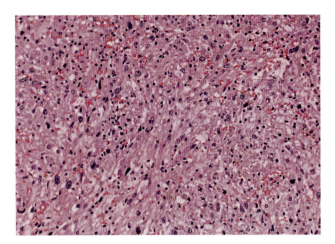

FIG. 2-14-9. Epithelioid angiomyolipoma: The patient is a 97-year-old man. Microhematuria led to the discovery of the tumor. Segmental resection was performed. In this field the tumor is made up of eosinophilic spindle and epithelioid cells. Note the scattered cells with atypical nuclei

have cytologic atypia (Fig. 2-14-9) such as variation in nuclear size, nucleomegaly, and occasional mitoses. Yet, most of these cases still behave in a benign fashion. However, there is ample evidence reported in the world literature to document that a small AML subset behaves in malignant fashion [49–56]. These cases are characterized by aggressive clinical behavior associated with spread of disease resulting in death.

Microscopically, malignant AMLs are made up of spindle to highly atypical round "epithelioid" cells with large nuclei, large nucleoli, and frequent mitotic figures, some of which are atypical, in addition to areas of typical AML. Furthermore, in a few of the purported cases of malignant AML, the fat cells and abnormal vessels characteristic of AML are absent [54]. They are referred to as "carcinoma-like monotypic epithelioid AML" [51]. It is important to point out that AML may be associated with clear cell RCC [51, 57]. Thus, differentiation from the sarcomatoid variant of RCC becomes necessary. Despite an epithelioid histologic appearance, epithelioid AML cells are negative for low/high-molecular-weight keratin (AE1/AE3), epithelial membrane antigen (EMA), and CAM 5.2 (markers of RCC) and positive for HMB4 and smooth muscle actin (markers of AML) (Fig. 2-14-2B). However, conflicting immunohistochemical results have been reported for epithelioid cells co-expressing epithelial cell markers and HMB45 [53, 58] or for tumors that have lost HMB45 reactiv-

ity after recurrence [51]. To account for this perplexing phenomenon, Cibas et al. [54] proposed that some true malignant AMLs may become HMB45-negative with antigenic drift seen when the tumor dedifferentiates. Furthermore, some even express paradoxical "linage-incorrect" antigens, such as EMA and cytokeratins. Nevertheless, the diagnosis of a malignant AML requires negative-staining epithelial markers and positive HMB45 staining [52] in addition to apparently malignant behavior.

Angiomyolipoma as a sporadic form is usually small and remains asymptomatic. AMLs in TSC patients are usually described as small, multiple, and bilateral. However, both forms may become large and symptomatic. The most common symptom is abdominal pain caused by hemorrhage in the tumor. This is not surprising because these tumors are highly vascular and have structurally highly abnormal vessels (vide supra). In 10% of the cases, the bleeding may be so severe that it leads to hypovolemic shock [59]. Steiner et al. [60] of Johns Hopkins University made a prospective study of 24 patients with AML, both sporadic and TSC-associated. Those with tumors <4 cm were less likely to be symptomatic (24%) whereas those with tumors >4 cm were more often symptomatic (52%). With a mean follow-up time of 4 years, all patients with tumors <4 cm (*n* = 15) remained asymptomatic, although one required nephrectomy. Among tumors >4 cm (*n* = 13), seven required surgical treatments (partial nephrectomy in two patients and total nephrectomy in five). The indications for surgery were pain in six patients, hematuria/hemorrhage in three, to rule out RCC in two, and shock in one. Altogether, 27% of AMLs < 4 cm and 46% of tumors >4 cm grew during the study period. Patients with TSC and AMLs are different from patients with sporadic AMLs; they tended to present at a younger age, had a higher incidence of bilateral renal tumors, were more symptomatic, and had larger tumors that were more likely to grow and require surgical interventions. Based on the study, their recommendation was as follows: Patients with an isolated AML that is <4 cm may be followed conservatively with yearly CT or US study. It is not clear, however, if RCC can be reliably excluded from this group of patients carrying an AML diagnosis. Patients with an isolated AML > 4 cm can be divided into two groups. Those who are asymptomatic or mildly symptomatic may still be followed conservatively with semiannual CT or US study. If any significant growth is seen, even without symptoms, embolization of the tumor or nephron-sparing surgery should be considered. Those with an AML > 4 cm, and with severe symptoms (bleeding or uncontrollable pain) should undergo nephron-sparing surgery or embolization. Van Baal et al. [61], based on a 5-year follow-up, came to a similar conclusion: AMLs > 3.5 cm have a substantial risk for severe hemorrhage, and therefore an aggressive approach is advised.

In summary, renal angiomyolipoma is a benign tumor with many histologic appearances. The malignant variant is rare. Angiomyolipomas >4 cm, even with benign histology, can cause massive hemorrhage and should be treated surgically.

References

1. Bonetti F, Pea M, Martrigoni G, Zamboni G, Manfrin E, Clombari R, Mariuzzi E (1997) The perivascular epithelioid cell related lesions. Adv Anat Pathol 4:343–358.
2. Sadeghi S, Krigman H, Maluf H (2004) Perivascular epithelioid clear cell tumor of the common bile duct. Am J Surg Pathol 28:1107–1110.
3. Folpe AL, Goodman ZP, Ishak KG, Paulino AFG, Taboada EM, Meehan SA, Weiss SW (2000) Clear cell myomelanocytic tumor of the falciform/ligamentum teres. Am J Surg Pathol 24:1239–1246.
4. Tazelaar HD, Batts KP, Srigely JR (2001) Primary extrapulmonary sugar tumor (PEST): a report of four cases. Mod Pathol 14:615–622.
5. Cheng L, Gu JN, Eble JN, Bostwick DG, Younger C, MacLennan GT, Abdul-Karim FW, Geary WA, Koch MO, Zhang S, Ulbright TM (2001) Molecular genetic evidence for different clonal origin of components of human renal angiomyolipomas. Am J Surg Pathol 25:1231–1236.
6. Paradis V, Laurendeau I, Vieillefond A, Blanchet P, Eshwege P, Benoit G, Vidaud M, Jardin A, Bedossa P (1998) Clonal analysis of renal sporadic angiomyolipoma. Hum Pathol 29:1063–1067.
7. Goodman ZD, Ishak KG (1984) Angiomyolipoma of the liver. Am J Surg Pathol 8:745–750.
8. Tsui WMS, Colombari R, Portmann BC, Bonetti F, Thung SN, Ferrel LD, Nakanuma Y, Snover DC, Bioulac-Sage P, Dhillon AP (1999) Hepatic angiomyolipoma: a clinicopathologic study of 30 cases and delineation of unusual morphologic variants. Am J Surg Pathol 23:34–48.
9. Terris B, Flejou J-F, Picot R, Belghiti J, Heninn D (1996) Hepatic angiomyolipoma: a report of four cases with immunohistochemical and DNA-flow cytometric studies. Arch Pathol Lab Med 1120:68–72.
10. Hruban RH, Bhagavan BS, Epstein JI (1989) Massive retroperitoneal angiomyolipoma: a lesion that may be confused with well-differentiated liposarcoma. Am J Clin Pathol 92:805–808.
11. Bloom DA, Scardino PT, Ehrlich RM, Waisman J (1982) The significance of lymph node involvement in renal angiomyolipoma. J Urol 128:1292–1295.
12. Guinee DG, Thornberry DS, Azumi N, Przygodzki RM, Koss MN, Travis WD (1995) Unique pulmonary presentation of an angiomyolipoma: analysis of clinical, radiographic, and histologic features. Am J Surg Pathol 19:476–480.
13. Shimizu M, Manabe T, Tazelaar HD, Hirokawa S, Moriya T, Ito J, Hamanaka S, Hata T (1994) Intramyocardial angiomyolipoma. Am J Surg Pathol 18:1164–1169.
14. Hulbert JC, Graf R (1983) Involvement of the spleen by renal angiomyolipoma: metastasis or multicentricity? J Urol 130:328–329.
15. Maluf H, Dieckgraefe B (1999) Angiomyolipoma of the large intestine: report of a case. Mod Pathol 12:1132–1136.
16. Folpe AL, McKenney JK, Li Z, Smith SJ, Weiss SW (2002) Clear cell myomelanocytic tumor of the thigh: report of a unique case. Am J Surg Pathol 26:809–812.
17. Zamboni G, Pea M, Martignoni G, Zancanaro C, Faccioli G, Gilioli E, Pederzoli P, Bonetto F (1996) Clear cell "sugar" tumor of the pancreas: a novel member of the family of lesions characterized by the presence of perivascular epithelioid cells. Am J Surg Pathol 20:722–730.
18. Pan CC, Yang AH, Chang H (2003A) Malignant perivascular epithelioid cell tumor ("PEComa") involving the prostate. Arch Pathol Lab Med 127:e96–e98.
19. Pan C-C, Yu I-T, Chang H (2003B) Clear cell myomelanocytic tumor of the urinary bladder. Am J Surg Pathol 27:689–692.

20. Vang R, Kempson RL (2002) Perivascular epithelioid cell tumor ("PEComa") of the uterus: a subset of HMB-45 positive epithelioid mesenchymal neoplasms with an uncertain relationship to pure smooth muscle tumors. Am J Surg Pathol 26:1–13.

21. Lehman NL (2004) Malignant PEComa of the skull base. Am J Surg Pathol 28:11230–1232.

22. Harris GC, McCulloch TA, Perks G, Fisher C (2004) Malignant perivascular epithelioid cell tumor ("PEComa") of soft tissue. Am J Surg Pathol 28: 1655-1658

23. Govender D, Sabaratnam RM, Essa AS (2002) Clear cell "sugar" tumor of the breast; another extrapulmonary site and review of the literature. Am J Surg Pathol 26:670–675.

24. Gomez MR (1991) Phenotypes of the tuberous sclerosis complex with a revision of diagnostic criteria. Ann NY Acad Sci 615:1–7.

25. Kwiatkowski DJ, Short MP (1994) Tuberous sclerosis. Arch Derm 130:348–354.

26. Fryer AE, Chalmers A, Conner JM, Fraser I, Povey S, Yates AD, Yates JRW, Osterling JP (1987) Evidence that the gene for tuberous sclerosis is on chromosome Lancet 1:659–661.

27. Kandt RS, Haines JL, Smith M, Northrup H, Gardner EJM, Short MP, Dumars K, Roach ES, Steingold S, Wall S, Blanton SH, Flodman P, Kwiat Kowski DJ, Jerwell A, Weber JL, Koses AD, Pericak-Vance MA (1992) Linkage of an important gene locus for tuberous sclerosis to a chromosome 16 marker for polycystic kidney disease. Nat Genet 2:37–41.

28. The European Chromosome 16 Tuberous Sclerosis Consortium (1993) Identification and characterization of the tuberous sclerosis gene on chromosome 16. Cell 75:1305–1315.

29. Carbonara C, Longa L, Grosso E, Borrone C, Garre MG, Brisigotti M, Bigone N (1994) 9q34 loss of heterozygosity in a tuberous sclerosis astrocytoma suggests a growth suppressor-like activity also for the TSC gene. Hum Mol Genet 3:1829–1832.

30. Green AJ, Johnson PH, Yates JRW (1994) The tuberous sclerosis gene on chromosome 9q34 acts as a growth-suppressor. Hum Mol Genet 6:1833–1834.

31. Green AJ, Smith M, Yates JRW (1994) Loss of heterozygosity on chromosome 16p13.3 in harmartomas from tuberous sclerosis patients. Nat Genet 6:193–196.

32. Henske EP, Neumann HPH, Scheitehauer BW, Herbst EW, Short MP, Kwiatkowski DJ (1995) Loss of heterozygosity in the tuberous sclerosis (TSC2) region of chromosomal band 16p13 occurs in sporadic as well as TSC-associated renal angiomyolipoma. Genes Chromosome Cancer 13:295–298.

33. Henske EP, Scheithauer BW, Short MP, Wollmann R, Nahmias J, Hornigold N, van Slegtenhorst M, Welsh CT, Kwiatkowski DJ (1996) Allelic loss is frequent in tuberous sclerosis kidney lesions but rare in brain lesions. Am J Hum Genet 59:400–406.

34. Plank TL, Logginidou H, Klein-Szanto A, Henske EP (1999) The expression of hamartin, the product of the TSC1 gene, in normal human tissues and in the TSC1-

35. Eble JN (1998A) Angiomyolipoma of kidney. Semin Diagn Pathol 15:21–40.

36. Rothenberg DM, Brandt TD, D'Cruz I (1986) Computed tomography of renal angiomyolipoma presenting as right atrial mass. J Comput Assist Tomogr 10:1054–1056.

37. Game X, Soule M, Moussouni S, Roux D, Escourrou G, Chevreau C, Aziza R (2003) Renal angiomyolipoma associated with rapid enlargement and inferior vena caval tumor thrombus. J Urol 170:918–919.

38. Farrow GM, Harrison EG Jr, Utz DC, Jones DR (1968) Renal angiomyolipoma: a clinicopathologic study of 32 cases. Cancer 22:564–570.

39. Bonsib SM (1996) HMB45 reactivity in renal leiomyomas and leiomyosarcomas. Mod Pathol 9:664–660.

40. Nonomura A, Minato H, Kurumaya H (1998) Angiomyolipoma predominantly composed of smooth muscles: problems in histological diagnosis. Histopathology 33:20–27.

41. L'Hostis H, Deminire C, Ferriere JM, Coindre J-M (1999) Renal angiomyolipoma; a clinicopathologic, immunohistochemical, and follow-up study of 46 cases. Am J Surg Pathol 23:1011–1020.

42. Wang LJ, Lim KE, Wong YC, Chen CJ (1997) Giant retroperitoneal angiomyolipoma mimicking liposarcoma. Br J Urol 79:1001–1002.

43. Eble JN, Amin MB, Young RH (1997) Epithelioid angiomyolipoma of the kidney: a report of five cases with a prominent and diagnostically confusing epithelioid smooth muscle component. Am J Surg Pathol 21:1123–1130.

44. Stillwell TJ, Logginidou H, Klein-Szanto A, Henske EP (1999) The expression of hamartin, the product of the TSC1 gene, in normal human tissues and in the TSC1- and TSC2-linked angiomyolipoma. Mod Pathol 12:539–545.

45. Carsillo T, Arstirinisis A, Henske EP (2000) Mutations in the tuberous sclerosis complex gene TSC2 are a cause of sporadic pulmonary lymphangioleiomyomatosis. Proc Natl Acad Aci U S A 97:6085–6090.

46. Gomez MR (1991) Phenotypes of the tuberous sclerosis complex with a revision of diagnostic criteria. Ann N Y Acad Sci 615:1–7.

47. Oesterling JE, Fishman EK, Goldman SM, Marshall FF (1986) The management of renal angiomyolipoma. J Urol 135:1121–1124.

48. Ferry JA, Malt RA, Young RH (1991) Renal angiomyolipoma with sarcomatoid differentiation and pulmonary metastasis. Am J Surg Pathol 15:1083–1088.

49. Yamamoto T, Ito k, Suzuki K, Yamanaka H, Ebihara K, Sasaki A (2002) Rapidly progressive malignant epithelioid angiomyolipoma of the kidney. J Urol 168:190–191.

50. Martignoni G, Pea M, Bonetti F, Zamboni G, Carbonara C, Longa L, Zancanaro C, Maran M, Brisigotti M, Mariuzzi GM (1998) Carcinoma-like monotypic epithelioid angiomyolipoma in patients without evidence of tuberous sclerosis. Am J Surg Pathol 22:663–672.

51. Martignoni G, Pea M, Rigaud G, Manfrin E, Colato C, Zamboni G, Scarpa A, Tardanico R, Roncalli M, Bonetti F (2000) Renal angiomyolipoma with epithelioid sarcomatous transformation and metastasis: demonstration of the same genetic defects in the primary and metastatic lesions. Am J Surg Pathol 24:889–894.

52. Pea M, Bonetti F, Martignoni G, Henske EP, Manfrin E, Colato C, Berstein J (1998) Apparent renal cell carcinomas in tuberous sclerosis are hereogeneous: the indication malignant epithelioid angiomyolipoma. Am J Surg Pathol 22:180–187.

53. Cibas ES, Goss GA, Kulke MH, Demetri GD Fletcher CD (2001) Malignant epithelioid angiomyolipoma ("sarcoma ex angiomyolipoma") of the kidney. Am J Surg Pathol 25:121–126.

54. Lowe BA, Brewer J, Houghston DC, Jacobson F, Pitre T (1992) Malignant transformation of angiomyolipoma. J Urol 147:1356–1358.

55. Kawaguchi K, Oda Y, Nakanishi K, Matsuoka H, Tsuneyoshi M (2002) Malignant transformation of renal angiomyolipoma: a case report. Am J Surg Pathol 26:523–529.

56. Jimenez Re, Eble JN, Reuter VE, Epstein JI, Folpe AL, de Peralta-Venturina M, Tamboli P, Ansell ID, Grignon DJ, Young RH, Amin MB (2001) Concurrent angiomyolipoma and renal neoplasia: a study of 36 cases. Mod Pathol 14:157–163.

57. Bjornsson J, Short MP, Kwiatkowski DJ, Henske EP (1996) Tuberous sclerosis-associated renal cell carcinoma: clinical, pathological, and genetic features. Am J Pathol 149:1201–1208.

58. Bosniak MA (1981) Angiomyolipoma (hamartoma) of the kidney: a preoperative diagnosis is possible in virtually every case. Urol Radiol 3:135–142.

59. Steiner MS, Goldman SM, Fishman EK, Marshall FF (1993) The natural history of renal angiomyolipoma. J Urol 150:1782–1786.

60. Van Baal JG, Smits NJ, Lindfout D, Verhoff S (1994) The evolution of renal angiomyolipoma in patients with tuberous sclerosis. J Urol 152:35–38.

Part 3. Urinary Bladder

Question 1

What are the advantages and disadvantages, if any, of the revised (2004) WHO classification of urinary bladder neoplasms?

Answer

The World Health Organization (WHO) classification system published in 1973 had been most commonly used in the world until several years ago when this system was challenged. In 1997, a consensus conference was organized by Dr. F.K. Mostofi. It consisted of pathologists, urologists, and oncologists. The meeting was followed by another in 1998 with participation of members of the International Society of Urogical Pathology (ISUP). Recommendations were made to the WHO committee on urothelial tumors. Papillary tumors were divided into four categories: papilloma; papillary urothelial neoplasm of low malignant potential (PUNLMP); carcinoma, low grade (CaLG); and carcinoma, high grade (CaHG). Subsequently, this classification was adopted as the 2004 WHO classification system. As a result, grade 1 carcinomas by the 1973 WHO classification were reclassified as PUNLMP or CaLG; grade 2 carcinomas were assigned to the CaLG and CaHG groups; and grade 3 carcinomas became CaHG. The major difference from the 1973 WHO system was the introduction of the new designation PUNLMP. The intent was to separate a group of noninvasive papillary neoplasms that behave in a benign fashion from the cancer designation.

Ever since, the 1998 WHO/ISUP classification has been a subject of contention. A drawback was that the proposed system did not have sufficient clinical validation or supportive molecular and biochemical evidence. Subsequently, however, manuscripts reporting clinical follow-up based on the WHO/ISUP system began to appear in the literature. The major dispute was on the designation PUNLMP. Some investigators gave support while others presented negative data regarding the new system. Despite some support for the designation PUNLMP, this entity has not been reproducibly diagnosed in daily practice.

In our opinion, the 1998 WHO/ISUP classification or the consequent 2004 WHO classification still is a "working classification" for three reasons. First, it needs more and stronger evidence to support that PUNLMP is indeed different from CaLG in its clinical behavior. Second, the currently available histologic criteria are not concrete enough to be useful for practicing pathologists. Finally, molecular evidence is needed to support the concept of PUNLMP.

Comments

Based on the clinical behavior and more recently on molecular differences, urothelial tumors can be divided into two major types: low grade and high grade. The low-grade tumor, which is more common, is always papillary and exhibits mild cellular and nuclear pleomorphism. The low-grade tumors are typically noninvasive or invasive only into the lamina propria. Although patients with this type of tumor may develop new lesions, often referred to as recurrences (mostly of monoclonal origin but some of oligoclonal origin), the prognosis is excellent except in up to 10% of patients in whom a higher-grade tumor develops and subsequently invades the muscle layer, metastasizes, and causes cancer death [1]. The high-grade type, which is less common, usually presents as either a papillary or solid muscle-invasive tumor and is associated with a poor prognosis.

Several classification systems have been published for grading urothelial tumors of the urinary bladder [2–5]. The most commonly used worldwide is the 1973 WHO grading system [6].

1973 World Health Organization Classification

The 1973 WHO grading system divides urothelial papillary tumors into four types: papilloma and carcinomas of grade 1, 2, or 3. This classification system has been well accepted by pathologists as well as urologists and oncologists. However, it is not without problems: Lack of detailed histologic criteria is the major weakness of the system. The generally accepted criteria are that grade 1 carcinomas are papillary neoplasms with epithelium that most closely resembles normal urothelium and shows only a limited degree of cellular atypia. At the extreme end, grade 3 carcinomas show pronounced atypia: loss of cellular polarity; variation in cell size; nuclear pleomorphism, with often hyperchromatic nuclei; increased nuclear/cytoplasmic ratio; and an increased number of mitotic figures including abnormal ones. Grade 2 carcinomas are an intermediate group, falling between the two extremes. These carcinomas are heterogeneous: Some of them fall into the gray zone bordering on either grade 1 or grade 3, and the decision is subject to the judgment of the pathologist. This results in lumping many cases in the middle. Grade 2 carcinomas consist of tumors with variable biologic potential that fall between grades 1 and 3. To define these tumors more clearly, several groups of investigators have attempted to divide grade 2 tumors into two subtypes [3, 4, 7]. As is true with any classification scheme, the more elaborate it is, the more the diagnostic reproducibility diminishes. Regardless of the classification system used, however, data reported in the literature seem to indicate that the prognosis is dependent on the tumor multiplicity, size, grade, and stage [8] at the initial diagnosis (although the last two are closely related), and mucosal changes elsewhere (normal/mild, moderate, or severe dysplasia/carcinoma in situ) [8, 9].

1998 World Health Organization/International Society of Urologic Pathology (WHO/ISUP) Classification

The WHO/ISUP system addressed the problems of the 1973 WHO grading system [10]. The aim was to develop a universally acceptable classification scheme for bladder lesions that could be used effectively by pathologists, urologists, and oncologists. The intent was to avoid overdiagnosis of cancer for lesions that take a benign clinical course. The WHO/ISUP system divides bladder urothelial lesions into five major categories: normal, hyperplasia, flat lesions with atypia, papillary neoplasms, and invasive neoplasms. When handling papillary lesions, the WHO/ISUP classification maintains the four subtypes of the 1973 WHO classification. How is the new classification translated to the WHO 1973 classification? The relationship is illustrated in Table 3-1-1. The definition of papilloma remains the same. Transitional cell carcinoma grade 1 is now divided into PUNLMP and CaLG [11], grade 2 carcinomas are divided into CaLG and CaHG, and grade 3 carcinomas correspond to CaHG. The system was published without validation of prognostic significance. The term PUNLMP was introduced to replace many of the grade 1 transitional cell carcinomas. It was defined as "a papillary urothelial lesion with an orderly arrangement of cells within papillae with minimal architectural abnormalities and minimal nuclear atypia irrespective of cell thickness" [10]. The variance in opinion continued, however, as demonstrated by the issuance of a slightly modified WHO/ISUP system [11, 12]. In this system, after assigning the most benign tumors to the PUNLMP category, the remaining, more aggressive tumors are divided to three classes: grade 1, 2, and 3 carcinomas. Nevertheless, the 1998 WHO system was the one adopted as the 2004 WHO classification [13] (Table 3-1-1).

TABLE 3-1-1. Classification of urothelial neoplasms

WHO 1973	WHO/ISUP 1998 (WHO 2004)	WHO 1999[a]
Papilloma	Papilloma	Papilloma
Grade 1 Ca	PUNLMP[2]	PUNLMP
Grade 2 Ca	Low-grade Ca	Grade 1 Ca
Grade 3 Ca	High-grade Ca	Grade 2 Ca
		Grade 3 Ca

PUNLMP, Papillary urothelial neoplasm of low malignant potential.
[a] WHO/ISUP 1998 (WHO [13]) and WHO 1999 (Holmang [11]) are identical other than that the latter subdivides high-grade Ca into two classes.

In the 2004 WHO classification [13], PUNLMP is defined as a papillary urothelial tumor that resembles the exophytic urothelial papilloma but shows increased cellular proliferation, exceeding the thickness of normal urothelium. It appears that this lesion represents the lower end of the 1973 WHO grade 1 transitional cell carcinoma. It is true that a subgroup of patients presenting with a low-grade papillary tumor has an extremely good prognosis in terms of progression of disease, and this subgroup may fall into the designation PUNLMP. This cumbersome term, PUNLMP, "evolved from a concerted effort to remove the word carcinoma" from histologically and biologically benign lesions previously called "grade 1" [14]. We have no objection to refining a subgroup of urothelial tumors as such if the patients with such lesions take an absolutely benign course.

Clinical Follow-up Data to Evaluate the Significance of the WHO/ISUP Classification System

As was stated earlier, the WHO/ISUP classification, now adopted as 2004 WHO classification [13] was proposed without validation. Subsequently, long-term follow-up data have appeared in the world literature. The major focus was on the clinical follow-up of patients with PUNLMP, the results of which are tabulated in Table 3-1-2. Most studies concluded that the PUNLMP concept is useful for predicting its benign course. In these studies, progression was defined as recurrence with a pT1 or higher-stage tumor, development of pTis, and/or metastasis/cancer death.

The study by Holmang et al. [11] is the only prospective study and involved all new bladder cases in Western Sweden during a 2-year period. It compared recurrence and progression rates of PUNLMP, CaLG, and CaHG. All microscopic slides were reviewed by one expert pathologist. After review, 81% of PUNLMPs were originally diagnosed as either papilloma or grade 1 carcinoma and 19% as grade 2 by the 1973 WHO classification. After a follow-up of 5–7 years, the recurrence rate was significantly lower in patients with PUNLMP compared with those with CaLG (35% vs. 71%, $P < 0.001$). Recurrence was three times more common ($P < 0.001$) at the 4-month cystoscopy in patients with CaLG than in those with PUNLMP. There was no case of progression in the PUNLMP group ($n = 95$)

compared with six in the CaLG group (6/160). The difference was, however, not statistically significant. There was a significant difference in the progression rate between CaLG and CaHG ($P < 0.0001$). It was concluded that WHO grade 1 tumors are benign in more than 90% of cases and that subdivision of grade 1 tumors as PUNLMP and CaLG seems to add valuable prognostic information.

The Oosterhuis group [15] classified 322 newly diagnosed Ta tumors by the 1998 WHO/ISUP and 1973 WHO classifications. After a mean of 79 months of follow-up, there was no difference in either the recurrence or progression rate among PUNLMP, CaLG, and CaHG groups. It was concluded that the prognostic value of the 1998 WHO/ISUP classification system is limited to predicting progression-free survival between PUNLMP and CaHG ($P = 0.04$, log-rank test).

Samaratunga et al. [16] had 29 PUNLMPs and 73 CaLGs, all newly diagnosed and in stage pTa. The cases were also classified by the 1973 WHO system. The 1973 WHO grade assigned was that on the original pathology report so as not to introduce a grading bias. After up to 90 months of follow-up, there was no significant difference in the recurrence rate among WHO/ISUP grades. The progression rates of PUNLMP and CaLG groups were 6.9% and 9.6%, respectively, whereas grade 1 and grade 2 groups by the WHO classification had a progression rate of 7.1% (3/42) and 13.9% (11/79), respectively. It was concluded that the 1973 WHO grade ($P = 0.03$) and WHO/ISUP grade ($P = 0.002$) both independently predicted progression. Despite a lack of their own supportive data, these authors stated in the discussion that on the basis of published reports PUNLMP tumors have a negligible risk of progression compared with the low but increased risk of progression with CaLG.

Pich et al. [17] compared the recurrence and progression rates of PUNLMP and CaLG cases with median follow-up duration of 76 months for the former and 15 months for the latter. The recurrence rate was significantly higher in the CaLG group than in the PUNLMP group (76.7% vs. 47.4%, $P = 0.04$). None of the PUNLMP cases showed progression, whereas 5 patients (11.6%) of the CaLG group had tumor progression, all of whom died of bladder cancer. A significant difference between the two groups was also found when comparing the pathologic parameters: mitosis count ($P = 0.006$), MIB-1

TABLE 3-1-2. Progression of papilloma, PUNLMPs, and urothelial carcinomas, low-grade and high-grade

Investigator	Classification	No.	No. of tumors at initial diagnosis 1	2–3	≥4	Follow-up	Recurrence	Progression[a]	Comments/conclusions
Holmang [12], 2001	WHO/ISUP								1. All slides reviewed by one pathologist.
	PUNLMP[b]	95	81	10	4	5–7 years	33 (35%)	6 (4%) ⎫	2. Recurrence: a tumor identified at cystoscopy that was fulgurated (no histologic material) or resected (histologically studied).
	CaLG	160	124	23	13		88 (71%)	⎬ $P < 0.001$	3. A significant difference in progression rate between CaLG and CaHG ($P < 0.001$) as was between grade 2 and grade 3 of 1973 WHO system ($P < 0.0011$).
	CaHG	108	80	17	11		58 (73%)	25 (23%) ⎭	4. 1998 WHO/ISUP system seems to have advantage compared with 1973 WHO classification.
									5. There seems to be no significant difference in progression rate between PUNLMP and CaLG.
Osterhuis [15], 2002	WHO/ISUP								1. Five-year recurrence-free survival is not significantly different between groups ($P = 0.12$).
	PUNLMP[b]	116				79 mos. (mean)	30 (26%)	3 (3%)[c]	2. Five-year progression-free survival shows a small but significant difference ($P = 0.04$) between PUNLMP and CaHG.
	CaLG	141					43 (30%)	6 (4%)	3. The prognostic value of 1998 WHO/ISUP classification system is limited to predicting progression-free survival, especially between PUNLMP and CaHG ($P = 0.04$).
	CaHG	45					18 (40%)	4 (8%)	
	WHO 1973								
	G1	31				79 mos. (mean)	Not available	Not available	
	G2	286							
	G3	1							
Samaratunga [16], 2002	WHO/ISUP								1. Diagnoses based on group review.
	PUNLMP[b]	29				≤90 mos.	No. for each type not available but statistically no different among groups	2 (6.9%)	2. Progression: recurrence with pT1, T2, Tis or their combination.
	CaLG	73				≤90 mos.		7 (9.6%)	3. Recurrence rates among WHO/ISUP statistically not significant. WHO 1973 G3 recurrence rate is significantly different from those of G1 ($P = 0.0001$) and G2 ($P = 0.00001$).
	CaHG	29				≤90 mos.		10 (34.5%)	4. WHO 1973 grade ($P = 0.003$) and tumor size ($P = 0.03$) independently predicted progression, as did WHO/ISUP grade ($P = 0.002$) and tumor size ($P = 0.04$).
	WHO 1973								5. One of PUNLMP tumors that progressed required cystectomy for muscle-invasive carcinoma.
	G1[b]	42				≤90 mos.	No. for each type not available, but G1 vs. G3, $P = 0.0001$, G2 vs. G3, $P = 0.00001$	3 (7.1%) ⎫	6. PUNLMPs have a negligible risk of progression compared with the low but increased risk of progression of CaLG.
	G2	79				≤90 mos.		11 (13.9%) ⎬ $P = 0.003$	
	G3	6				≤90 mos.		4 (66.7%) ⎭	

TABLE 3-1-2. *Continued*

Investigator	Classification	No.	No. of tumors at initial diagnosis			Follow-up (years)	Recurrence	Progression[a]	Comments/conclusions
			1	2-3	≥4				
Pich [17], 2001	WHO/ISUP PUNLMP[b] CaLG	19 43				76 mos. (median) 15 mos. (median)	9 (47.4%) 33 (76.7%) *P* = 0.04	0 5 (11.6%)	1. Diagnosis by one pathologist. 2. Five-year recurrence-free survival: 68% for PUNLMP and 21% for CaLG (*P* = 0.002). 3. All 5 patients in whom cancer progressed died of bladder cancer. 4. Significant difference is found between PUNLMP and CaLG in mitotic count (*P* = 0.006), tumor recurrence (*P* = 0.04), MIB-1 (cell proliferation index, *P* = 0.002), positive staining for p53 (*P* = 0.03). 5. Distinction between PUNLMP and CaLG reflects a different biologic activity and clinical behavior.
Desai [18], 2000	WHO/ISUP Papilloma PUNLMP[b] CaLG CaHG	8 (all pTa) 8 (all pTa) 42 (1 pT1) 62 (31 pT1)				7.4 (mean)	33% ⎫ 64% ⎬ *P* = 0.02 56% ⎭	0%[d] ⎫ 10.5%[e] ⎬ *P* = 0.031 27.1%[f] ⎭	1. WHO/ISUP grade correlates with tumor stage (*P* < 0.005), recurrence (*P* = 0.02), and progression in stage (*P* = 0.031). 2. Loss of CD44 (cell surface binding protein to hyaluronidate collagen) immunohistochemical staining and increasing CK20 (cytokeratin-associated intermediate filaments) reactivity are significantly correlated with increasing tumor grade and stage (*P* < 0.005, each comparison).
Fujii [19] 2003	WHO/ISUP PUNLMP[b]	50				>5 years or until death. 11.7 years (mean)	30 (60%); 68% of patients disease-free after 5 years	17 (34%)	1. All cases reviewed and diagnosed by two pathologists. 2. In all case, progression was to CaLG/ pTa or pT1. 3. Despite a high recurrence rate, PUNLMP carries a very low malignant potential.

CaLG and CaHG, low-grade and high-grade carcinoma, respectively.

[a] Progression defined as recureence with pT1 or higher stage, CaLG, CaHG, pTis, or/and metastasis/death.

[b] All new cases without prior history of bladder tumor.

[c] One patient died as a result of bladder carcinoma 44 months after the diagnosis of the primary tumor.

[d] Total number for each category not available.

[e] PTa to pT1 in 2.6%, pTa to pT2 in 5.3%, death from cancer in 5.3%.

[f] PTa to pT1 in 8.3%, pTa to pT2 in 6.3%, death from cancer in 16.7%.

(proliferative index) ($P = 0.002$), and positive staining for p53 ($P = 0.03$). They concluded that distinction between PUNLMP and CaLG reflects different biologic activity and clinical behavior.

The patients of Desai et al. [18] consisted of 8 cases of papilloma, 8 of PUNLMP (all pTa), 42 of CaLG (1 pT1), and 62 of CaHG (31 pT1). Progression analysis was based on 106 of 120 total cases for whom follow-up data were available. None of the 16 combined papilloma/PUNLMP cases demonstrated progression. Progression in stage was observed in 10.5% of the CaLG group and 27.1% of the CaHG group. The difference between the combined papilloma/PUNLMP vs. CaLG vs. CaHG was significant ($P = 0.031$). It was concluded that WHO/ISUP grading correlated with tumor stage ($P < 0.005$), recurrence ($P = 0.02$), and progression in stage ($P = 0.031$).

Finally, the study by Fujii et al. [19] consisted of a relatively large number of cases of PUNLMP ($n = 50$) with a respectable follow-up period (although the study was retrospective). The study was limited to PUNLMP patients, all of them without a previous history of urothelial tumor. With a mean follow-up of 11.7 years, the recurrence rate was 60%, and the progression rate was 34%. All cases showing progression were limited to pT1, and none of the cases had tumor extending to the muscle layer or upper urinary tract tumors. An important observation was that 34 patients (68%) were disease-free for more than 5 years (18 after initial treatment and 16 after treatment for recurrent tumors). The authors concluded that despite a high rate of recurrence PUNLMP carried very low malignant potential. It is regrettable that the authors did not include the cases of CaLG for comparison, without which the biologic potential of PUNLMP cannot be fully evaluated as an independent tumor category.

Advantages and Disadvantages and Interobserver Agreement When Using the WHO/ISUP System

There is no disagreement in the definition of papilloma. Lesions so diagnosed are benign and not associated with disease progression. The data described above and summarized in Table 3-1-2 appear to indicate that tumors classified as PUNLMP are associated with a minimal risk of future development of higher-stage tumors. Data for five of the six studies depicted in Table 3-1-2 are summarized in Table 3-1-3. Assuming that there is no geographic difference in the frequency of these two types of neoplasm and that there is no bias in the selection of cases for study, the reported PUNLMP/CaLG ratio ranges from 1:1.68 to 1:1.21 to 1:2.52 to 1:5.25 with a more than fourfold difference. The differences most likely reflect the variability in defining and interpreting PUNLMP and CaLG. In other words, one lesion defined as PUNLMP by one pathologist may be diagnosed as CaLG by another pathologist. This discrepancy listed in Table 3-1-3 heavily discounted the validating power of these studies. The other problem is that some of the patients with a long-term follow-up of recurrent diseases may go back and forth between PUNLMP and CaLG because of the poorly defined criteria. In reality, they may have only one disease of low-grade urothelial neoplasm. Furthermore, the behavioral difference (in terms of progression) between PUNLMP and CaLG is slight. There were so few cases assigned to each category that none of the investigator groups was able to demonstrate a statistically significant difference in the progression rate. Because of the subtle difference and the difficulty of distinguishing the two entities microscopically (vide infra), general acceptance among pathologists, urologists, and oncologists has been slow [14, 20–25].

TABLE 3-1-3. Frequency of PUNLMP and CaLG cases incorporated in the study to evaluate the biologic potential

Investigator	No. PUNLMP	No. CaLG	PUNLMP/CaLG ratio
Holmang [12], 2001	95	160	0.59
Osterhuis [15], 2002	116	141	0.82
Samaratunga [16], 2002	29	73	0.40
Pich [17], 2001	19	43	0.44
Desai [18], 2000	8	42	0.19

PUNLMP, papillary urothelial neoplasm of low malignant potential; CaLG, carcinoma, low grade.

Bostwick and Mikuz [26] summarized the work carried out by most of the members of Committee No. 1 at the International Conference on the Diagnosis of Non-Invasive Urothelial Neoplasms held in Ancona, Italy (May 2001). An international multidisciplinary team of experts was assembled. The purpose of the conference was to discuss and reach consensus regarding the optimal contemporary diagnosis and classification of noninvasive and early invasive urothelial carcinoma (pTa and pT1). Although a diverse group of pathologists participated, several prominent contributors to this ongoing debate were notably absent. The meeting consensus was that the 1973 WHO classification for papillary urothelial neoplasms (papilloma and grade 1, grade 2, and grade 3 carcinoma) is still superior to all existing alternatives (including the 1998 WHO/ISUP system), with some refinement of diagnostic criteria. According to the participants, the advantages of the 1973 WHO classification are as follows: It has been used widely for a long time and is successful for stratifying patients for therapy. The disadvantages are imprecise criteria; high interobserver variability; heterogeneity of grade 1 and 2 tumors; and use of "carcinoma" for a neoplasm with minimal biologic consequences (grade 1). They also recognized advantages of the 1998 WHO/ISUP system: relatively precise histologic criteria, possibly solving the problem of heterogeneity of grades 1 and 2 of the 1973 WHO classification; and utility for therapy the same as the 1973 WHO system. The disadvantages are the following: not validated (as noted above, although since then clinical data based on the new classification system are accumulating); associated with uncertain reproducibility; introduced an unwanted term, "low malignant potential"; and the use of "high grade" may induce the performance of cystectomy by some urologists.

Arguing against Bostwick and Mikuz, Busch and Algaba [27] claimed that the 1973 WHO classification should be replaced by the WHO/ISUP classification for the following reasons: Less than 5% of grade 1 carcinomas progressed or killed the patients (thus more than 95% of these tumors did not appear to be cancers); imprecise criteria for grading (poor definition of differences between grades 1 and 2 and between grades 2 and 3); the poor interobserver reproducibility of the 1973 WHO system [11, 28, 29, Busch et al., unpublished observation, cited in 27]. The advantages of the WHO/ISUP system are the following: several recent studies (vide supra) verifying differences in the recurrence rate, progression rate, and mortality by grades; the WHO/ISUP classification providing a slightly simpler and possibly more reproducible stratification of low- and high-grade cases, which is of practical value in the clinical decision process.

Clearly, each side presents arguments in its favor. In our opinion, the 1998 WHO/ISUP should receive credit for describing the histologic criteria in more detail. Nevertheless, a major difficulty still exists in distinguishing PUNLMP from CaLG.

In their 1998 publication, Epstein et al. [10] defined PUNLMP as a papillary urothelial lesion with an orderly arrangement of cells in papillae with minimal architectural abnormalities and minimal nuclear atypia irrespective of cell thickness. Mitotic figures are found but are infrequent and usually limited to the basal layer. The major distinction from urothelial papilloma is that papilloma has no architectural or cytologic atypia and has no more than seven layers of urothelial cells lining a fibrovascular core. CaLG is defined as a papillary neoplasm with an overall orderly appearance but with easily recognizable variation of architectural and/or cytologic features, even at scanning magnification. Variation of polarity and nuclear size, shape, and chromatin texture comprise the minimal but definitive cytologic atypia. Mitotic figures are infrequent and usually seen in the lower half, although they may be seen at any level of the urothelium. Although principal features for the differential diagnosis are described in reasonable detail, they did not elaborate on what is meant by "architectural" abnormality.

Busch and Algaba [27], who supported the 1998 WHO/ISUP classification, proposed a decision tree for refined grading of bladder carcinoma based on recognizing the distinction of order/disorder and variation/no variation in the architectural pattern and cellular features. In their proposal, if predominant order is present, it is a PUNLMP; if it is not present, CaLG or CaHG is diagnosed. Again, they fail to explain what is meant by "predominant order." To practicing pathologists, these descriptions are inadequate, highly subjective, confusing, and not practical enough to be useful for a differential diagnosis.

Consultation was obtained with Dr. Busch and Dr. Sonny Johansson of the University of Nebraska Medical Center, who are coauthors discussing

PUNLMP in the book entitled *World Organization Classification of Tumours* [13]. In his letter, Dr. Busch kindly explained the differential scheme as follows.

"Under a medium magnification, an overview impression is important in decision. If the impression is that of very orderly pattern where the individual cells are very similar and relate to one another similarly throughout the specimen, the lesion falls in the category PUNLMP (Fig. 3-1-1). If the architecture still gives an overall impression of order, but variation in nuclear size, form, internuclear distance, and nuclear texture etc. exists, the tumor falls in the category of CaLG (Figs. 3-1-2, 3-1-3, 3-1-4). If the architecture

(pattern) gives a predominantly disordered impression, but it is easy to find areas with attempts to organize, it is referred to as CaHG (WHO 1999 grade 2) [11, 12], Fig. 3-1-4), and if the pattern is completely chaotic, it is still CaHG but is classified as WHO 1999 grade 3."

Despite criteria set by detailed description, interobserver variability is unavoidable due to the subjectivity of pathologists' interpretation of the histologic picture. Yorukoglu et al. [21] tested the intraobserver and interobserver reproducibility with six expert uropathologists. Fifteen cases each considered to represent classic examples of PUNLMP, CaLG, and CaHG

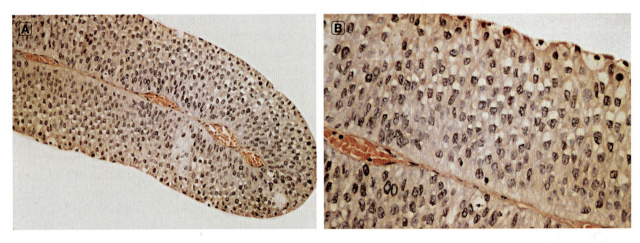

FIG. 3-1-1. **A, B** Papillary urothelial neoplasm of low malignant potential (PUNLMP). The papilla is composed of multiple layers of orderly urothelial cells of uniform size. The long axes of the nuclei parallel each other and are perpendicular to the stromal core. The nuclei are uniform in size, and mitosis is not found in this field. (Courtesy of Sonny L. Johansson, MD, PhD, University of Nebraska Medical Center, Omaha)

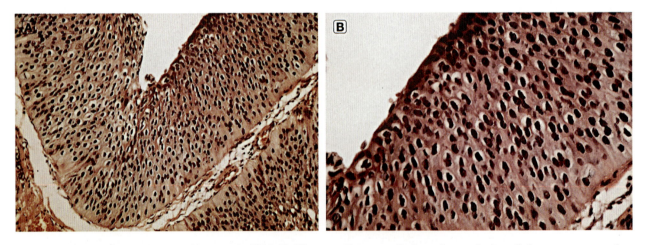

FIG. 3-1-2. Urothelial carcinoma of low grade (CaLG). The overall pattern is that of an orderly cellular arrangement, but even at low power (**A**) one can appreciate some variation in size and intercellular space and focal disarray in the cell axis. These changes become apparent at high power (**B**). Note some overlapping nuclei. (Courtesy of Sonny L. Johansson, MD, PhD, University of Nebraska Medical Center, Omaha)

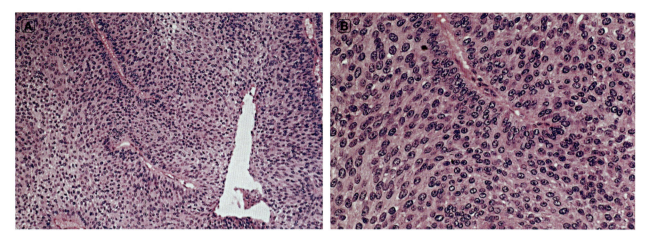

FIG. 3-1-3. **A, B** Another example of urothelial carcinoma of low grade

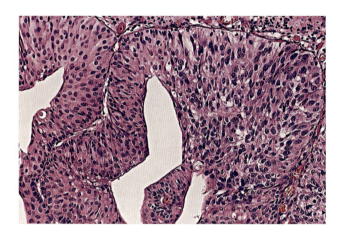

FIG. 3-1-4. Another urothelial carcinoma with two patterns. The tumor in the left half of the field satisfies the criteria for CaLG, and the tumor on the right side satisfy the criteria for CaHG by the WHO/ISUP classification scheme

were selected. Five cases randomly selected from each category were sent to each participant together with the WHO/ISUP guidelines [10]. After the first review, the results and the study sets were collected; and the labels were then changed and returned to the participants together with the remaining 10 cases. The mean intraobserver reproducibility was 78% (k = 0.67),[1] and individual participant's reproducibility (intraobserver) varied from 63% to 93% (k = 0.45–

---

1 K values are a measure of the level of agreement: 0–0.2, slight; 0.21–0.40, fair; 0.41–0.60, moderate; 0.61–0.80, substantial; and 0.81–1.00, almost perfect.

0.89). Moderate interobserver agreement was achieved for both the 1998 WHO/ISUP and 1973 WHO classification systems (k = 0.56 and 0.48, respectively), and the difference was not significant (p > 0.05). Despite the "clearly defined" histologic criteria, the 1998 WHO/ISUP system provided a slight but statistically insignificant increase in both intraobserver and interobserver reproducibility. There was agreement for PUNLMP in only 48% of cases, and agreement was 56% for the 1973 grade 1 tumors. They concluded that the newly proposed classification system for noninvasive urothelial neoplasms does not increase the reproducibility.

Murphy et al. [22] reported the reproducibility of the 1998 WHO/ISUP system in a community practice setting. A series of specimens was divided into a learning set and a study set and independently examined by three pathologists. Specimens in the learning set were interpreted without previous education, whereas the study set was diagnosed immediately after intensive education. Agreement was slight to moderate (k = 0.12–0.50) in distinguishing PUNLMP from CaLG. Education did not result in increased interpretive conformity. In view of the difficulty for practicing pathologists when applying the 1998 WHO/ISUP system, Murphy et al. [5, 22] recommended that PUNLMP and CaLG should be combined as a single entity to represent a low-grade bladder tumor group. The rationale is that urologists base the treatment of low-grade urothelial neoplasms primarily on stage and that they usually treat low-grade noninvasive papillary neoplasms the same way regardless of whether these tumors are interpreted as PUNLMP, papilloma, or low-grade or grade 1 carcinoma [22, 25]. By combining PUNLMP and CaLG as a single entity of low-grade tumors, the ability of pathologists to distinguish this group from the CaHG group improved markedly (discrepancy rate 9%) [22].

Bol et al. [23] drew a similar conclusion that interobserver disagreement was substantial using the WHO/ISUP classification scheme with potentially strong implications for patients. In the discussion, they questioned the usefulness of this classification system in urologic practice and noted that the three entities (papilloma, PUNLMP, CaLG) with a relatively indolent course as to progression do not necessarily help improve therapeutic decision-making by clinicians.

In summary, when the WHO/ISUP classification was published in 1998, some of the expert pathologists were against its use, including one of the authors, because it was proposed without validation [25]. Since then, some follow-up data have emerged either to give some support to or oppose the classification. Although data appear favorable for the concept of PUNLMP, the difference from the CaLG is so slight that statistically significant difference has not been demonstrated by any study. We recommend continuing to watch for further clinical data and molecular and biochemical evidence to emerge before we make a final decision regarding the usefulness of the 1998 WHO/ISUP classification. Conceptually, the 1998 WHO/ISUP system sounds reasonable in that low-grade urothelial tumors that behave nonaggressively have been removed from the cancer category. Nevertheless, the WHO/ISUP system is still a "working classification." Clear clinical data are required to demonstrate that PUNLMP is indeed different from the CaLG in its biologic potential. Furthermore, the currently available histologic criteria [10, 27] are not concrete enough to be useful for practicing pathologists. The histologic criteria should be provided with a more detailed descriptive guideline with multiple photographic illustrations. Even with that information, however, interobserver agreement may not reach an acceptable level. Then, as Murphy et al. [22] suggested, a two-tier system—low-grade and high-grade urothelial tumors—may actually be a practical alternative because interobserver agreement can be significantly improved [22]. This system should not compromise patients' care by clinicians.

References

1. Greene LF, Hanash KA, Farrow GM (1973) Benign papilloma or papillary carcinoma of the urinary bladder? J Urol 110:205–207.
2. Bergkvist A, Ljungqvist A, Moberger G (1965) Classification of bladder tumours based on cellular pattern: preliminary report of a clinical-pathological study of 300 cases with minimal follow-up of eight years. Acta Chir Scand 130:371–378.
3. Pauwels RPE, Scharpers RFM, Smeets AWGB, Debruyne FMJ, Geraedts JPM (1988) Grading in superficial bladder cancer. 1. Morphological criteria. Br J Urol 61:129–134.
4. Malmstrom P-U, Busch C, Norlen BJ (1987) Recurrence, progression and survival in bladder cancer: a retrospective analysis of 232 patients with 5-year follow-up. Scand J Urol Nephrol 21:185–195.
5. Jordan AM, Weingarten J, Murphy WM (1987) Transitional cell neoplasms of the urinary bladder: can biological potential be predicted from histologic grading? Cancer 60:2766–2774.
6. Mostofi FK, Sorbin LH, Torloni H (1973) Histological typing of urinary bladder tumours: international histological classification of tumours. No. 10. World Health Organization, Geneva.
7. Carbin B, Eckman P, Gustafson H, Christensen NJ, Sandsedt B, Silfversward C (1991) Grading of human urothelial carcinoma based on nuclear atypia and mitotic frequency. I. Histological description. J Urol 145:968–971.
8. Millan-Rodriguez F, Chechile-Toniolo G, Salvador-Bayarri J, Palou J, Vicente-Rodriguez J (2000) Multivariate analysis of the prognostic factors of primary superficial bladder cancer. J Urol 163:73–78.
9. Heney NM, Ahmed S, Flanagan MJ, Frable W, Gorder MP, Hafermann MD, Hawkins IR for National Bladder Cancer Collaborative Group A (1983) Superficial bladder cancer: progression and recurrence. J Urol 130:1083–1086.
10. Epstein JI, Amin MB, Reuter VR, Mostofi FK, and the Bladder Consensus Conference Committee (1998) The World Health Organization/International Society of Urological Pathology consensus classification of urothelial (transitional cell) neoplasms of the urinary bladder. Am J Surg Pathol 22:1435–1448.
11. Holmang S, Hedelin H, Anderstrom C, Holmberg E, Busch C, Johansson SL (1999) Recurrence and progression in low grade papillary urothelial tumors. J Urol 162:702–707.
12. Holmang S, Andius P, Hedelin H, Wester K, Busch C, Johansson SL (2001) Stage progression in Ta papillary urothelial tumors: relationship to grade, immunohistochemical expression of tumor markers, mitotic frequency and DNA ploidy. J Urol 165:1124–1130.
13. WHO (2004) WHO histological classification of tumours of the urinary tract. In: Eble JN, Sauter G, Epstein JI, Sesterhenn IA (eds) Pathology and genetics

of tumors of the urinary system and male genital organs: World Health Organization classification of tumours. IARS Press, Lyon, p 90.

14. Murphy WM (2001) Editorial comments. In: Holmang S, Andius P, Hedelin H, Wester K, Busch C, Johansson SL. Staging progression in Ta papillary urothelial tumors; relationship to grade, immunohistochemical expression of tumor markers, mitotic frequency and DNA ploidy. J Urol 165:1124–1130.

15. Oosterhuis JWA, Schapers RFM, Janssen-Heijnen MLG, Pauwels RPE (2002) Histological grading of papillary urothelial carcinoma of the bladder: prognostic value of the 1998 WHO/ISUP classification system and comparison with conventional grading system. J Clin Pathol 55:900–905.

16. Samaratunga H, Makarov, Epstein JI (2002) Comparison of WHO/ISUP and WHO classification of non-invasive papillary urothelial neoplasms for risk of progression. Urology 60:315–319.

17. Pich A, Chiusa L, Formiconi A, Galliano D, Bortolin P, Novone R (2001) Biologic differences between non-invasive papillary neoplasms of low malignant potential and low-grade (grade 1) papillary carcinomas of the bladder. Am J Surg Pathol 25:1528–1533.

18. Desai S, Lim SD, Jimenez RE, Chun T, Keane TE, McKenney JK, Zavala-Pompa A, Cohen C, Young RH, Amin MB (2000) Relationship of cytokeratin 20 and CD44 protein expression with WHO/ISUP grade in pTa and pT1 papillary urothelial neoplasia. Mod Pathol 13:1315–1323.

19. Fujii Y, Kawakami S, Koga F, Nemoto T, Kihara K (2004) Long-term outcome of bladder papillary urothelial neoplasms of low malignant potential. BJU Int 92:559–562.

20. Lopez-Beltran A, Montironi R (2004) Non-invasive urothelial neoplasms: according to the most recent WHO classification. Eur Urol 46:170–176.

21. Yorukoglu K, Tuna B, Dikicioglu E, Duzcan E, Isisag A, Sen S, Mungan U, Kirkali Z (2003) Reproducibility of the 1998 World Health Organization/International Society of Urologic Pathology classification of papillary urothelial neoplasms of the urinary bladder. Virchows Arch 443:734–740.

22. Murphy WM, Takezawa K, Maruniak NA (2002) Interobserver discrepancy using the 1998 World Health Organization/ International Society of Urologic Pathology classification of urothelial neoplasms: practical choices for patient care. J Urol 168:968–972.

23. Bol MGW, Baak JPA, Buhr-Wilghagen S, Kruse A-J, Kjellevold KH, Janssen EAM, Mestad O, Ogreid P (2003) Reproducibility and prognostic variability of grade and lamina propria invasion in stages Ta, T1 urothelial carcinoma of the bladder. J Urol 169: 1291–1294.

24. Jones TD, Cheng L (2006) Papillary urothelial neoplasm of low malignant potential (PUNLMP): evolving terminology and concepts. J Urol 175:1995–2003.

25. Oyasu R (2000) World Health Organization and International Society of Urological Pathology classification and two-number grading system of bladder tumors (editorial counter point). Cancer 88:1509–1512.

26. Bostwick DG, Mikuz G (2002) Urothelial papillary (exophytic) neoplasms. Virchows Arch 441:109–116.

27. Busch C, Algaba F (2002) The WHO/ISUP 1998 and WHO 1999 systems for malignancy grading of bladder cancer: scientific foundation and translation to one another and previous systems. Virchows Arch 441: 105–108.

28. Ooms ECM, Andersen WAAD, Alons CL, Boon ME, Veldhuizen RW (1983) Analysis of the performance of pathologists in the grading of bladder tumors. Hum Pathol 14:140–143.

29. Robertson AJ, Swanson Beck J, Burnett RA, Howatson SR, Lessels AM, McLaren KM, Moss SM, Simpson JG, Smith GD, Tavadia HB, Walker F (1990) Observer variability in histopathological reporting of transitional cell carcinoma and epithelial dysplasia in bladders. J Clin Pathol 43:17–21.

Question 2

What are the features of inverted papilloma of the urinary tract? How does it differ from papillary urothelial carcinoma? Is there a malignant counterpart of inverted papilloma? What are the differential diagnoses?

Answer

Inverted papilloma of the urothelial tract is a benign tumor that affects men more frequently than women. More than 90% of inverted papillomas are located in the trigone, bladder neck, and prostatic urethra; and they seldom recur after surgical removal. They may also occur in the upper urinary tract including the renal pelvis and ureters. An intimate association with the proliferative disorders, including von Brunn's nests, cystitis cystica, and cystitis glandularis, suggests their close histogenetic relationship. It is not clear whether inverted papilloma is indeed a neoplasm. Occasionally, inverted papilloma shows some histologic atypias, such as nuclear enlargement, prominent nucleoli, and mitotic figures, or exophitic papillary growth; but their clinical significance remains unknown. Although uncommon, urothelial carcinomas may exhibit an endophytic growth pattern (carcinoma with inverted growth pattern). It is imperative to distinguish inverted papilloma from urothelial carcinoma with an inverted growth pattern. The features suggesting carcinoma are desmoplastic invasion, extension into the muscularis propria, and diffuse cytologic atypia compatible with high-grade urothelial carcinoma.

The low frequency of FGF-receptor 3, a marker of low-grade urothelial cell carcinoma, and a low Ki 67 proliferation index seem to indicate that inverted papilloma is a neoplasm with a molecular mechanism different from that of urothelial carcinoma.

Comments

An inverted papilloma (IP) is an uncommon, benign polypoid lesion of urothelial origin first reported in 1963 [1]. It comprises less than 1% of urothelial neoplasms. IP typically presents in old adults, and far more commonly in men than in women. Clinically, IP most commonly manifests with hematuria or obstructed urine flow because of its frequent location in the trigone or the bladder neck. IP may also occur in the upper urinary tract.

Pathologic Features of Inverted Papilloma

In contrast to the exophytic growth pattern of the conventional urothelial tumors, the epithelial growth is directed into its own stroma from the normal-appearing surface urothelium. This growth pattern is reflected in the endoscopic appearance; it is typically a dome-shaped mass or a pedunculated mass with a smooth surface Fig. 3-2-1). Histologically, islands or cords of epithelium, 7–10 cells in width, invert from the normal-appearing surface urothelium and extend

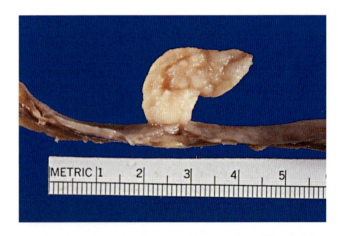

FIG. 3-2-1. Pedunculated ureteral inverted papilloma, 0.8 × 1.5 × 2.0 cm. It has a relatively smooth surface. Note it is bent 90° cranially while adapting to grow in the limited space of the ureter

into the stroma; there may be a cystic space in the center cell nests that may contain eosinophilic secretion. The peripheral basal cells are frequently arranged perpendicular to their long axis, described as "palisading," and the inner cells are spindle and streaming Fig. 3-2-2). The tumor cells are uniform, and mitotic activity is rare. Foci of squamous differentiation are frequent. Although rare, IPs may exhibit a pseudoglandular or truly glandular pattern, which is made up of mucus-producing columnar cells [2]. This pattern often coexists with the ordinary urothelial-type cells. The stroma is loose fibrous and contains numerous thin-walled blood vessels.

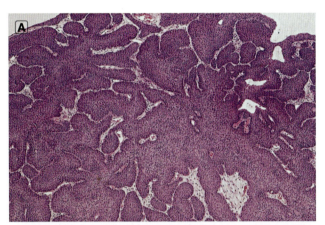

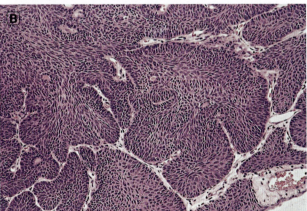

FIG. 3-2-2. **A** Inverted papilloma. Branching trabeculae of urothelial cells arise directly from the normal-appearing attenuated surface urothelium and extend deeply into the loose paucicellular stroma. **B** At a higher power, the peripheral basal cells are in areas arranged perpendicular to their long axis, and the inner cells are spindle and streaming. The tumor cells are uniform and show no mitosis

Is there a malignant counterpart of IP? Does an IP become malignant?

There have been a number of reports claiming that malignant alterations developed in an otherwise typical IP. Before accepting their claim, it is necessary to review the reported data critically. The claim may be justified only when both inverted IP and carcinoma are present in addition to a recurrent tumor taking an aggressive course. It is important to note that some cytologic and architectural variants can be seen in an otherwise typical IP. Finally, it is necessary to realize that urothelial carcinoma can grow in an inverted (endophytic) growth pattern. These topics are discussed below.

IP with Nuclear Atypia, Mitotic Activity, or Broad Cores Resulting in Nodular Epithelial Cell Nests (Fig. 3-2-3)

In the report by Kunze et al. [2], cytologic atypia (prominent nucleoli and mitotic activity) was found in 6 of 40 cases. Their significance remains unknown as clinical follow-up data were not presented. The case reported by Kimura et al. [3] was a polypoid ureteral tumor that had a typical histologic appearance of IP except for some cytologic atypia. Because an intraoperative diagnosis of "transitional cell carcinoma of the inverted type" was rendered, nephroureterectomy was performed. The postoperative course of the known 2 years was uneventful. Cases reported by Stower et al. [4] and Uyama and Moriwaki [5] as IP with malignant changes show similar cytologic atypia but lacked clinical evidence of malignancy. Uyama's patient was alive and well for the known 5 years after nephroureterectomy, irradiation, and chemotherapy. As with the case reported by Kimura et al. [3], the aggressive therapy makes assessment of malignancy impossible.

The 11 cases of IP with cytologic atypia reported by Broussard et al. [6] were accompanied with the clinical follow-up ranging from 5 months to 7 years. In all cases, the atypical areas were focal and consisted of cells with prominent nuclei, cells showing atypical squamous metaplasia, dysplastic cells approaching the level of carcinoma in situ, and multinucleated giant cells. Ki-67 was slightly increased in some cases. The two cases with prominent nucleoli demonstrated an increase in p53 staining. Clinical follow-up revealed no history of prior or subsequent bladder neoplasms. Thus, their data indicate that a

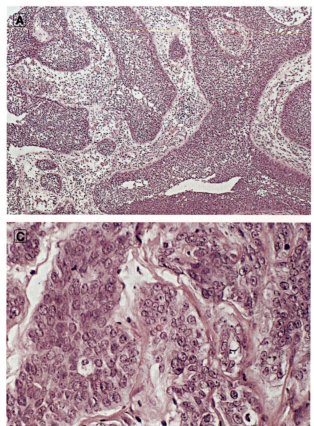

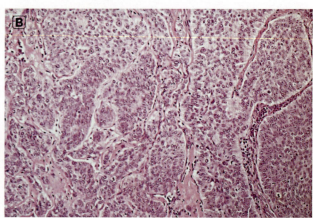

FIG. 3-2-3. Inverted papilloma with atypia. This inverted papilloma, in general, shows the usual histology (**A**) but has an area with cytologic atypia including nucleomegaly and nucleolomegaly (**B, C**). Clinical follow-up of 3 years showed no evidence of recurrence or progression of the disease

certain degree of cytologic atypia can be tolerated as IP.

IP with Focal Surface Papillary Proliferation

Kyriakos and Royce [7] described, in 10% of ureteral IPs, a few papillary fronds overlying or adjacent to an IP lesion. They resembled those of a conventional urothelial papilloma or grade 1 papillary urothelial carcinoma. However, the authors were noncommittal as to the possible biologic significance of the papillary component; they did suggest, however, that it might represent proliferative activity similar to cystitis cystica and von Brunn's nests, which are commonly observed in the adjacent mucosa.

IP with Foci of Distinct Exophytic Papillary Growth, Reported to Represent a Papillary Urothelial Carcinoma Accompanying an IP

Several reports describe a papillary (exophytic) urothelial cell component. These lesions were described as a transitional cell carcinoma growing within an IP [2, 8–11]. However, invasive growth was not observed

in any of these lesions. To be convincing that it indeed represents a carcinoma, it would be necessary to demonstrate undisputable cytologic atypia, invasiveness, recurrence as carcinoma at the same site, or metastasis. Risio et al. [12] reported two cases of combined IP and exophytic lesions. One of them, from a 75 year-old man, had a papillary lesion with areas of IP histology. The papillary lesion was unequivocally invasive to the lamina propria. Based on these observations, it appears that on rare occasions an exophytic papillary urothelial carcinoma may occur within an IP.

What is the histogenesis of the combined IP and exophytic papillary lesion? Three possible mechanisms may be offered. (1) If an exophytic component is composed of cells with a low nuclear grade (grade 1 of the 1973 WHO classification scheme) and shows no microscopic evidence of invasive growth, one could consider such cases as a morphologic variant of IP. (2) Should we consider that these cases represent a growth of dual differentiation—i.e., a benign tumor (IP) and a malignant tumor (albeit of low-grade malignancy)? (3) Could they represent a collision tumor? IP most commonly occurs without concurrent or past exophytic bladder carcinoma, suggesting that its pathogenesis differs from that of urothelial carcinomas. In fact, Kunze et al. [2] suggested that IP may be derived from the proliferative lesions originating in von Brunn's nests. However, IPs are also known to occur in patients with an exophytic urothelial carcinoma, developing simultaneously or metachronously [12, 13].

Nested Variant of Urothelial Carcinoma, Which Could Be Mistakenly Reported as Malignant Alteration Involving IP (Fig. 3-2-4)

Talbert and Young [14] were the first to report a peculiar urothelial carcinoma with a deceptively benign appearance in its cytologic and architectural appearance (Fig. 3-2-4A). The invasive nests resembled von Brunn's nests, cystitis cystica, cystitis glandularis, or nephrogenic metaplasia. This variant occurs predominantly in elderly men and is commonly located around the ureteral orifice [15], the site that is favored by both urothelial carcinoma and IP. Microscopically, anastomosing cords and nests arise from a generally intact surface urothelium. The cells show only mild cytologic atypia, resembling those of IP [15–17]. Some of the nests may show central cyst formation (Fig. 3-2-4B) or squamous differentiation, again having features in common with IP. However, irregular distribution of the nests, irregularly shaped nests, the presence of numerous closely packed nests, and focal cytologic atypia (Fig. 3-2-4B) [14] should raise the suspicion of carcinoma rather than von Brunn's nests or IP. Obvious invasion of the muscle fibers (Fig.3-2-4C), if found, would

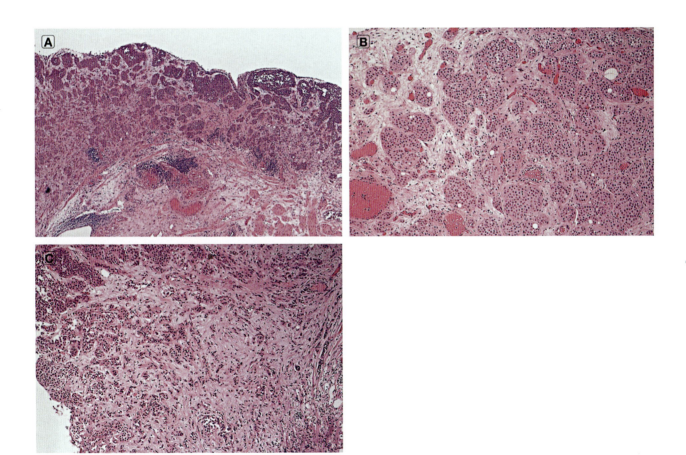

FIG. 3-2-4. Nested variant of urothelial carcinoma. Deceptively benign-looking nests of varying size are located underneath the bladder mucosa (thus resembling von Brunn's nests). However, as the nests move downward, they become smaller and more irregular in size and shape and invade the tunica muscularis mucosae muscle (**A**). Under a higher power (**B**), tumor nests vary in size, but cellular pleomorphism is minimal. **C** Note that the tumor shows an invasive growth pattern as it invades smooth muscle fibers of the tunica muscularis mucosae. Note also the desmoplastic reaction

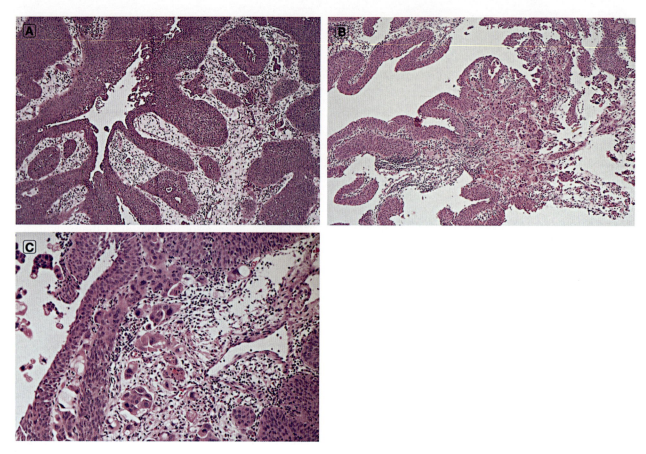

FIG. 3-2-5. Urothelial carcinoma of high grade with both exophytic and endophytic growth patterns. This tumor is unusual in that it is made up of both exophytic and endophytic (inverted) growth patterns and of cells with nuclear grade 2 and 3 (1973 WHO classification system). **A** In this field, the tumor exhibits an endophytic growth pattern and comprises grade 2 carcinoma. Small invasive nests are present in the right half of the field. **B, C** In this field, both exophytic and endophytic growth patterns are found with multiple grade 3 carcinoma nests invading the lamina propria

establish the diagnosis of carcinoma. Desmoplasia, if found, clearly supports the cancer diagnosis. Murphy and Deana [18] stated that some areas in every case are composed of cells with small but pleomorphic nuclei, slightly irregular chromatin, and large nucleoli. Of interest and of use is a tendency toward increasing cellar anaplasia with increasing depth of invasion (Fig. 3-2-4C) [18]. Despite the minimal cytologic atypia, the tumor is aggressive and has potential for invasion and metastasis.

Urothelial Carcinoma of Inverted Pattern, Which Could Be Mistakenly Reported as a Malignant Variant of IP

It is well recognized that occasionally cell growth in a urothelial carcinoma is directed inward (endophytic), thereby producing an inverted growth pattern (Figs. 3-2-5, 3-2-6). Therefore, differentiation from IP

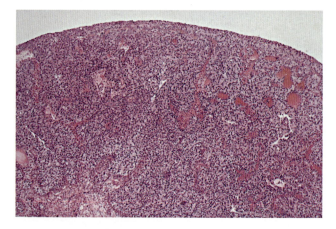

FIG. 3-2-6. This nodular urothelial carcinoma of high grade, endophytic type is sending multiple fused invasive nests into the lamina propria

becomes crucial. Amin et al. [19] stated that, "distinction from IP requires attention to architectural and cytological features of the lesions. Transitional cell carcinoma with an inverted growth pattern has thicker columns, with irregularity in the width of the columns, and transition of cords and columns into more solid areas. The characteristic orderly maturation, spindling, and peripheral palisading seen in IP are generally absent or inconspicuous in carcinoma with an inverted growth pattern. Unequivocal invasion into the lamina propria or the muscularis propria rules out the diagnosis of IP" (Figs. 3-2-5, 3-2-6). Unfortunately, these criteria may be inadequate when deciding whether the lesion is an IP or a urothelial carcinoma, inverted type. The features suggestive of urothelial carcinoma are the following: (1) obvious invasion with or without desmoplastic reaction—the diagnosis of lamina propria invasion requires the unquestionable presence of irregularly shaped nests or single cells in the lamina propria that may be accompanied with desmoplastic or inflammatory reaction, or tumor cells clearly invading the muscularis propria [19]; (2) cytologic atypia—nuclear pleomorphism, irregularities of the nuclear borders and chromatin distribution, prominent nucleoli; and (3) brisk mitotic figures. The presence of a surface papillary component, as well as other architectural features cited above can be used to establish the diagnosis of carcinoma. The only proof of malignancy depends on aggressive behavior during the follow-up.

Molecular Changes that Distinguish IP from Urothelial Carcinoma

In the 2005 United States and Canadian Academy of Pathology (USCAP) annual meeting, the gene expression pattern of IP in comparison to that of urothelial carcinoma with an inverted pattern was reported [20]. Although the mutation of fibroblast growth factor receptor 3 (FGFR3; a marker of low-grade urothelial carcinoma) was found at a low frequency (5/51), significantly different was the higher frequency in carcinomas of inverted pattern, of mutation of receptor *FGFR3* ($P < 0.0001$) [21, 22], and expression of Ki-67 (a proliferation marker) ($P < 0.0001$). Increased Ki-67 ($\geq 5\%$) expression and mutated *FGFR* status allowed one to distinguish IP from carcinoma of inverted pattern with a sensitivity of 68.9% [95% confidence interval (CI95): 53.4%–

81.8%] and a specificity of 90.5% (CI95: 69.6%–98.8%). However, it was also concluded that inverted tumors without clear features of malignancy should not be classified as malignant because of the limitation of molecular studies.

In summary, an inverted papillary tumor is a distinct benign entity and behaves in a benign fashion. About 15% of them show cytologic atypia as characterized by nuclear atypia, nucleomegaly, and some mitotic figures. Some IPs show a focal area of exophytic growth pattern, and such lesions have been considered a combined IP and papillary urothelial carcinoma. If invasion is present, a tumor with an endophytic pattern should be considered urothelial carcinoma. Finally, IPs may rarely coexist with an overt invasive carcinoma. If an inverted lesion demonstrates a diffuse nuclear atypia (> grade 2), it may be classified as a carcinoma and should not be classified as malignant conversion of the IP. Further molecular study is necessary to demonstrate the differences between IP and carcinoma of inverted pattern.

References

1. Potts IF, Hirst E (1963) Inverted papilloma of the bladder. J Urol 90:175–179.
2. Kunze E, Schauer A, Schmitt M (1983) Histology and histogenesis of two different types of inverted urothelial papillomas. Cancer 51:348–358.
3. Kimura G, Tsuboi N, Nakajima H, Yoshida k, Masugi Y, Akimoto M (1987) Inverted papilloma of the ureter with malignant transformation: a case report and review of the literature: importance of the recognition of he inverted papillary tumor of the ureter. Urol Int 42:30–36.
4. Stower MJ, MacIver AG, Gingell JC, Clarke E (1990) Inverted papilloma of the ureter with malignant change. Br J Urol 65:13–16.
5. Uyama T, Moriwaki S (1981) Inverted papilloma with malignant change of renal pelvis. Urology 17:200–201.
6. Broussard JN, Tan PH, Epstein JI (2004) Atypia in inverted urothelial papilloma: pathology and prognostic significance. Hum Pathol 35:1499–1504.
7. Kyriakos M, Royce RK (1989) Multiple simultaneous inverted papillomas of the urinary tract: a case report with a review of ureteral and renal pelvic inverted papillomas. Cancer 63:368–380.
8. Lazarevic B, Garret R (1978) Inverted papilloma and papillary transitional cell carcinoma of urinary bladder: report of four cases of inverted papilloma, one showing papillary malignant transformation and review of the literature. Cancer 42:1904–1911.

9. Palvio DHB (1985) Inverted papillomas of the urinary tract: a case of multiple, recurring inverted papillomas of the renal pelvis, ureter and bladder associated with malignant change. Scand J Urol Nephrol 19:299–302.

10. Stein BS, Rosen S, Kendall AR (1984) The association of inverted papilloma and transitional cell carcinoma of the urothelium. J Urol 131:751–752.

11. Stower MJ, MacIver AG, Gingell JC, Clarke E (1990) Inverted papilloma of the ureter with malignant change. Br J Urol 65:13–16.

12. Risio M, Coverlizza S, Lasaponara F, Vercesi E, Giaccone G (1988) Inverted urothelial papilloma: a lesion with malignant potential. Eur Urol 14:333–338.

13. Anderstrom C, Johansson S, Petterson SV (1982) Inverted papilloma of the urinary tract. J Urol 127:1132–1134.

14. Talbert ML, Young RH (1989) Carcinoma of the urinary bladder with deceptively benign-appearing foci: a report of three cases. Am J Surg Pathol 13:374–381.

15. Drew PA, Furman J, Civantos F, Murphy WM (1996) The nested variant of transitional cell carcinoma: an aggressive neoplasm with innocuous histology. Mod Pathol 9:989–994.

16. Terai A, Tamaki M, Hayashida H, Tomoyoshi T, Takeuchi H, Yoshida O (1996) Bulky transitional cell carcinoma of bladder with inverted proliferation. Int J Urol 3:316–319.

17. Lin O, Cardillo M, Dalbagni G, Linkov I, Hutchinson B, Reuter VE (2003) Nested variant of urothelial carcinoma: a clinicopathologic and immunohistochemical study of 12 cases. Mod Pathol 16:1289–1298.

18. Murphy WM, Deana DG (1992) The nested variant of transitional cell carcinoma: a neoplasm resembling proliferation of Brunn's nests. Mod Pathol 5:240–243.

19. Amin MB, Gomez JA, Young RH (1997) Urothelial transitional cell carcinoma with endophytic growth patterns: a discussion of patterns of invasion and problems associated with assessment of invasion in 18 cases. Am J Surg Pathol 21:1057–1068.

20. Eiber M, Blaszyk H, van Oers JMM, Zwarthoff E, van der Kwast T, Stoer R, Burger M, Cheville JC, Sauter G, Amin M, Hofstaedter F, Hartman A (2005) Molecular analysis of inverted urothelial tumors. Mod Pathol 18 (suppl 1):138A.

21. Van Rhijn BWG, Lurkin I, Radvanyi F, Kirkels WJ, van der Kwast TH, Zwarthoff EC (2001) The fibroblast growth factor receptor 3 (FGFR3) mutation is a strong indicator of superficial bladder cancer with low recurrence rate. Cancer Res 61:1265–1268.

22. Van Rhijn BWG, van der Kwast TH, Vis AN, Kirkels WJ, Boeve ER, Jobsis AC, Zwarthoff EC (2004) FGFR3 and p53 characterize alternative genetic pathways in the pathogenesis of urothelial carcinoma. Cancer Res 64:1911–1914.

Question 3

What is small cell carcinoma of the urinary bladder? What are the biologic behaviors of this tumor and its relationship to the conventional urothelial carcinoma?

Answer

Small cell carcinoma is a rare, highly aggressive form of urothelial cancer that affects elderly men more often than women. The urinary bladder is the most common site of its development in the urinary tract. The initial manifestation commonly is hematuria. At the time of diagnosis, most of the tumors have invaded the muscularis propria. As the name implies, the tumor is composed of small round or oval cells and occasionally spindle-shaped cells with "salt and pepper" chromatin and inconspicuous nucleoli. The tumors are indistinguishable from metastatic small cell carcinoma of the lung. Most of the tumors express some sort of neuroendocrine markers. The prognosis is dismal regardless of the mode of treatment. Cystectomy versus noncystectomy does not seem to affect the prognosis. Cisplatinum-based chemotherapy may be applied to prolong lives.

Comments

General Features

Among lung cancers, small cell carcinoma is a common variant, accounting for about 25% of malignant pulmonary tumors. Although extrapulmonary small cell carcinomas are rare, they have been reported with increasing frequency at locations such as the esophagus, breast, head and neck, skin, lower gastrointestinal tract, and genitourinary tract [1]. In the genitourinary tract, a collective review showed that it is most frequent in the urinary bladder followed, in descending order of frequency, by the prostate, renal pelvis, and ureter [2].

Small cell carcinoma of the urinary bladder is a rare tumor, accounting for less than 1% of all bladder tumors [1–6]. Although it has been considered a tumor of neuroendocrine differentiation, not all the tumors expressing markers are considered small cell carcinoma. Neuroendocrine cells are found in the normal urothelium [7], but its origin via dedifferentiation of neuroendocrine cells seems unlikely [8]. The most plausible source is the multipotential (stem) cell capable of differentiating in more than one cell type. This hypothesis is supported by the observation that nearly 50% of small cell carcinomas of the urinary bladder are associated with components of urothelial carcinoma, squamous cell carcinoma, or adenocarcinoma [3–5, 8–13].

Clinical Features of Small Cell Carcinoma of the Urinary Bladder

It affects the elderly. The male/female ratio is 3:1 [8]. The most common presenting symptom is gross or microscopic hematuria. Rarely, it is accompanied by paraneoplastic syndromes including symptoms due to hypercalcemia [14], ectopic adrenocortical hormone [15], or gonadotropin [16] release. At presentation, most of the patients have tumors invading the muscularis propria (81/85) [3], (63/64) [10]. Only 1 of the 64 cases in the Cheng series [10] was in pT1.

Pathologic Features

Gross appearance of the tumors is that of a polypoid to nodular mass frequently with a central ulcer (Fig. 3-3-1). Most of them occur in the bladder, but some develop in the upper urinary tract including the renal pelvis and ureter [12, 17].

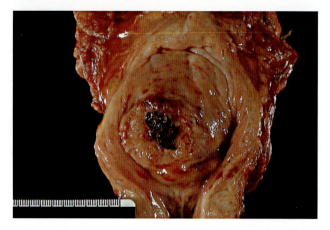

FIG. 3-3-1. Small cell carcinoma in a cystectomy specimen. The tumor is sessile, occupying the posterior wall. An ulcer at the dome of the tumor is covered with blood clot

Microscopically, the tumor consists of small, round cells (Figs. 3-3-2, 3-3-3, 3-3-5A), oat cells Fig. 3-3-4A), intermediate cells, or spindle cells growing in sheets. These cells are indistinguishable from those of pulmonary small cell carcinoma. Nucleoli are usually small or not apparent. In approximately 50% of the cases, small cell carcinoma is mixed with urothelial carcinoma (Figs. 3-3-3, 3-3-4B), squamous cell carcinoma, or even adenocarcinoma. Rarely, small cell carcinoma is accompanied by an area differentiating to carcinoid [12]. In radical cystectomy specimens, carcinoma in situ (Fig. 3-3-5C) is found in high frequency (16/20 cases by Quek et al. [18]).

Immunohistochemical reactions vary from case to case. Small cell carcinoma cells of the urinary bladder generally stain diffusely to epithelial markers, EMA

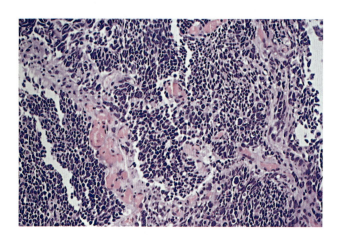

FIG. 3-3-2. Small cell carcinoma of the urinary bladder invading the muscularis propria. Small cells with round to oval nuclei are arranged in groups and invade the muscle layer

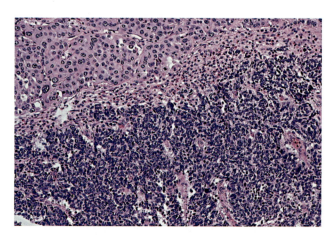

FIG. 3-3-3. Small cell carcinoma of the urinary bladder mixed with an area of high-grade urothelial carcinoma

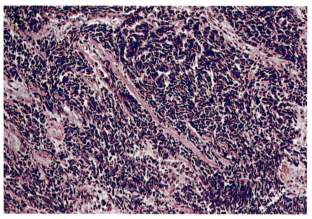

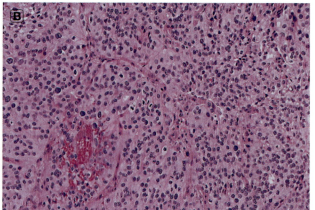

FIG. 3-3-4. Small cell carcinoma of the urinary bladder, oat cell type (**A**). This case also had an area of low-grade urothelial carcinoma (**B**)

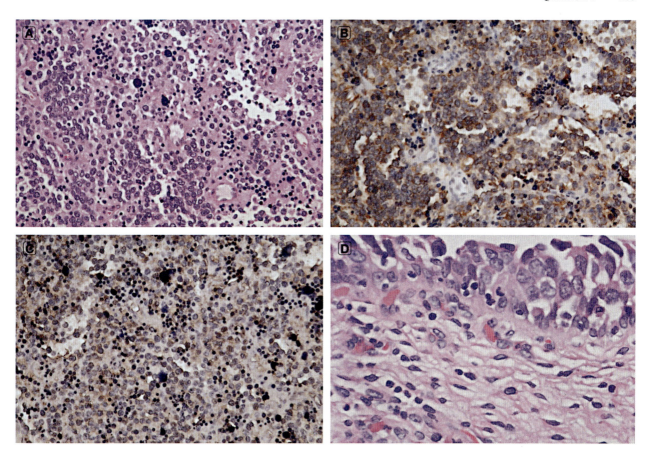

FIG. 3-3-5. Small cell carcinoma of the urinary bladder consisting of relatively uniform small cells (**A**). The tumor cells are reactive to neuron-specific enolase (**B**) and synaptophysin (**C**) but not to chromogranin A (not shown). This case was accompanied with the surface mucosa showing carcinoma in situ. Note that the carcinoma in situ consists of atypical large cells, not small cells (**D**)

[4, 11], Cam 5.2 [3], and/or AE1/3 [13]. Neuroendocrine markers are typically positive in small cell carcinoma. Neuron-specific enolase (NSE) is expressed in most of the cases [4, 13]. Synaptophysin and chromogranin are expressed in at least half of the cases [3, 4]. Positivity for at least one of these three neuroendocrine markers and one of the epithelial markers are required for establishing the diagnosis of small cell carcinoma of the urinary bladder. Compared to primary lung small cell carcinoma, which shows TTF1 immunoreactivity in more than 90% of cases, bladder small cell carcinomas express TTF1 at a lower frequency: approximately 38% of cases based on a study of 44 cases [19].

Treatment and Prognosis

Most patients have a locally advanced or metastatic cancer at the time of diagnosis. Several reports discuss the outcome based on a small number of cases. In the largest series of 64 cases by Cheng et al. [10], none of the clinicopathologic parameters studied (age, sex, presenting symptoms, smoking history, the presence of non-small-cell carcinoma component, chemotherapy, or radiation therapy) was associated with a survival advantage. No significant survival difference was found between patients who did or did not undergo cystectomy ($P = 0.65$). The overall 1-year, 18-month, 3-year, and 5-year disease-specific survival rates were 56%, 41%, 23%, and 16%, respectively.

Of the 23 patients with bladder small cell carcinoma reported by Trias et al. [3], 18 were dead within 18 months. Three were well without evidence of the disease at 36, 48, and 50 months, respectively. All three had a tumor at T2 and were treated by transurethral resection (TUR) followed by chemotherapy. It is of interest that all three surviving patients had tumors that were nonreactive to neuroendocrine markers (NSE and chromogranin A). They thus do not meet the current diagnostic criteria for small cell carcinoma. One of the remaining two patients was alive with the disease and the other was lost for follow-up.

Trias et al. [3] also summarized data reported in the world literature. In a review series of 93 patients, 63 were dead within 18 months, whereas 30 were alive without disease (17 patients >2 years and 11 patients >5 years). They concluded that cis-platinum-based chemotherapy appeared to improve the prognosis. Holmang et al. [6] made a similar observation; of 18 patients with stages T2M0 to T4M0 cancer treated surgically (cystectomy or TUR), 5 had no evidence of tumor after a median 10-year follow-up (6–18 years). They concluded that some patients can be cured by TUR or partial or radical cystectomy when combined with radiotherapy so long as there was no evidence of distant metastasis.

References

1. Christopher ME, Seftel AD, Sorenson K, Resnick MI (1991) Small cell carcinoma of the genitourinary tract: an immunohistochemical, electron microscopic and clinicopathological study. J Urol 146:382–388.
2. Mackey JR, Au HJ, Hugh J, Venner P (1998) Genitourinary small cell carcinoma: determination of clinical and therapeutic factors associated with survival. J Urol 159:1624–1629.
3. Trias I, Algaba F, Condom E, Espanol I, Segui J, Orsola I, Villavicencio H, Garcia del Muro X (2001) Small cell carcinoma of the urinary bladder: presentation of 23 cases and review of 134 published cases. Eur Urol 39:85–90.
4. Blomjous CE, Vos W, De Voogt HJ, Van der Valk O, Meijer CJ (1989) Small cell carcinoma of the urinary bladder: a clinicopathologic, morphometric, immunohistochemical and ultrastructural study of 18 cases. Cancer 64:1347–1357.
5. Grignon DJ, Ro JY, Ayala AG, Shum DT, Ordonez NG, Logothetis CJ, Johnson DE, Mackay B (1992) Small cell carcinoma of the urinary bladder. Cancer 69:527–536.
6. Holmang S, Borghede G, Johansson SL (1995) Primary small cell carcinoma: a report of 25 cases. J Urol 153:1820–1822.
7. Anonymous (1981) Bladder cancer In: Skrabanek P, Walsh A (eds) UICC technical report series, report no. 13. International Union Against Cancer, Geneva, 1981, p 38.
8. Murphy WM, Grignon DJ, Perlman EJ (2004) Tumors of the kidney, bladder, and related urinary structures. In: AFIP Atlas of Tumor Pathology Series 4. American Registry of Pathology, Washington, DC, pp 259–260.
9. Algaba F, Sauter G, Schoenberg MP (2004) Small cell carcinoma: WHO histological classification of tumours of the urinary tract. In: Eble JN, Sauter G, Epstein JI, Sesterhenn IA (eds) Pathology and genetics of tumors of the urinary system and male genital organs: World Health Organization classification of tumours. IARS Press, Lyon, p 135.
10. Cheng L, Pan C-X, Yang XY, Lopez-Beltran A, MacLennan GT, Lin H, Kuzel TM, Papavero V, Tretiakova M, Nigro K, Koch MO, Eble JN (2004) Small cell carcinoma of the urinary bladder: a clinicopathologic analysis of 64 cases. Cancer 101:957–962.
11. Mills SE, Wolfe III JT, Weiss MA, Swanson PE, Wick MR, Fowler JE Jr, Young RH (1987) Small cell undifferentiated carcinoma of the urinary bladder: a light-microscopic, immunocytochemical, and ultrastructural study of 12 cases. Am J Surg Pathol 11:606–617.
12. Ordonez NG, Khorsand J, Ayala AG, Sneige N (1986) Oat cell carcinoma of the urinary tract. Cancer 58:2519–2530.
13. Podesta AH, True LD (1989) Small cell carcinoma of the bladder: report of five cases with immunohistochemistry and review of the literature with evaluation of prognosis according to stage. Cancer 64:710–714.
14. Reyes CV, Soneru I (1985) Small cell carcinoma of the urinary bladder with hypercalcemia. Cancer 56:2531–2533.
15. Partanen S, Askainen U (1985) Oat cell carcinoma of the urinary bladder with ectopic adrenocorticotropic hormone production. Hum Pathol 16:313–315.
16. Kawamura J, Machida S, Yoshida O, Oseko F, Imura H, Hattori M (1978) Bladder carcinoma associated with ectopic production of gonadotropin. Cancer 42:2773–2780.
17. Guillou L, Duvoisin B, Chobaz C, Chapius G, Costa J (1993) Combined small-cell and transitional cell carcinoma of the renal pelvis. Arch Pathol Lab Med 117:239–243.
18. Quek ML, Nichols PW, Yamzon J, Daneshmand S, Mirand G, Cai J, Groshen S, Stein JP, Skinner DG (2005) Radical cystectomy for primary neuroendocrine tumors of the bladder: the University of Southern California experience. J Urol 174:93–96.
19. Jones TD, Kernek KM, Yang XJ, Lopez-Beltran A, MacLennan GT, Eble JN, Lin H, Pan CX, Tretikova M, Baldridge LA, Cheng L (2005) Thyroid transcription factor-1 expression in small cell carcinoma of the urinary bladder: an immunohistochemical profile of 44 cases. Hum Pathol 36:718–723.

Question 4

What is nephrogenic adenoma? What is the histogenesis of nephrogenic adenoma? What is the immunohistochemical profile of the lesion? Is there any relation between the development of a nephrogenic adenoma and kidney transplant?

Answer

Nephrogenic adenoma is a relatively common reactive process. Many of these lesions, if not all, are proliferative autotransplants of renal tubular cells shed in urine and implanted on a traumatized urothelial lining. Nephrogenic adenoma typically occurs in persons with a history of injury to the urothelial mucosa, including surgical manipulation, catheterization, calculi, and chronic inflammation. Immunosuppression associated with renal transplantation may enhance its development. However, most nephrogenic adenomas are not associated with organ transplant.

The urinary bladder is the most commonly affected site, followed by the urethra, ureter, and renal pelvis. The clinical history of some sort of trauma to the urinary tract is a frequent finding. Grossly, the nephrogenic adenoma is a small lesion <1 cm in diameter. The characteristic microscopic findings are (1) presence of glandular or tubular structures resembling renal tubules; (2) variation of tubular structures with cystic dilatation; (3) presence of a hyaline basement sheath around these tubules; and (4) a background of edematous granulation-type tissue associated with inflammation. It is important to distinguish this lesion from bladder and prostate cancers as there are morphologic similarities. The diagnosis should be established based primarily on morphologic features. The immunohistochemical profiles of nephrogenic adenoma is identical to that of renal tubules, including positivity for PAX2, keratins, and α-methylacyl coenzyme A racemase (AMACR) and negative for prostate-specific antigen (PSA), high-molecular-weight keratin (34βE12), and p53.

Comments

Nephrogenic adenoma (NA), also known as nephrogenic metaplasia, is a common reactive lesion of the urinary tract that was first reported by Davis under the designation "hamartoma." [1]. One year later, Friedman and Kuhlenbeck [2] characterized the lesion in detail and proposed the name "nephrogenic adenoma" because of its similarity to renal tubules. NA typically occurs in patients with a history of trauma to the urothelial mucosa, which includes surgical manipulation, catheterization, previous resection of a tumor, presence of calculi, and chronic urinary tract inflammation. Immunosuppression may enhance the development of NA. Although a high incidence of NA has been reported in renal transplant recipients, most NAs are seen in patients without an organ transplant.

Clinical Presentation

Nephrogenic adenoma is more common in males than in females (2:1), occurs in patients ranging in age from 15 to 94 years, and involves the urinary bladder most commonly (55%) followed by the urethra (41%) and the ureter (4%) [3]. An authentic case of malignant transformation has not been reported.

The clinical manifestation is nonspecific. Most patients present with gross and microscopic hematuria, increased urinary frequency, or dysuria [4]. The NAs developing in the ureter may be associated with stones, multiple episodes of cystitis, chronic pyelonephritis, ureteral obstruction, and hydronephrosis, which raises the suspicion for carcinoma [5].

Endoscopic Findings

Endoscopic examination most characteristically reveals either a friable strawberry-like or papillary lesion. The average diameter of the lesions is 2–3 mm. The largest lesion in our study of 38 cases was 8 mm [6]. For any lesion >1 cm, a diagnosis other than NA should be seriously considered. In kidney recipients, NA frequently develops at multiple sites with no preferential location in the bladder [7, 8].

Pathologic Findings

Based on their detailed analysis of 80 cases, Young and Scully summarized the pathologic features as follows [3, 9]: Approximately 56% are papillary, 34% sessile, and 10% polypoid. Microscopically, the lesion can be divided to four patterns: tubular, cystic, papillary-polypoid, and diffuse.

The most common pattern present in 96% of the cases was tubular (Fig. 3-4-1A). The tubules were generally small, hollow, and round, although some were solid and occasionally elongated. Tubules in the lamina propria were focally arranged in an irregular pattern and suggested infiltrating tubules of adenocarcinoma (Fig. 3-4-1B). Some of the tubules were elongated and branching, forming a complex network of channels [3] (Fig. 3-4-1C). The lining cells were cuboidal and had eosinophilic to pale, slightly granular cytoplasm (Fig. 3-4-1B). The lumen often contained eosinophilic secretion. The basement membrane around tubules was thickened in 20 cases. In 12 of 80 cases, some of the cells had clear cytoplasm.

A cystic pattern (Fig. 3-4-1D) was observed in 58 of 80 cases, and in 6 it was striking. The lining cells were flattened but may be lined by hobnail cells (Fig. 3-4-1D).

The third pattern was papillary to polypoid, projecting to the bladder lumen (Fig. 3-4-1E,F). Papillae were observed in 9 cases and a polypoid pattern in 43 cases. They are almost always associated with areas of tubular differentiation.

The fourth pattern, diffuse, was present in 11 cases and was almost always focal. Cells were closely arranged in thin cords, which made it difficult to differentiate it from invasive carcinoma. NA nests could be found within the lamina propria (Fig. 3-4-1A) and occasionally within the muscularis propria. Mitosis was infrequent, and variation in the nuclear size was common.

Differential Diagnoses

It is important for the pathologist to distinguish NA from neoplastic and proliferative lesions occurring in the lower urinary tract, especially when only a small biopsy sample is available. Such lesion are clear cell adenocarcinoma of the urethra, prostatic adenocarcinoma, atypical adenomatous hyperplasia of the prostate, clear cell adenocarcinoma of the bladder, and clear cell variant of urothelial carcinoma. These lesions share several features in common with NA: location (urethra), clear cells, diffuse and papillary growth pattern, even signet cells, and involvement of the prostate tissue.

Clear Cell Adenocarcinoma of the Lower Urinary Tract

Clear cell adenocarcinoma of the lower urinary tract is a distinct entity that has been considered of Müllerian duct origin. It is far more common in females than in males and occurs most commonly in the urethra. Furthermore, more than 50% of the tumors occur in a diverticulum (Fig. 3-4-2A,B). A past history of surgical manipulation of the urinary tract, trauma, calculi, or urinary tract infection points to the diagnosis of NA. Conversely, the absence of such a history raises an index of suspicion for clear cell adenocarcinoma, especially in females [9]. Cells with abundant clear cytoplasm are unusual in NA. There are significant cytologic atypia and mitotic activity in most clear cell adenocarcinomas [9, 10]. According to the Gilcrease group [10], only mild cytologic atypia and a single mitotic figure were observed in 2 of 13 NAs, whereas 4 of 5 clear cell adenocarcinomas showed severe atypia, and the mitotic rate ranged from 2 to 12 per 10 high-power fields. Immunohistochemical analysis was not helpful other than strong staining for p53 in each of five cases and high MIB-1-positive cells (average 47/200 cells) in clear cell adenocarcinoma compared with 5.5 in NA. It is noteworthy that NA can develop in a diverticulum of the urinary bladder

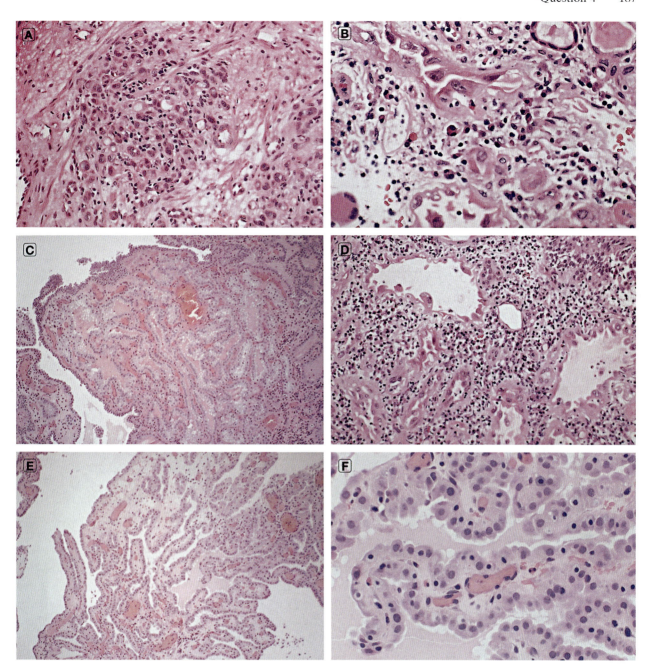

Fig. 3-4-1. Nephrogenic adenoma. **A** Typical tubular pattern. Small packed tubules are in the lamina propria, separating tunica muscularis mucosae muscle fibers. **B** Tubules are irregular in size and shape, as are the lining cells, which have eosinophilic cytoplasm, moderately enlarged nuclei, and occasional prominent nucleoli. Note that some nuclei are smudged, indicating degenerative changes. Lymphocytes and plasma cells infiltrate the stroma. **C** Branching tubules are lined by cuboidal cells with clear cytoplasm. **D** Some tubules are cystically dilated and lined by cells whose nuclei are pushed to the lumen (hobnail cells). **E** (low power), **F** (high power) Papillary pattern of nephrogenic adenoma. The papillary fronds are lined by a cuboidal cell layer with small uniform nuclei

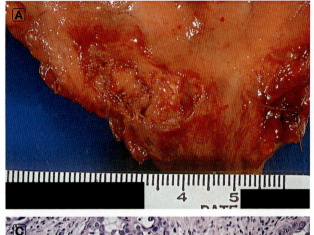

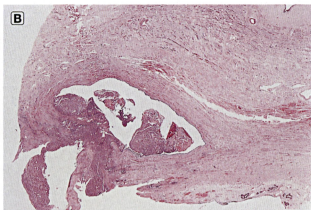

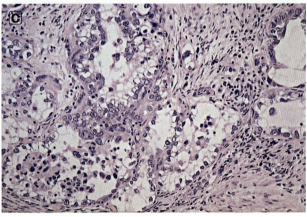

FIG. 3-4-2. Clear cell adenocarcinoma of female urethra. **A** Cystectomy specimen. A polypoid carcinoma is in a diverticulum of proximal urethra. **B** Adenocarcinoma growing in a diverticulum. **C** Well-differentiated tubular adenocarcinoma with clear cytoplasm and nuclei showing moderate pleomorphism

and the urethra [11]. Thus, in female patients, differentiating it from clear cell adenocarcinoma becomes a major problem. Again, the presence of nuclear atypia and common mitotic figures help establish the diagnosis of clear cell adenocarcinoma. Immunohistochemical nuclear staining of PAX2 protein ensures the diagnosis of NA (see the histogenesis for details).

Urothelial Carcinoma with Clear Cell Features

Urothelial carcinoma may exhibit areas with clear cytoplasm (Fig. 3-4-3), a tubulocystic or a striking micropapillary pattern [12–15]. Marked cytologic atypia and areas showing the typical urothelial carcinoma differentiation should aid in the differential diagnosis from NA.

Prostatic Adenocarcinoma

Nephrogenic adenoma occasionally develops in the urethra and can become a serious diagnostic challenge in distinguishing it from prostatic adenocarcinoma because of the presence of small tubules and clusters of cells in the fibromuscular stroma of the

prostate [16]. In both lesions, the tubular structure is lined by a single layer of cuboidal cells that may have clear cytoplasm and even prominent nucleoli. This pitfall in the diagnosis has been discussed by Epstein and Yang [17]. They stressed the importance of variation in the size of the tubules (which range from tiny tubules to cysts), hobnail-like cells, and the hyaline sheath of the basement membrane, features that are distinctly unusual for prostate cancer. When these features are present, the pathologist should raise suspicion for the diagnosis of prostate cancer and order some immunohistochemical markers to rule it out. NA is negative to PSA and prostate-specific acid phosphatase. It is important to stress, however, that 58% of NAs are positive for AMACR, a positive marker for prostate cancer, with staining ranging from patchy to focal to diffuse. Meanwhile, the reaction to 34βE12, a negative marker for prostate cancer, was positive in 38% of the NA cases [6].

Atypical Adenomatous Hyperplasia of the Prostate

Atypical adenomatous hyperplasia (AAH) commonly develops in the transition zone of the prostate

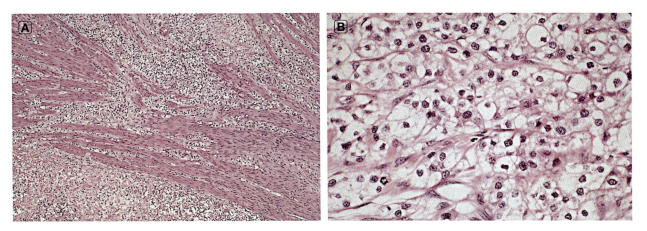

FIG. 3-4-3. **A, B** Urothelial carcinoma with clear cell features in a 71-year-old man. It is deeply invasive to the muscularis propria (**A**). A cystectomy specimen revealed foci of urothelial cell carcinoma in situ. The patient died 20 months later with wide spread metastasis

and therefore may be detected in a TUR specimen. AAH consists of aggregates of uniform-sized tubules lined by cuboidal clear cells with round nuclei. The basal cell layer is present but may be inconspicuous. The columnar cells and basal cells should stain positively for PSA and 34βE12, respectively, while NA is negative for PSA, positive or negative for 34βE12 [6].

Histogenesis

The idea that NA represents a metaplastic reaction of the urothelium has been widely accepted without proof despite an unusual finding against the metaplasia hypothesis: NA has developed in a sigmoid neobladder and an ileal conduit (where no urothelial cells are present) after cystectomy [18, 19].

As stated earlier, NA is not uncommon in kidney transplant recipients [7, 20, 21]. In 2002, a novel report came from a group of Austrian investigators: Mazal et al. [22] presented compelling evidence that NA developing in renal transplant recipients originated from tubular cells of the donor kidney. Using the fluorescence in situ hybridization (FISH) technique, they showed that all NAs in 14 female recipients of transplants from male donors and 10 male recipients from female donors showed the same sex-chromosome status as the donor kidney but not the same sex-chromosome status as the recipients' surrounding bladder tissue. The Mazal study with kidney markers aquaporin 1 (a membrane protein of water channels expressed in the proximal tubule and the descending thin limb of Henle's loop, but

not in other nephron segments, the collecting duct, or urothelial cells), PAX2 (a transcription factor expressed during organogenesis) [22], and binding to lectins all pointed to an origin from renal tubular cells. More recently, Tong et al. [23] confirmed the Mazal group findings by showing that PAX2 was likewise expressed in all NAs that were unrelated to kidney transplants ($n = 39$: 21 in the urinary bladder, 16 in the prostatic urethra, 2 in the distal urethra) but not in the normal prostate and urothelium, adenocarcinomas of the prostate ($n = 100$), or invasive urothelial carcinomas ($n = 47$). Thus, these studies have conclusively demonstrated that NAs express renal tubular cell markers and thus strongly suggest that NAs are an autotransplant-associated proliferation of renal tubular cells.

A pertinent question is why NA occurs in association with a history of urothelial tract trauma. Ingelfinger offered a decent histogenetic explanation for the NAs in renal transplant recipients: Normally, thousands of renal tubular cells are shed daily in the urine. These include viable cells as shown by successful growth in vitro of shed renal tubular cells [24]. Dysfunctional or injured urothelial lining may favor the "take" of shed viable tubular cells in immunocompromised hosts with a transplanted kidney [7]. It is reasonable to assume that denuded bladder mucosa, even in immunologically intact hosts, may take an autotransplant albeit rare. NA commonly occurs in a diverticulum of the urinary bladder and the urethra. Stagnation of urine may favor the growth of detached renal tubular cells [25].

References

1. Davis TA (1949) Hamartoma of the urinary bladder. Northwest Med 48:182–185.
2. Friedman NB, Kuhlenbeck H (1950) Adenomatoid tumor of the urinary bladder reproducing renal structure (nephrogenic adenoma). J Urol 64:657–670.
3. Oliva E, Young RH (1995) Nephrogenic adenoma of the urinary tract: a review of the microscopic appearance of 80 cases with emphasis on unusual features. Mod Pathol 8:722–730.
4. Bhagavan BS, Tiamason EM, Weenk RE, Berger BW, Hamamoto G, Eggleston JC (1981) Nephrogenic adenoma of the urinary bladder and urethra. Hum Pathol 12:907–916.
5. Gokaslan ST, Krueger JE, Albores-Saavedra J (2002) Symptomatic nephrogenic metaplasia of ureter: a morphologic and immunohistochemical study of four cases. Mod Pathol 15:765–772.
6. Gupta A, Wang HL, Policarpio-Nicolas ML, Tretiacova MS, Papavero V, Pins MR, Jiang Z, Humphrey PA, Cheng L, Yang X J (2004) Expression of alpha-methylacyl-coenzyme A racemase in nephrogenic adenoma. Am J Surg Pathol 28:1224–1229.
7. Beaudry C, Bertrand PE, Leplante L, Houde M, Lamoureux C, Laverdiere M, Dandavino R (1983) Nephrogenic adenoma of the bladder after kidney transplantation; surgical trauma and cytomegalovirus infection as possible etiologic factors. J Urol 130:1183–1185.
8. Fournier G, Menut P, Moal M-C, Hardy E, Volant A, Mangin P (1996) Nephrogenic adenoma of the bladder in renal transplant patients: a report of 9 cases with assessment of deoxyribonucleic acid ploidy and long-term follow-up. J Urol 156:41–44.
9. Young RH, Scully RE (1986) Nephrogenic adenoma: a report of 15 cases, review of the literature, and comparison with clear cell adenocarcinoma of the urinary tract. Am J Surg Pathol 10:268–275.
10. Gilcrease MZ, Delgado R, Vuich F, Albores-Saavedra J (1998) Clear cell adenocarcinoma and nephrogenic adenoma of the urethra and urinary bladder: a histologic and immunohistochemical comparison. Hum Pathol 29:1451–1456.
11. Medeiros LJ, Young RH (1989) Nephrogenic adenoma arising in urethral diverticulum. Arch Pathol Lab Med 113:125–128.
12. Kotliar SN, Wood CG, Schaeffer AJ, Oyasu R (1995) Transitional cell carcinoma exhibiting clear cell features: a differential diagnosis from clear cell adenocarcinoma of the urinary tract. Arch Pathol Lab Med 119:79–81.
13. Young RH, Zukerberg LR (1991) Microcystic transitional cell carcinomas of the urinary bladder: a report of four cases. Am J Clin Pathol 96:635–639.
14. Amin MB, Ro JY, El-Sharkawy T, Lee Km, Troncoso P, Silva EG, Ordonez NG, Ayala AG (1994) Micropapillary variant of transitional cell carcinoma of the urinary bladder. Am J Surg Pathol 13:1224–1232.
15. Johansson SL, Borghede G, Holmang S (1999) Micropapillary bladder carcinoma; a clinicopathological study of 20 cases. J Urol 161:1798–1802.
16. Young RH (1992) Nephrogenic adenomas of the urethra involving the prostate gland: a report of two cases of a lesion that may be confused with prostate adenocarcinoma. Mod Pathol 5:617–620.
17. Epstein JI, Yang XJ (2002) Prostate biopsy interpretation. Lippincott Williams & Wilkins, Baltimore, pp 277–283.
18. Redondo Maertinez R, Rey Lopez A (1998) Adenoma nefrogenica en mucosa intestinal: un caso en una anastomosis uretero-sigmoidea. Arch Esp Urol 51:284–286.
19. Strand WR, Alfert HJ (1987) Nephrogenic adenoma occurring in an ileal conduit. J Urol 137:491–492.
20. Gordon HL, Kerr SG (1975) Nephrogenic adenoma of bladder in immunosuppressed renal transplantation. Urology 5:275–277.
21. Behesti M, Morales A (1982) Nephrogenic adenoma of bladder developing after renal transplantation. Urology 20:298–299.
22. Mazal PR, Schaufler R, Alten-Huber Muller R, Haitel A, Watschinger B, Kratzik C, Krupitza G, Regele H, Meisl FT, Zechner O, Kerjaschki D, Susani M (2002) Derivation of nephrogenic adenomas from renal tubular cells in kidney-transplant recipients. N Engl J Med 347:653–659.
23. Tong G-X, Melamed J, Mansukhani M, Memeo L, Hernanzdez O, Deng F-M, Chiriboga L, Waisman J (2006) PAX2: a reliable marker for nephrogenic adenoma. Mod Pathol 19:356–363.
24. Dorrenhaus A, Muller JI, Golka K, Jedrusik P, Schulze H, Follman W (2000) Cultures of exfoliated epithelial cells from different locations of the human urinary tract and the renal tubular system. Arch Toxicol 74:618–626.
25. Ingelfinger JR (2002) Nephrogenic adenomas as renal tubular outposts. N Engl J Med 347:684–686.

Question 5

What are the clinical and pathologic features needed for the diagnosis of interstitial cystitis? What are the most important entities that should be considered in the differential diagnosis?

Answer

Although called "cystitis" for years, interstitial cystitis currently is regarded as a painful bladder syndrome because it does not always demonstrate an inflammatory picture microscopically. It is an enigmatic condition of unknown etiology and pathogenesis. The diagnosis is established based on clinical features, which consist of irritative voiding symptoms including urgency, frequency, pain, and absence of objective evidence of other disease (including negative urine culture and cytology) as well as characteristic endoscopic findings, which generally are demonstrated after overdistension of the bladder. Because the presenting symptoms of interstitial cystitis are suggestive of an inflammatory process, infectious disease, or a urothelial neoplasm, especially carcinoma in situ must be excluded by urine culture and microscopic examination of urine sediment/biopsy specimens. The etiology and pathogenesis and therapy are discussed under Questions 6 and 7, respectively.

Comments

At a meeting of the New England Branch of the American Urological Association in 1914, Hunner reported eight cases of women with a long-standing "bladder problem" as a "rare type of bladder ulcer" and described the cystoscopic and microscopic find-

ings in detail [1]. According to the currently accepted diagnostic criteria, Hunner's ulcer actually is seen in only 10% of patients with interstitial cystitis. Although the term interstitial cystitis (IC) has been commonly used for years, it is not necessarily accompanied by inflammatory changes. In 2002, The Interstitial Continence Society (ICS) defined IC as painful bladder syndrome (PBS)[1] [3]. The ICS prefers this term to IC, and the diagnosis of IC requires confirmation by typical cystoscopic and histologic features. Because of its popular use, "IC" is used in the present discussion. The IC affects women more frequently than men at a 5:1 ratio, with a peak prevalence at age 41–45 years for women and at a later age (late sixties) for men [4]. Depending on the diagnosis criteria used, the prevalence ranges from 45 to 197/100,000 for women and 8 to 41/100,000 for men [4]. IC is reportedly far more common among whites than in other races [5]. The prevalence in Japan is much lower, estimated to be 4.5/100000 women [6]. However, this may be an underestimate because only 10% of Japanese urologists reported using the National Institutes of Health criteria to aid the diagnosis [7]. As awareness of IC by the public as well as urologists increases, so does the prevalence. It is commonly assumed that many patients with IC are undiagnosed [8].

The syndrome is characterized by three criteria: (1) chronic voiding symptoms (suprapubic pain partially alleviated by bladder emptying, urgency, and frequency); (2) no objective evidence of other diseases (e.g., urinary tract infection or neoplasia); and (3) characteristic findings at cystoscopy [2, 9].

Two subtypes of IC are recognized based on cystoscopic findings: Type 1 (nonulcer type) is far more

---

[1] PBS is the complaint of suprapubic pain related to bladder filling accompanied by other symptoms such as increased daytime and nighttime frequency, in the absence of proven urinary infection or other obvious pathology [2].

common (about 90%) than type 2 (classic or ulcer type). The two types appear different regarding patient demographics, cystoscopic and histologic findings, age at onset, and response to treatment, further suggesting that they may be distinct entities [10–12].

What are the symptoms and how is the diagnosis made?

The patients often complain of multiple symptoms not only related to the bladder but non-bladder symptoms, suggesting that pathophysiological process may involve multiple organ systems beside the bladder. The University of Wisconsin interstitial cystitis scale (Table 3-5-1) was created to quantify IC symptoms [13] and has been used to evaluate changes in symptoms during follow-up [13–15]. It includes seven symptoms directly related to the bladder and 18 non-bladder reference symptoms.

Another commonly used system, the O'Leary system [16] created by the Harvard Medical School group, has gained popularity and in fact may be being used more commonly than the University of Wisconsin interstitial cystitis scale. The questionnaire consists of six sections: A, urinary symptoms; B, pain symptoms; C, sexual function; D, general health; E, symptom relationship with menstrual cycle; and F, quality of life.

Because there is no decisive diagnostic test, IC remains a diagnosis by exclusion. The symptoms are nonspecific. To exclude the known causes, such as infection and carcinoma, microbial culture and cytologic examination of urine must be performed, and the results should be negative. In an effort to ensure that patients entered for IC study would be homogeneous, the National Institute of Arthritis, Diabetes,

TABLE 3-5-1. University of Wisconsin interstitial cystitis scale

The scale for grading the severity of symptoms is completed by the patient within the context of the question, "How often did you experience the following symptoms today?"
- Interstitial cystitis items—expressed in rating scale of 0 (not at all) to 6 (a lot): discomfort, bladder pain, nocturia, day frequency, sleeping, urgency, burning
- Reference items—pelvic pain (discomfort), headache, backache, dizziness, feelings of suffocation, chest pain, ringing in ears, aches in joints, swollen ankles, nasal congestion, "flu," abdominal cramps, tingling in fingers and toes, nausea, blind spots in vision or blurred vision, heart pounding, sore throat, coughing

From Goin et al. [15].

Digestive and Kidney Diseases (NIDDK) in the United States held workshops in 1987 [17] and 1988 [18], and the consensus criteria were adopted (Table 3-5-2) [19]. Cystoscopy with hydrodistention was required to document inclusion or exclusion. Subsequently, however, the NIDDK criteria were judged to be too restrictive for clinical use as they exclude 60% of patients from the diagnosis [20]. In 2003, three international consensus conferences attempted to update the IC diagnostic criteria [21]. Because cystoscopy with hydrostatic distention was judged to lack specificity and correlated poorly with symptoms [22–24], thus providing little useful information above and beyond the history and physical examination, it is indicated only to exclude bladder cancer [25]. The Interstitial Cystitis Data Base (ICDB) Study sponsored by the NIDDK is a typical ongoing multicenter observational study designated to determine the treated history of IC and identify common patient characteristics [26]. In this study, endoscopic study was optional and was at the discretion of the study investigators. The eligibility criteria were to include

TABLE 3-5-2. Interstitial cystitis patient accrual form

Automatic exclusions
<18 years old
Benign or malignant bladder tumors
Radiation cystitis
Tuberculous cystitis
Bacterial cystitis
Vaginitis
Cyclophosphamide cystitis
Symptomatic urethral diverticulum
Uterine, cervical, vaginal, or urethral Ca
Active herpes
Bladder or lower ureteral calculi
Waking frequency < 5 times in 12 h
Nocturia < 2 times
Symptoms relieved by antibiotics, urinary antiseptics, urinary analgesics (e.g., phenazopyridine hydrochloride)
Duration < 12 months
Involuntary bladder contractions (urodynamics)
Capacity > 400 cc; absence of sensory urgency

Automatic inclusions
Hunner's ulcer

Positive factors
Pain on bladder filling relieved by emptying
Pain (suprapubic, pelvic, urethral, vaginal or perineal)
Glomerulations on endoscopy
Decreased compliance on cystometrography

From Gillenwater and Wein [17]. Bladder distention is defined arbitrarily as 80 cm water pressure for 1 min. Two positive factors are necessary for inclusion in the study population. Substratication at the conclusion of the study by bladder capacity with the patient under anesthesia was less than or greater than 350 ml.

all IC-like patients (the eligibility criteria are listed in Table III of Simon et al. [26]). Enrolled patients were predominantly females (91.5%) and white (91.0%), with an average age at enrollment of 44.3 years. Approximately 45% of patients underwent cystoscopic examination at baseline screening with or without hydrodistention and with or without biopsy. A statistically significant association ($P < 0.01$) was found between pain and urgency and the presence of Hunner's ulcer (see below for pathology discussion), but there was no association of these symptoms with the cystoscopic findings, including glomerulations [27] (see pathology section for detail).

What are the cystoscopic findings?

A detailed clinical pathologic study was reported by Hand in 1949 [28], but it was Messing and Stamey [27] who in 1978, based on cystoscopic findings after distention, proposed dividing IC into two types: ulcerative (classic) and nonulcerative. They considered the latter type an early lesion, but subsequent studies indicate that they probably represent two types of disease: Patients with classic IC are older (26–84 years old, mean age 64 years) than patients with the nonulcer type (19–71 years old, mean age of 39 years) [10, 29]. In the classic type, cystoscopic examination under general anesthesia and inspected under 70 cm of water pressure reveals reduced bladder capacity [10, 27, 29], so-called Hunner ulcers, and pinpoint hemorrhages. These changes become more striking on the second distention of the bladder. Red strawberry-like dots called glomerulations (a term coined by Walsh [30]) (Fig. 3-5-1), often coalesce to become hemorrhagic spots as a result of cracks and fissures. Glomerulations are generally prominent in the dome, posterior wall, and lateral walls of the bladder and are rarely seen or are absent on the trigone [12, 27]. The nonulcer type presents with symptoms similar to those of the classic type, but the cystoscopic findings are unremarkable until after overdistention, when glomerulations become apparent. By definition, Hunner's ulcers are absent.

What are the histologic findings?

An excellent correlative study between the cystoscopic findings and the microscopic findings was reported by Johansson and his colleagues [29, 31, 32]. The following findings are based primarily on their observations and are summarized as follows. In essence, there are no findings specific for or diagnostic of IC of either the classic or the nonulcer type.

Striking histologic changes are found only in the classic type: Multiple foci of mucosal ulcer are covered with blood and fibrinous exudates (Hunner's ulcer) (Fig. 3-5-2A,B). The underlying lamina propria contains granulation tissue infiltrated primarily with lymphocytes and plasma cells. Occasionally, lymphoid tissue with germinal centers is observed (Fig. 3-5-2A). Neutrophils are rare. Petechial hemorrhages corresponding to glomerulations

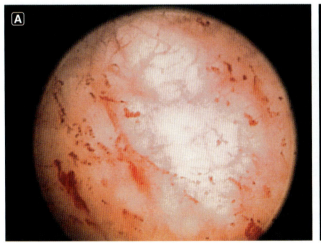
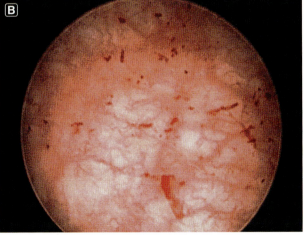

FIG. 3-5-1. **A, B** Endoscopic findings in an interstitial cystitis bladder, nonulcer type. Glomerulation developed after overdistention of the bladder. Note scattered petechial hemorrhages, either spotty or linear, along dilated capillaries in the lamina propria. The patient is a 49 year-old woman with a more than 5-year history of irritable urinary tract symptoms. (Courtesy of Quentin Clemens, MD, Northwestern University Feinberg School of Medicine, Chicago)

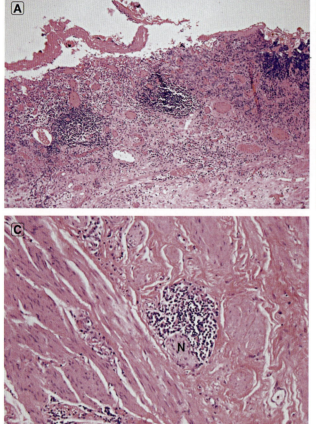

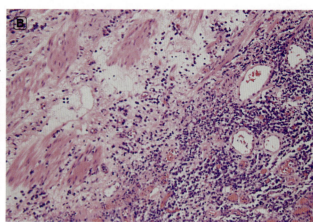

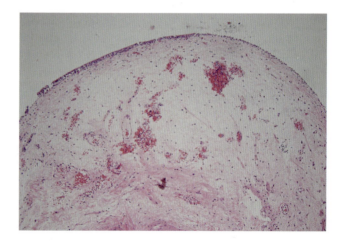

FIG. 3-5-2. Interstitial cystitis, ulcer type in an 81-year-old woman. She underwent cystectomy. An extensively ulcerated mucosa is covered with fibrin layer. The lamina propria contains numerous dilated capillaries and postcapillary venules and a number of lymphocytes, plasma cells, and mast cells (**A, B**). Two lymphoid follicles with a germinal center are present (**A**). Chronic inflammation has extended to the muscularis propria (**B**). Perineural (*N*) mononuclear leukocytes are present in **C**

on endoscopy are found in the lamina propria, and these foci increase with hydrostatic distention. Eosinophilic leukocytes are rare. Mast cells are found scattered in the lamina propria as well as in the muscularis propria. (See below for further discussion on the significance of mast cell infiltration.) Biopsy specimens taken from cystoscopically normal areas often showed mucosal denudation with detached epithelium floating. Perineural mononuclear cell infiltrates (Fig. 3-5-2C) were seen in 79% of the patients with the classic disease but not in patients with the nonulcer type or in controls [29].

In contrast to the classic type, the light microscopic findings in nonulcer type patients are meager. The only noteworthy findings are diffuse edema and foci of fresh hemorrhage in the lamina propria observed only after overdistention (Fig. 3-5-3). The inflammatory reaction is minimal (Fig. 3-5-4). Some of these inflammatory foci could represent the glomerulations observed on endoscopy. Mucosal cracks were observed only in the nonulcer type by the Johansson group [29], but the Erickson group observed them in both mildly as well as severely

FIG. 3-5-3. Interstitial cystitis, nonulcer type in a 78-year-old man. The lamina propria shows diffuse edema and perivascular fresh hemorrhages (glomerulations). The inflammatory reaction is minimal

inflamed bladders, the latter probably including the classic type [12].

Neither the ruptures nor the glomerulations were associated with any significant degree of inflammatory response. Biopsies from normal-appearing

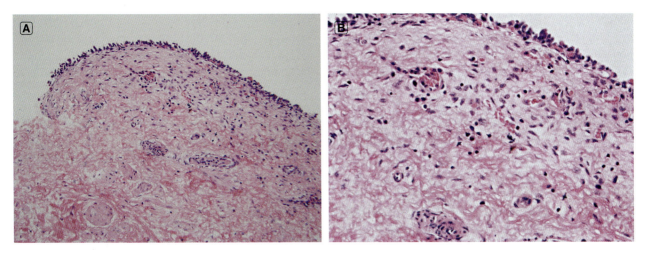

FIG. 3-5-4. **A,B** Interstitial cystitis, nonulcer type in a 25 year-old woman. Only minimal mononuclear cell infiltration is seen in the lamina propria

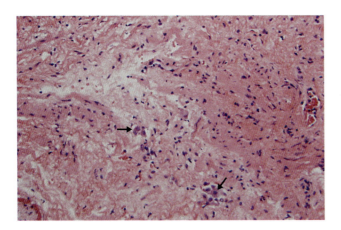

FIG. 3-5-5. Interstitial cystitis, nonulcer type in a 21-year-old woman. The bladder biopsy shows no notable abnormality except for a few mononuclear cells, most likely mast cells (*arrows*)

mucosa in nonulcer patients did not show significant changes except for slight edema. In approximately 10% of cases, biopsy specimens taken from the most diseased areas may be classified as normal (Fig. 3-5-5), implying that these patients of either type present with neither a Hunner's ulcer nor glomerulations at any level of severity [24]. Based on our experience, we agree with these assessments. In contrast to the classic type, mast cells were not increased in either the lamina propria or the muscularis propria [31].

What are the important differential diagnoses?

Because the presenting symptoms of IC are suggestive of an inflammatory process, infectious diseases, including viral, microbial, and parasitic infections,

must be excluded. The latter two can be ruled out by urine culture and microscopic examination of urine sediment or biopsy tissue. The possibility of IC being due to viruses and microbes that are undetectable by the routine culture technique remains. Another important disease category that must be ruled out is neoplasms including carcinoma in situ. The latter characteristically presents with microscopic hematuria and irritable bladder symptoms. Here, negative urine cytology and biopsy are crucial before the diagnosis of IC is entertained.

Are mast cells increased in interstitial cystitis?

A number of reports describe the presence of mast cells in the urinary bladder of IC patients. While evaluating reported data, several facts should be kept in mind, including the anatomic location of mast cells in the biopsy, a possible difference in their number by histologic type (nonulcer versus classic type), and the fact that two types of mast cells exist, one of which requires a specific fixation technique for its demonstration. Theoharides et al. [33] and Pang et al. [34] reported a mast cell increase without specifying their location. Others specifically mentioned an increase only in the detrusor muscles compared with the controls [35–37]. Some other groups demonstrated a significantly increased number of mast cells in both the mucosa/urothelium and detrusor muscles [38, 39]. However, the number and the range of mast cells in the normal bladder remain in question. Other investigators compared mast cell number between the classic type and nonulcer type and found an increase only in the former [40, 41]. Dundore et al. [42]

concluded that there was no increase of mast cells in IC biopsies from nonulcer type IC. This study, however, had a problem in the selection of control cases. Feltis et al. [39] reported a significant increase in mast cells in both the lamina propria (P < 0.01) and the detrusor muscles (P < 0.001) in biopsies that were a mixture of classic and nonulcer types. Their control groups were excellent, consisting of a large number of biopsies of normal histology and of autopsy bladders obtained from heart-beating organ donors.

As has been stated above, two types of mast cell can be found in the bladder: mucosa-type mast cells and connective tissue-type mast cells. Demonstration of mucosal-type mast cells requires a specific fixation and staining technique [40]. Aldehyde fixatives (e.g., formalin solution) block the specific binding sites of mucosal mast cell granules [43]. This blocking may be overcome by either a prolonged staining time [43] or use of special fixatives, such as an iso-osmotic mixture of 0.6% formaldehyde in 0.5% acetic acid [44]. Mast cells are identified as metachromatic granules with toluidine blue at pH 0.5. Fall et al. [31] used, as fixative, both an iso-osmotic mixture of 0.6% formaldehyde and 0.5% acetic acid, and conventional 4% formaldehyde. In classic IC, iso-osmotic formaldehyde and acetic acid (which stains both mucosa- and connective tissue-type mast cells) revealed a significant increase (twofold) in mast cell counts, and increase was due to mucosa-type mast cells located not only in the lamina propria but also in the urothelium, a finding unique to the classic type. In contrast, there was no increase in mast cells in the lamina propria of the nonulcer-type cases. In the detrusor muscle, a significant increase in mast cells was observed only in the classic type due to connective tissue-type mast cells.

It is concluded that mast cells are increased in IC biopsies. The increase is predominantly in the detrusor muscle, especially in the classic type. Furthermore, mast cell increase in the detrusor muscle was of the connective tissue type, whereas an increase in the lamina propria was due to mucosa-type mast cells, some of which migrated to the overlying urothelium. At this time, the significance of recognizing two types of cell in the pathogenesis of IC remains unknown. We do know, however, that they respond to different types of pharmacologic agents and release different mediators [45]. For instance, in response to neuropeptides, connective tissue mast cells secrete by compound exocytosis (release of secretory granule contents by explosion as seen with anaphylaxis). In contrast, mucosal mast cells secrete by intragranular or "piecemeal" activation (slow release with an intact core membrane) [46] (for further discussion, refer to Question 6).

Another question is that mast cells can undergo degranulation when they respond to stimuli. Special stains may not work for detecting degranulated mast cells. Histamine [41, 47], methylhistamine (the major metabolite of histamine), and the specific mast cell marker tryptase [48], were shown to be increased in the urine of IC patients, suggesting that mast cells in IC patients are activated. Thus, not only mast cell number but, more importantly, the status of mast cell granules is critically important in the pathogenesis of IC [33, 46, 48–50]. The Theoharides group [39] found more than 90% of the mast cells in IC samples were degranulated to varying degrees, whereas nearly all were intact in the controls. Similar observations had been made previously by Lynes et al. [37]. Mast cells were not only activated but were located in the vicinity of neuronal processes [46, 48–50], suggesting their functional association. Possible significance is discussed under Question 6.

In summary, interstitial cystitis is characterized by the presence of typical clinical pictures, negative findings for infection and neoplasm, cystoscopic findings such as glomerulations and ulceration, and histologic findings such as mucosal edema and increased mast cells. Pathologically, interstitial cystitis is a diagnosis by exclusion.

References

1. Hunner GL (1918) A rare type of bladder ulcer in women; report of cases. Boston Med Surg J 172:660–668.
2. Abrams P, Cardozo L, Fall M, Griffiths D, Rosier P, Ulmsten U, van Kerrebroeck P, Victor A, Wein A (2002) The standardization of terminology of lower urinary tract function: report from Standardization Sub-Committee of the International Continence Society. Neurourol Urodyn 21:167–178.
3. Warren JW, Meyer WA, Greenberg P, Horne L, Diggs C, Tracy JK (2006) Using the International Continence Society's definition of painful bladder syndrome. Urology 67:1138–1143.
4. Clemens JQ, Meenan RT, Rosetti MC, Gao SY, Calhoun EA (2005) Prevalence and incidence of interstitial cystitis in a managed care population. J Urol 173:98–102.

5. Simon LJ, Landis J, Erickson DR, Nyberg LM, the ICDB Study Group (1997) The Interstitial Cystitis Database Study: concepts and preliminary baseline descriptive statistics. Urology 49(suppl 5A): 64–75.

6. Ito T, Miki M, Yamada T (2000) Interstitial cystitis in Japan. BJU Int 86:634–637.

7. Kusek JW, Nyberg LM (2001) The epidemiology of interstitial cystitis: is it time to expand our definition? Urology 57(suppl 6A):95–99.

8. Ueda T (2003) The legendary beginning of the international consultation on interstitial cystitis. Intern J Urol 10:S1–S2.

9. Hanno PM (1998) Interstitial cystitis and related diseases. In: Walsh PC, Retic AD, Vaughn ED Jr, Wein AJ (eds) Campbell's urology, vol 1. Saunders, Philadelphia, pp 631–662.

10. Peeker R, Fall M (2002) Toward a precise definition of interstitial cystitis: further evidence in differences of classic and nonulcer disease. J Urol 167:2470–2472.

11. Buffington CA (2004) Comorbidity of interstitial cystitis with other unexplained clinical conditions. J Urol 172:1242–1248.

12. Erickson DR, Belchis DA, Dabbs DJ (1997) Inflammatory cell types and clinical features of interstitial cystitis. J Urol 158:790–793.

13. Keller ML, McCarthy DO, Neider RS (1994) Measurement of symptoms of interstitial cystitis: a pilot study. Urol Clin North Am 21:67–71.

14. Erickson DR, Morgan KC, Ordille S, Keay SK, Xie SX (2001) Nonbladder related symptoms in patients with interstitial cystitis. J Urol 166:557–562.

15. Goin JE, Olaleye D, Peters KM, Steinert B, Habicht K, Wynant G (1998) Psychometric analysis of the University of Wisconsin interstitial cystitis scale: implications for use in randomized clinical trials. J Urol 159:1085–1090.

16. O'leary MP, Sant GR, Fowler FJ Jr, Whitmore KE, Spolarich-Kroll J (1997) The interstitial cystitis symptom index and problem index. Urology 49(suppl 5A):58–63.

17. Gillenwater JY, Wein AJ (1988) Summary of the National Institute of Arthritis, Diabetes, Digestive and Kidney Diseases Workshop on Interstitial Cystitis, National Institutes of Health, Bethesda, Maryland, August 28–29, 1987. J Urol 140:203–206.

18. Wein AJ, Hanno PM, Gillenwater JY (1990) Interstitial cystitis: an introduction to the problem. In: Hanno PM, Staskin DR, Krane RJ, Wein AJ (eds) Interstitial cystitis. Springer-Verlag, London, pp 3–15.

19. Hanno PM (1994) Diagnosis of interstitial cystitis. Urol Clin North Am 21:63–66.

20. Hanno PM, Landis JR, Matthews-Cook Y, Kusek J, Nyberg L Jr, The Interstitial Database Study Group (1999) The diagnosis of interstitial cystitis revisited: lessons learned from the National Institutes of Health Interstitial Cystitis Database Study. J Urol 161:553–557.

21. Nickel JC (2004) Interstitial cystitis: the paradigm shifts. International consultations on interstitial cystitis. Rev Urol 6:200–202.

22. Waxman JA, Sulak PJ, Kuehl TJ (1998) Cystoscopic findings consistent with interstitial cystitis in normal women undergoing tubal ligation, J Urol 160:1663–1667.

23. Denson MA, Griebling TL, Cohen MB, Kreder KJ (2000) Comparison of cystoscopic and histological findings in patients with suspected interstitial cystitis. J Urol 164:1908–1911.

24. Tomaszewski JE, Landis JR, Russack V, Williams TM, Wang L-P, Hardy C, Brensinger C, Matthews YL, Abele ST, Kusek JW, Nyberg LM; The Interstitial Cystitis Database Study Group (2001) Biopsy features are associated with primary symptoms in interstitial cystitis: results from the interstitial cystitis database study. Urology 57(suppl 6A):67–81.

25. Ottem DP, Teichman JM (2005) What is the value of cystoscopy with hydrodistention for interstitial cystitis? Urology 66:494–499.

26. Simon LJ, Landis JR, Erickson DR, Nyberg LM, the ICDB Study Group (1997) The Interstitial Cystitis Data Base Study: concepts and preliminary baseline descriptive statistics. Urology 49(suppl 5A): 64–75.

27. Messing EM, Stamey TA (1978) Interstitial cystitis: early diagnosis, pathology, and treatment. Urology 12:381–392.

28. Hand JR (1949) Interstitial cystitis: report of 223 cases (204 women and 19 men). J Urol 61:291–310.

29. Johansson SL, Fall M (1990) Clinical features and spectrum of light microscopic changes in interstitial cystitis. J Urol 143:1118–1124.

30. Walsh A (1978) Interstitial cystitis. In: Harrison JH, Gittes RF, Perlmutter AD, et al (eds) Campbell's urology, vol 1. Saunders, Philadelphia, pp 693–707.

31. Fall M, Johansson SL, Aldenborg F (1987) Chronic interstitial cystitis; a heterogeneous syndrome. J Urol 137:35–38.

32. Johansson SL, Fall M, Peeker R (2004) Interstitial cystitis. In: Foster CS, Ross JS (eds) Pathology of the urinary bladder. Saunders, Philadelphia, pp 91–101.

33. Theoharides TC, Sant GR, El-Mansoury M, Letourneau R, Ucci AA Jr, Meares EM Jr (1995) Activation of bladder mast cells in interstitial cystitis: a light and electron microscopic study. J Urol 153:629–636.

34. Pang X, Marchand J, Sant GR, Kream RM, Theoharides TC (1995) Increased number of substance P positive nerve fibers in interstitial cystitis. Br J Urol 75:744–750.

35. Larsen S, Thompson SA, Hald T, Barnard RJ, Gilpin CJ, Dixon JS, Gosling JA (1982) Mast cells in interstitial cystitis. Br J Urol 54:283–286.

36. Kastrup J, Hald T, Larsen S, Nielsen VG (1983) Histamine content and mast cell count of detrusor muscle in patients with interstitial cystitis and other types of chronic cystitis. Br J Urol 55:495–500.

37. Lynes WL, Flynn SD, Shortliffe LD, Lemmers M, Zipser R, Roberts J II, Stamey TA (1987) Mast cell involvement in interstitial cystitis. J Urol 138:746–752.

38. Christmas TJ, Rode J (1991) Characteristics of mast cells in normal bladder, bacterial cystitis and interstitial cystitis. Br J Urol 68:473–478.

39. Feltis JT, Perez-Marrero R, Emerson LE (1987) Increased mast cells of the bladder in suspected cases of interstitial cystitis: a possible disease marker. J Urol 138:42–43.

40. Aldenborg F, Fall M, Enerback L (1986) Proliferation and transepithelial migration of mucosal mast cells in interstitial cystitis. Immunology 58:411–416.

41. Lundeberg T, Liedberg H, Nordling L, Theodorsson E, Owzarski A, Ekman P (1993) Interstitial cystitis: correlation with nerve fibers, mast cells and histamine. Br J Urol 71:427–429.

42. Dundore PA, Schwartz AM, Semerjian H (1996) Mast cell counts are not useful in the diagnosis of nonulcerative interstitial cystitis. J Urol 155:885–887.

43. Wingren U, Enerback L (1983) Mucosal mast cells of the rat intestine: a re-evaluation of fixation and staining properties, with special reference to protein blocking and solubility of the granular glycosaminoglycan. Histochem J 15:571–582.

44. Enerback L (1966) Mast cells in rat gastrointestinal mucosa. I. Effect of fixation. Acta Pathol Microbiol Scand 66:289–302.

45. Galli SJ (1993) New concepts about the mast cells. N Engl J Med 328:257–265.

46. Letourneau R, Pang X, Sant GR, Theoharides TC (1996) Intragranular activation of bladder mast cells and their association with nerve processes in interstitial cystitis. Br J Urol 77:41–54.

47. Yun SK, Laub DJ, Weese DL, Lad PM, Leach GE, Zimmern PE (1992) Stimulated release of urine histamine in interstitial cystitis. J Urol 148:1145–1148.

48. Pang X, Boucher W, Triadafilopoulos G, Sant GR, Theoharides TC (1996) Mast cell and substance P-positive nerve involvement in a patient with both irritable bowel syndrome and interstitial cystitis. Urology 47:436–438.

49. Elbadawi AE, Light JK (1996) Distinctive ultrastructural pathology of nonulcerative interstitial cystitis: new observations and their potential significance in pathogenesis. Urol Int 56:137–162.

50. Elbadawi A (1997) Interstitial cystitis: a critique of current concepts with a new proposal for pathologic diagnosis and pathogenesis. Urology 49(suppl 5A): 14–40.

Question 6

What are the possible etiology and pathogenesis of interstitial cystitis?

Answer

Several hypotheses have been proposed, none of which is completely satisfactory. There has been no report that specifically addresses the possible pathogenetic difference between the ulcer and nonulcer types. Several significant proposals have been presented in literature: increased urothelial permeability to urine contents due to the defective urothelial barrier; stress-induced heightened autonomic nervous system sharing co-morbidity with another vaguely defined disease complex; and neurogenic inflammation/activation of mast cells initiating the chain of events. These possibilities are not necessarily mutually exclusive but may be closely interrelated. Of the proposed mechanisms, the most attractive is the neurogenic inflammation hypothesis. Overactive sensory nerve fibers in the bladder send urge signals to the pontine micturition center, which in turn stimulates detrusor muscle contraction via the parasympathetic nerve. Locally, at the same time, the intrinsically abnormal urothelium exhibits a heightened neurosensory-like action by excessive release of adenosine triphosphate. It, in turn, stimulates the nearby sensory nerve fibers and induces them to release neurokinins, such as substance P and calcitonin gene-related peptide. These neurokinins stimulate mast cells that have migrated close to sensory nerve fibers. From their granules, mast cells release inflammatory cytokines in a piecemeal fashion. As a result, vasodilatation, edema, and chronic inflammation ensue, the features of interstitial cystitis. Although evidence points to the importance of mast cells in this process, the possibility of the neurokinins acting directly on endothelial cells should be kept open at least in some cases. Infectious disease and a genetic factor might be the trigger of interstitial cystitis.

Comments

The following are hypotheses supported by clinical and experimental studies.

Increased Urothelial Permeability

Parsons and his colleagues are the proponents of the hypothesis that, at least in a sizable number of patients, the irritable voiding symptoms are due to the defective mucosal barrier caused by the deficient glycosaminoglycan (GAG) layer on the urothelial surface [1–6]. According to them, GAG (mucus) present on the normal urothelial surface binds water molecules tightly to the oxygen of the sulfate group. Thus, water molecules trapped and interposed at the boundary act as a physical barrier to the bladder content (urine) [7]. In one of the studies, a group of normal subjects and patients with interstitial cystitis (IC) were challenged with 40 ml of 40 mEq KCl, and subjective responses of urgency or pain stimulation was recorded [5]. There was a marked sensitivity to intravesical KCl in 75% of patients with IC versus 4% of control ($P < 0.01$). Normal subjects who previously had demonstrated minimal sensitivity to KCl had markedly increased sensitivity after intravesical protamine treatment (to remove GAG) (11% vs. 79%). The irritative symptoms were reversed in 42% of subjects after heparin (a type of GAG) instillation. However, potassium sensitivity was also found in patients with acute urinary tract infection, the data indicating the GAG barrier becomes defective in association with acute urinary tract infection [5]. In clinical studies, Parsons' hypothesis was supported at least in part by objective alleviation of the irritative symptoms with an oral heparinoid (sodium pentosan polysulfate[1]) (given orally for at least 4 months) [8, 9]. Subsequent similar studies by other groups resulted in mixed results. The data by Chelsky et al. [10] with intravesically administered radionuclide, [99m]technetium-diethyl-enetriaminepentaacetic acid (^{99m}Tc-DTPA) were not supportive. Later, however, this report was criticized by Teichman and Nielsen-Omeis [11], who attributed their conclusion to the small statistical power of the study cases. Erickson et al. [12] instilled 100 ml of 5% rhamnose solution into the bladder of six IC patients and eight controls. The mean rhamnose absorption was much greater by bladders of IC patients than by bladders of eight controls ($P = 0.008$). However, rhamnose absorption varied greatly among IC patients. Teichman et al. [11] used the potassium leak test before heparin or oral pentosan polysulfate sodium treatment. The potassium leak test was positive in 23 and negative in 15. After a minimum of 6 months of therapy, patients with a positive leak test were more likely to show improvement than those with a negative test, as evidenced by a decrease in the pain score of more than 25% (78% vs. 40%, $P = 0.01$), frequency (83% vs. 47%, $P = 0.02$), and nocturia (83% vs. 53%, $P = 0.05$).

Whatever the barrier function studies may show, the ultimate significance is determined by clinical studies based on prospective randomized placebo controls. Several studies have been conducted. The data are discussed later in the therapy section (Question 7).

Ultrastructural study has demonstrated conflicting results. Dixon et al. [13] saw no differences between IC and control biopsies regarding the appearance of the surface urothelial cells and glycocalyx as demonstrated with ruthenium red. Using scanning electron microscopy, Anderstrom et al. [14] observed only nonspecific findings to indicate an increased urothelial cell turnover. The IC patients had a reduced mucin layer. In contrast, Elbadawi and Light [15] found substantial alterations in all structures in the biopsies from nonulcer-type patients; urothelial cells were noncohesive with wide intercellular spaces, and masses of cell debris were often found on the surface of the urothelium. The unique asymmetrical unit membrane of normal umbrella cells could not be

demonstrated with certainty. In the lamina propria, capillaries were engorged, and the stroma was diffusely edematous and had a variable number of lymphocytes and mast cells that were mostly activated. The detrusor muscle showed distinctive and consistent changes; intracellular edema resulted in bloating and displayed an "oak leaf" appearance of muscle cells. Degenerative changes were also demonstrated in the nerves and vessels. These authors concluded that the changes were distinctive enough for the diagnosis of IC, nonulcer type and did not support the GAG deficiency hypothesis. The striking findings reported by Elbadawi and Light are impressive but should be confirmed by others.

Immunologic Mechanism

Evidence for abnormal immunologic mechanisms as a cause of IC is meager, and all findings appear to be nonspecific or of dubious significance [16–18]. However, as will be discussed later, intravesical bacillus Calmette-Guerin treatment appeared effective in ameliorating symptoms at least in a study reported by one group [19]. Erickson et al. [20] demonstrated that severely inflamed bladders were associated with an increase in T cells ($P < 0.0003$) and B cells ($P < 0.0001$) as compared with less inflamed IC bladders.

Urothelial cells normally do not express HLA class II antigen. However, abnormal expression of the HLA DR molecule was immunohistochemically demonstrated in the urothelium in 18 of 20 biopsies from IC patients but not in biopsies of bacterial cystitis and normal bladders [21]. Inappropriate expression of HLA class II molecules, particularly HLA-DR products, is a feature of a number of tissues affected by the autoimmune process [22]. This raises the possibility of autoimmunity as a pathogenetic mechanism. However, another question is what triggers HLA class II molecule expression. The fact that active chronic inflammation is infrequent suggests that it is an unlikely mechanism of disease induction.

Stress-Induced Heightened Autonomic Nervous System, Sharing Co-morbidity with Other Vaguely Defined Chronic Disease Complexes

Interstitial cystitis is a multifactorial syndrome. Epidemiologic studies have shown that IC patients share co-morbidity with other vaguely defined symptoms [23, 24] such as chronic pelvic pain syndrome (defined

---

[1] It is also referred to as pentosanpolysulfate sodium.

as lower abdominal pain unrelated to pregnancy that has lasted more than 6 months) [25, 26], irritable bowel syndrome [23, 24, 27–29], fibromyalgia (defined as a chronic condition of diffuse musculoskeletal pain associated with specific tender points on examination) [30], and chronic pain and fatigue syndrome (defined as persistent or prolonged fatigue of more than 6 months without a medical or psychiatric condition that can account for the symptoms [31,3 2]. Association is more common in patients with classic-type IC [33]. These associations suggest that at least in some cases of IC the pathophysiologic process affects other organ systems as well. More recently, Kusek and Nyberg [25] considered IC as part of chronic pelvic pain syndrome, and Gunter [34] proposed that patients with chronic pelvic pain should be investigated for the presence of IC as well as for various gynecologic, gastrointestinal, musculoskeletal, and neurologic disorders. Their proposal is based on the assumption that pelvic pain may be either nociceptive or nonnociceptive (neuropathic), the former from injury to a pain-sensitive organ/tissue that is somatic or visceral in origin. Somatic pain originates from skin, muscles, bone, and joints and is transmitted along sensory fibers; it is generally described as sharp or dull and is usually discrete [34]. Visceral pain, on the other hand, is transmitted through the sympathetic fibers and could be described as poorly localized, dull, or crampy. Visceral pain is frequently associated with autonomic phenomena such as nausea, vomiting, sweating, and strong emotional reactions. Neuropathic pain is the result of an insult to the central or peripheral nervous system and typically produces burning pain, paresthesia, and lancinating pain [34]. Based on different responses to the treatment, Buffington [33] stated that the cause of pain in patients with the classic (ulcer) type may be nociceptic, whereas pain in patients with nonulcer type may be neuropathic. It is noteworthy that the symptoms cited above appear to share a dysregulated autonomic nervous system or emotional stress as common denominators.

The symptoms of IC wax and wane over the course. Stress is known to aggravate the symptoms [35]. The trigger may originate from two sources. First, chronic inflammation in the bladder and urine reaching the subepithelial areas, a consequence of the defective urothelial barrier, may stimulate the sensory nerves (Fig. 3-6-1), which induces a premature urge to urinate. Micturition requires coordinated contraction of the bladder detrusor muscle mediated via para-

sympathetic input from the preganglionic neurons in the lumbosacral spinal cord, whereas sphincter relaxation is mediated by the sympathetic nerve via hypogastric plexuses (Fig. 3-6-1). In patients with IC, the urge to urinate is prematurely relayed to the locus coeruleus (LC), a micturition center in the pons. Neurophysiologic investigations on micturition are conducted primarily in rats and cats. Barrington's nucleus in the pons is one of the micturition centers in the rat and lies ventromedial to the LC [36]. Areas corresponding to the pontine micturition center described in the rat and cat have been identified in humans through brain imaging [36]. Barrington's nucleus is an extra hypophyseal site of corticotropin-releasing factor (CRF) release, suggesting that it serves as a neuromodulator/neurotransmitter. Evidence for stress-induced activations in CRF expression in Barrington's nucleus has been demonstrated in rats [37, 38]. Barrington's neurons synapse with the LC using CRF as a neurotransmitter [36]. The LC, with norepinephrine as its neurotransmitter, sends a message to the forebrain and limbic nuclei as arousal (desire to urinate). Activation of the LC has been demonstrated by artificial distention of the bladder [39, 40] or colon [39, 41] in the rat and cats with the feline interstitial cystitis model [42]. For the efferent pathway, axons of Barrington's neurons terminate onto preganglionic parasympathetic neurons. Thus, diverging projections of Barrington's nucleus (caudal and cranial) to the LC and spinal cord can serve as a substrate for the coordination of central and peripheral responses to the pelvic visceral stimuli [36].

The second source of trigger for urgency (Fig. 3-6-1) is environmental stress (visual, physical, psychological). It leads to release of the hypothalamic neurohormone CRF, which initiates pituitary adenocorticotropin release and activation of CRF in Barrington's nucleus.

The pathogenetic mechanism of the closely related irritable bowel syndrome could be explained by a similar pathogenetic mechanism: Stress, as a precipitating factor, increases CRF expression in Barrington's neurons [37, 38]. For the colon, Barrington's CRF projection to the spinal cord has been postulated to be mediated via the vagus nerve [36].

The role of the pituitary-adrenal axis has been investigated by several groups. It is uncertain if it plays a significant role. According to Lutgendorf et al. [43], patients with morning urinary cortisol levels of <12.5 nmol/l were 12.8 times more likely to report urinary urgency than those with values above this

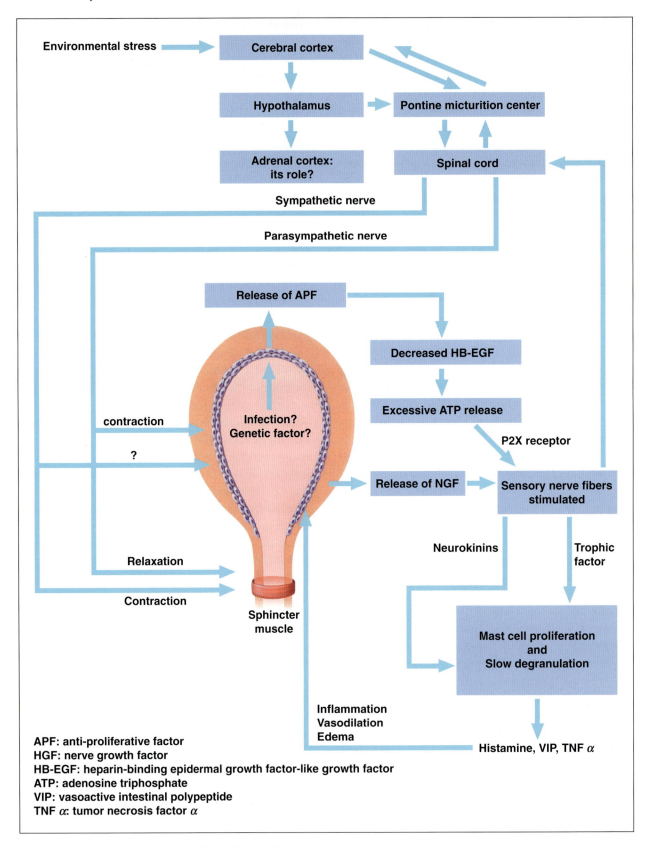

Fig. 3-6-1. Postulated mechanism of interstitial cystitis

cutoff point. Studies of cats with the feline interstitial cystitis model indicate that the cortisol response to ACTH stimulation during stressful circumstances was decreased. Additionally, adrenal glands were smaller in cats with feline interstitial cystitis than in healthy cats [44]. Buffington suggested that the decreased adrenocortical response could be due to a genetic disorder [33].

The following observations support the contention that a heightened sympathetic nervous system in response to stress has some role in IC. Irwin et al. [45] reported abnormal vasomotor tone (contraction) in the pedal skin in response to isolated cold stress in IC patients. Sympathetic neuron density was significantly increased near urothelial cells ($P < 0.01$) and detrusor muscles ($P < 0.01$) and around vessels ($P < 0.05$) of IC patients [46].[2] The increase was more prominent in the ulcer-type IC. Enhanced innervation of the bladder was also observed in the submucosa and the detrusor muscle by Lundeberg et al. [47] and Hohenfellner et al. [48]. By immunofluorescence microscopy, the latter investigators concluded that the increase was of sympathetic, not cholinergic (parasympathetic), neurons.[3] Increased urinary excretion of norepinephrine, indicative of adrenergic sympathetic transmission, has been described in patients with IC [49].

How could these findings be tied to the clinical picture of IC? Hohenfellner et al. [48] suggested that enhanced sympathetic outflow increases local mast cell population, citing the reported finding in rat synovium by Levine et al. [50] (see the following section for the possible pharmacologic mechanism), whereas the Peeker group [46] failed to offer a persuasive explanation.

---

[2] This conclusion is based on an immunohistochemical reaction of nerve fibers located near epithelial cells, detrusor muscle, and around vessels reacting primarily to neuropeptide Y and tyrosine hydroxylase [46], markers of sympathetic fibers, and low reactivity to substance P, a sensory fiber marker.

[3] This conclusion is based on the increased immunofluorescent reaction of submucosal neurons to the antibodies against the neuropeptides vasoreactive intestinal peptide and neuropeptide Y, both of which are contained in sympathetic fibers, and not to substance P or calcitonin-gene-related peptide, primary sensory afferent fiber markers. These conclusions were challenged by later investigators who concluded that most proliferative neural fibers in the submucosa are sensory fibers as they immunohistochemically react to antibodies against substance P and calcitonin-gene-related peptide, sensory nerve fiber markers. Refer to the following section.

Activation of Mast Cells and Subsequent Induction of Neurogenic Inflammation

Activation of mast cells and subsequent induction of neurogenic inflammation has become the most attractive hypothesis based on the currently available data. The salient features to support the hypothesis are that in the IC bladders: (1) neural fibers, probably predominantly sensory type, are increased, especially in the lamina propria; (2) mast cells are increased in the lamina propria [51, 52] and the detrusor muscle [51–56] and are topographically closely associated with vessels and neural fibers; and (3) mast cells are in various stages of activation. These salient features are discussed below.

A close spatial relation between mast cells and nerves has been reported for a number of species and many organs [57]. Frequent perivascular localization of mast cells was also reported in the urinary bladder submucosa [58, 59]. In a study with normal guinea pig bladder, mast cells were found not only juxtaposed to, but often completely wrapped around, nerve fibers that were immunoreactive with the antibodies against neuropeptides substance P (SP) and calcitonin gene-related peptide (CGRP)—neuropeptides secreted by sensory nerves [57]. Their distribution was primarily in the submucosa near capillaries and other vessels but occasionally in the detrusor muscle. Moreover, mast cells could be found in intramural autonomic ganglia. Electron microscopy revealed that mast cell lamellipodia were in contact with a neurite process. Keith et al. [57] concluded that most of the nerve fibers in contact with mast cells are primary sensory nerves based on their lack of myelin (consistent with C fibers[4]) and the presence of sensory fiber neuropeptides. The Theoharides group [61] found that mast cells in bladder biopsies from IC patients averaged 40/mm^2 in contrast to 10/mm^2 in controls (urinary incontinence and chronic bacterial cystitis) or 50/mm^2 in bladder cancer patients. A striking finding was that 90% of mast cells in IC biopsies were activated (degranulated), whereas almost all of these cells were intact in the controls and cancer patients. In biopsies from IC patients,

---

[4] Sensory fibers are divided into A (alpha, beta, gamma, delta), B, and C fibers by the size, and conduction velocity. A delta is 3–5 μM in size and 6–30 m/s in velocity, and C fibers are 0.4–1.2 μm in size and 0.5–2.0 m/s in velocity [60].

SP-containing nerve fibers were increased in the submucosa and were frequently in juxtaposition to mast cells [62]. Electron microscopy demonstrated that these mast cells contained secretory granules at various stages of dissolution. This is a significant observation, indicating that mast cells in the IC bladder have a unique mode of differential release of mediators, unlike the explosive release of mediators typically seen during anaphylaxis [63].

Inevitably, this raises a number of questions. What attracts mast cells to nerve fibers (mostly sensory but perhaps others such as sympathetic)? What triggers mast cell activation, and what is the significance? What follows mast cell activation? What causes proliferation of nerve fibers?

Trophic substances are released to attract mast cells. Levine et al. [50] found in the rat synovium that the mast cell population was positively affected by the density of both sympathetic and afferent sensory nerve fibers. In this study, selective damage to sensory neurons with capsaicin and postganglionic sympathetic neurons with guanethidine resulted in a significant reduction in mast cell counts. Thus, the data suggested that nerve fibers exerted a trophic influence on mast cell infiltration.

What causes nerve fiber proliferation? In response to inflammation, nerve growth factor (NGF) production is upregulated in many tissues including the urinary bladder. Lowe et al. [64] assayed the NGF level in bladder biopsies from 16 women with chronic cystitis, idiopathic sensory urgency, or IC using an enzyme-linked immunosorbent assay (ELISA). In all patients the levels were significantly elevated compared to those of four controls of genuine stress incontinence ($P < 0.05$). An immunofluorescence study demonstrated NGF in the urothelium, and the intensity was most marked in the bladder with idiopathic sensory urgency. In an acute cystitis model in Wistar rats, increased NGF was observed 3 weeks after initiation of cystitis. The increase was demonstrated in the bladder and pelvic ganglia ($P < 0.05$), as were enlargement of peripheral neurons ($P < 0.05$) and the dorsal root ganglia (L1-S1) ($P < 0.05$) and an increase in mast cells in the submucosa and the muscle layer (approximately sevenfold, $P < 0.05$) [65]. NGF sensitizes nociceptive sensory neurons [66], which in turn release SP and CGRP, as previously discussed. It has been proposed that NGF reaches the major pelvic and dorsal root ganglia through retrograde axon transport [67, 68].

It must be pointed out, however, that these animal studies [64, 65, 69] are based on acute cystitis models, which could elicit a host response that is entirely different from the one that can be observed in human IC. Nevertheless, the animal studies seem to provide support for what may occur in human IC bladders. The only notable difference is that the inflammation associated with IC is chronic and in most cases mild. Yet, that NGF is involved is supported by the increase in nerve fibers, accumulation of degranulating mast cells, edema, and vascular engorgement in the lamina propria in the IC bladder.

What triggers mast cell activation? Spanos et al. [70] demonstrated in rats that psychological stress (induced by immobilizing animals as a nontraumatic acute stress) activated more than 70% of resident mast cells in the bladder within 30 min, as evidenced by degranulation shown by light microscopy and electron microscopy. Furthermore, stress-induced bladder mast cell activation was substantially reduced in weanling rats treated with capsaicin (to destroy sensory nerve termini), with the data suggesting that mast cell activation was due, in part, to the release of neuropeptides such as SP and CGRP stored in sensory nerve endings.

The afferent bladder pathway consists of small myelinated Aδ and unmyelinated C fibers. Aδ fibers transmit signals mainly from mechanoreceptors, which detect bladder fullness or wall tension, whereas the C fibers signal when there is infection or an irritative condition. C afferent fibers have reflux function also to facilitate or trigger voiding [71]. When the sensory nerve endings are stimulated (by noxious substances in urine as a result of a leaky urothelial barrier or by acute and chronic inflammation), they release neurokinins (SP, neurokinin [NK] A, neurokinin B). SP directly activates nearby mast cells [57, 69, 72]. Involvement of mast cells in the subsequent reaction was clearly demonstrated in an experiment with mast cell-deficient mice [69]; intravesical instillation of SP or *Escherichia coli* lipopolysaccharide (LPS) induced an inflammatory reaction, edema, and hemorrhage only in the congenic normal mice and not in mast cell-deficient mice. The activated mast cells released a number of cytokines including histamine, vasoactive intestinal peptide (VIP), and tumor necrosis factor-α (TNFα). VIP is responsible for the vasodilation of postcapillary veins and extravasation [69, 73]. Because the action of neurokinins is mediated by their receptor (NK1-receptor), and the receptor is expressed by postcapillary venules, SP can also act directly on the vessels [74, 75]. At this time, it remains unclear whether mast cell activation by SP is mediated by its NK1 receptor. It appears, though, that the NK1 receptor is involved in this process as intravenous administration of the NK1 receptor-specific antagonists RP 67580 [74] and CP-96,345 inhibited tachykinin-induced neurogenic inflammation (plasma extravasation) [75].

Synthesis of Antiproliferative Factor/Low-Heparin-Binding Epidermal Growth Factor-like Growth Factor (AFP/HB-EGF) in IC Urothelium and Amplified Purinergic Receptor Expression in the Subepithelial Sensory Nerve Endings

A recent hypothesis proposed by the University of Maryland group led by Keay and Chai is that antiproliferative factor/low heparin-binding epidermal growth factor-like growth factor (HB-EGF) is synthesized in IC urothelium, and purinergic receptor expression is amplified in the subepithelial sensory nerve endings. According to their study, epithelial cells that line hollow organs, including the bladder, have neurosensory-like functions as the epithelial cells release adenosine triphosphate (APT) in response to stretch (mechanical deformation). Human urothelial cells can release ATP in response to stretch. This release was more pronounced in patients with IC than in controls [76, 77]. Released ATP, in turn, acts on purinergic receptors (P2X) of subepithelial sensory nerve terminals [78]. Furthermore, extracellular ATP stimulates ATP release from IC urothelium and therefore may play an autocrine role in mediating further release of ATP through activation of the P2X receptor [79]. In 1996, the Keay group reported that urine samples from IC patients contained an antiproliferative factor when tested with normal urothelial cells in culture. It was rare or absent in urine samples from various controls [80, 81]. Furthermore, it was produced by the urothelium and was found to inhibit the production of HB-EGF [82]. Sun and Chai [79] subsequently determined that the low level of HB-EGF was responsible for the augmented ATP release from the IC urothelium, that ATP release could be reduced by adding HB-EGF to the culture medium prior to ATP release assay, and that treatment of cells with suramin, a nonspecific P2 receptor antagonist, also reduced ATP release. Thus, suramin could be considered as a drug for IC patients.

The pathogenetic mechanism is illustrated in Fig. 3-6-1.

In summary, a significant contribution of this innovative group was to offer a pathogenetic mechanism to increase our understanding of sensory signaling pathways—that the urothelium of IC patients have augmented extracellular ATP signaling that could be blocked by suramin and HB-EGF.

Based on the available information, the following is a reasonable working hypothesis to account for the pathogenesis of IC. The trigger may originate from two sources: first, environmental stress in susceptible persons and record, an insult to the bladder, which could be infection or possibly genetic basis (Keay, 2000), and alter urothelial cell function, leading to synthesis of an antiproliferative factor and subsequent decreased synthesis of HB-EGF. This results in augmented ATP signaling, stimulating the sensory nerves (Fig. 3-6-1). This signals a premature urge to urinate via the micturition center. Activation of the parasympathetic system via the micturition center results in contraction of the detrusor muscle and relaxation of the bladder neck sphincter. Because of lingering chronic inflammation, NGF release in the bladder is constantly upregulated, and it stimulates neurokinin release from the sensory fibers and also causes nerve fiber proliferation. Trophic factor(s) released from the nerve endings attract mast cells. Mast cells respond to neurokinins and release the contents of granules in a piecemeal fashion. Released mast cell contents dilate the postcapilary venules and induce edema.

As was stated under Question 5, bladder biopsy may not show any recognizable abnormality in the lamina propria (without an increase in mast cells). In such cases, how can one explain the pathogenesis of the irritable voiding symptom? As stated earlier, because endothelial cells express the NK1 receptor, SP or CGRP (products of sensory nerve fibers), may directly stimulate venules, thus bypassing the involvement of mast cells.

References

1. Parsons CL, Stauffer C, Schmidt JP (1980) Bladder surface glycosaminoglycans: an efficient mechanism of environmental adaptation. Science 208:605–607.
2. Parsons CL, Boychuk D, Jones S, Hurst R, Callahan H (1990) Bladder surface glycosaminoglycans: an epithelial permeability barrier. J Urol 143:139–142.

3. Parsons CL, Lilly JD, Stein P (1991) Epithelial dysfunction in nonbacterial cystitis (interstitial cystitis). J Urol 145:732–735.

4. Parsons CL, Stein PC, Bidair M, Lebow D (1994) Abnormal sensitivity to intravesical potassium in interstitial cystitis and radiation cystitis. Neurourol Urodyn 13:515–520.

5. Parsons CL, Greenberger M, Gabal L, Bidair M, Barme G (1998) The role of urinary potassium in the pathogenesis and diagnosis of interstitial cystitis. J Urol 159:1862–1866.

6. Parsons CL, Greene RA, Chung M, Stanford EJ, Singh G (2005) Abnormal urinary potassium metabolism in patients with interstitial cystitis. J Urol 173:1182–1185.

7. Parsons CL (1996) Interstitial cystitis. Int J Urol 3:415–420.

8. Parsons CL, Schmidt JD, Pollen JJ (1983) Successful treatment of interstitial cystitis with sodium pentosanpolysulfate. J Urol 130:51–53.

9. Parsons CL, Mulholland SG (1987) Successful therapy of interstitial cystitis with pentosanpolysulfate. J Urol 138:513–516.

10. Chelsky MJ, Rosen SI, Knight LC, Maurer AH, Hanno PM, Ruggieri MR (1994) Bladder permeability in interstitial cystitis is similar to that of normal volunteers; direct measurement by transvesical absorption of ^{99m}technetium-diethylenetriaminepentaacetic acid. J Urol 151:346–349.

11. Teichman JM, Nielsen-Omeis BJ (1999) Potassium leak test predicts outcome in interstitial cystitis. J Urol 161:1791–1796.

12. Erickson DR, Herb N, Ordille S, Harmon N, Bhavanandan VP (2001) A new direct test of bladder permeability. J Urol 165:914–915.

13. Dixon JS, Holm-Bentzen M, Gilpin CJ, Gosling JA, Bostofte E, Hald T, Larsen S (1986) Electron microscopic investigation of the bladder urothelium and glycocalyx in patients with interstitial cystitis. J Urol 135:621–625.

14. Anderstrom CR, Fall M, Johansson SL (1989) Scanning electron microscopic findings in interstitial cystitis. Br J Urol 63:270–275.

15. Elbadawi AE, Light JK (1996) Distinctive ultrastructural pathology of nonulcerative interstitial cystitis: new observations and their potential significance in pathogenesis. Urol Int 56:137–162.

16. Said JW, Van de Velde R, Gillespie L (1989) Immunopathology of interstitial cystitis. Mod Pathol 2:593–602.

17. Wilson CB, Leopard J, Nakamura RM, Cheresh DA, Stein PC, Parsons CL (1995) Selective type IV collagen defects in the urothelial basement membrane in interstitial cystitis. J Urol 154:1222–1226.

18. Ochs RL, Stein TW Jr, Peebles CL, Gittes RF, Tan EM (1994) Autoantibodies in interstitial cystitis. J Urol 151:587–592.

19. Peters KM, Diokno AC, Steinert BW, Gonzalez JA (1998) The efficacy of intravesical bacillus Calmette-Guerin in the treatment of interstitial cystitis: long-term follow-up. J Urol 159:1483–1486.

20. Erickson DR, Belchis DA, Dabbs DJ (1997) Inflammatory cell types and clinical features of interstitial cystitis. J Urol 158:790–793.

21. Christmas TJ, Bottazzo GF (1992) Abnormal urothelial HLA-DR expression in interstitial cystitis. Clin Exp Immunol 87:450–454.

22. Kumar V, Abbas AK, Fausto N (eds) (2004) Robbins: pathologic basis of disease. Elsevier Saunders, Philadelphia, pp 193–267.

23. Alagiri M, Chottiner S, Ratner V, Slade D, Hanno PM (1997) Interstitial cystitis: unexplained associations with other chronic disease and pain syndrome. Urology 49(suppl 5A):52–57.

24. Erickson DR, Morgan KC, Ordille S, Keay SK, Xie SX (2001) Nonbladder related symptoms in patients with interstitial cystitis. J Urol 166:557–562.

25. Kusek JW, Nyberg LM (2001) The epidemiology of interstitial cystitis: is it time to expand our definition? Urology 57(suppl 6A):95–99.

26. Zondervan KT, Yudkin PL, Vessey MP, Jenkinson CP, Dawes MG, Barlow DH, Kennedy SH (2001) Chronic pelvic pain in the community: symptoms, investigations, and diagnosis. Am J Obstet Gynecol 184:1149–1155.

27. Whitehead WE, Palsson O, Jones KR (2002) Systematic review of the comorbidity of irritable bowel syndrome with other disorders: what are the causes and implications? Gastroenterology 122:1140–1156.

28. Lynn RB, Friedman LS (1993) Irritable bowel syndrome. N Engl J Med 329:1940–1945.

29. Azpiroz F, Dapoigny M, Pace F, Muller-Lissener S, Coremans G, Whorwell P, Stockbrugger RW, Smout A (2000) Nongastrointestinal disorders in the irritable bowel syndrome. Digestion 62:66–72.

30. Clauw DJ, Chrousos GP (1997) Chronic pain and fatigue syndromes: overlapping clinical and neuroendocrine features and potential pathogenetic mechanisms. Neuroimmunomodulation 4:134–153.

31. Holmes GP, Kaplan JE, Gantz NM, Komaroff AL, Schonberger LB, Straus SE, Jones JF, Dubois RE, Cunningham-Rundles C, Pahwa F (1988) Chronic fatigue syndrome: a working case definition. Ann Intern Med 108:387–389.

32. Straus SE, Komaroff AL, Wedner HJ (1994) Chronic fatigue syndrome: point and counterpoint. J Infect Dis 170:1–6.

33. Buffington CAT (2004) Comorbidity of interstitial cystitis with other unexplained clinical conditions. J Urol 172:1242–1248.

34. Gunter J (2003) Chronic pelvic pain: an integrated approach to diagnosis and treatment. Obstet Gynecol Surv 58:615–623.

35. Rothrock NE, Lutgendorf SK, Kreder KJ (2003) Coping strategies in patients with interstitial cystitis: relationships with quality of life and depression. J Urol 169:233–236.

36. Valentino RJ, Miselis RR, Pavcovich LA (1999) Pontine regulation of pelvic viscera: pharmacological target for pelvic visceral dysfunctions. Trends Pharmacol Sci 20:253–260.

37. Imaki T, Nahan JL, Sawchenko PE, Rivier C, Vale W (1991) Differential regulation of corticotropin-releasing factor mRNA in rat brain regions by glucocorticoids and stress. J Neurosci 11:585–599.

38. Imaki T, Vale W, Sawchenko PE (1992) Regulation of corticotropin-releasing factor mRNA in neuroendocrine and autonomic neurons by osmotic stimulation and volume loading. Neuroendocrinology 56:633–640.

39. Elam M, Thoren P, Svensson TH (1986) Locus coeruleus neurons and sympathetic nerves: activation by visceral afferents. Brain Res 375:117–125.

40. Page ME, Akaoka H, Aston-Jones G, Valentino RJ (1992) Bladder distention activates noradrenergic locus coeruleus neurons by an excitatory amino acid mechanism. Neuroscience 51:555–563.

41. Lechner SM, Curtis AL, Brons R, Valentino RJ (1997) Locus coeruleus activation by colon distention: role of corticotropin-releasing factor and excitatory amino acids. Brain Res 756:114–124.

42. Reche A Jr, Biffington CAT (1998) Increased tyrosine hydroxylase immunoreactivity in the locus coeruleus of cats with interstitial cystitis. J Urol 159:1045–1048.

43. Lutgendorf SK, Kreder KJ, Rothrock NE, Hoffman A, Kirschbaum C, Sternberg EM, Zimmerman MB, Ratliff TL (2002) Diurnal cortisol variations and symptoms in patients with interstitial cystitis. J Urol 167:1338–1343.

44. Westropp JL, Welk KA, Buffington CAT (2003) Small adrenal glands in cats with feline interstitial cystitis. J Urol 170:2494–2497.

45. Irwin PP, James S, Watts L, Fleming LL, Galloway NT (1993) Abnormal pedal thermoregulation in interstitial cystitis. Neurourol Urodyn 12:139–144.

46. Peeker R, Aldenborg F, Dahlstrom A, Johansson SL, Li J-Y, Fall M (2000) Increased tyrosine hydroxylase immunoreactivity in bladder tissue from patients with classic and nonulcer interstitial cystitis. J Urol 163:1112–1115.

47. Lundeberg T, Liedberg H, Nordling L, Theodorsson E, Owzarski A, Ekman P (1993) Interstitial cystitis: correlation with nerve fibers, mast cells and histamine. Br J Urol 71:427–429.

48. Hohenfellner M, Nunes L, Schmidt RA, Lampel A, Thuroff JW, Tanagho EA (1992) Interstitial cystitis: increased sympathetic innervation and related neuropeptide synthesis. J Urol 147:587–591.

49. Stein PC, Torri A, Parsons CL (1999) Elevated urinary norepinephrine in interstitial cystitis. Urology 53:1140–1143.

50. Levine JD, Coderre TJ, Covinsky K, Basbaum AI (1990) Neural influences on synovial mast cell density in rat. J Neurosci Res 26:301–307.

51. Johansson SL, Fall M (1990) Clinical features and spectrum of light microscopic changes in interstitial cystitis. J Urol 143:1118–1124.

52. Christmas TJ, Rode J (1991) Characteristics of mast cells in normal bladder, bacterial cystitis and interstitial cystitis. Br J Urol 68:473–478.

53. Fall M, Johansson SL, Aldenborg F (1987) Chronic interstitial cystitis; a heterogeneous syndrome. J Urol 137:35–38.

54. Feltis JT, Perez-Marrero R, Emerson LE (1987) Increased mast cell of the bladder in suspected cases of interstitial cystitis: a possible disease marker. J Urol 138:42–43.

55. Kastrup J, Hald T, Larsen S, Nielsen VG (1983) Histamine content and mast cell count of detrusor muscle in patients with interstitial cystitis and other types of chronic cystitis. Br J Urol 55:495–500.

56. Lynes WL, Flynn SD, Shortliffe LD, Lemmers M, Zipser R, Roberts J II, Stamey TA (1987) Mast cell involvement in interstitial cystitis. J Urol 138:746–752.

57. Keith IM, Jin J, Saban R (1985) Nerve-mast cell interaction in normal guinea pig urinary bladder. J Comp Neurol 363:28–36.

58. Christensen MM, Keith I, Rhodes PR, Graziano FM, Madsen PO, Bruskewitz RC, Saban R (1990) A guinea pig model for study of bladder mast cell function: histamine release and muscle contraction. J Urol 144:1293–1300.

59. Saban R, Christensen M, Keith M, Graziano M, Undem BJ, Agaard J, Bjorling D, Bruskewitz RC (1991) Experimental model for the study of bladder mast cell degranulation and smooth muscle contraction. Sem Urol 9:88–101.

60. Snell RS (2006) Clinical neuroanatomy. Lippincott Williams & Wilkins. Baltimore, pp 69–131.

61. Theoharides TC, Sant GR, El-Mansoury M, Letourneau R, Ucci AA Jr, Meares EM Jr (1995) Activation of bladder mast cells in interstitial cystitis: a light and electron microscopic study. J Urol 153:629–636.

62. Pang X, Marchand J, Sant GR, Kream RM, Theoharides TC (1995) Increased number of substance P positive nerve fibers in interstitial cystitis. Br J Urol 75:744–750.

63. Letourneau R, Pang X, Sant GR, Theoharides TC (1996) Intragranular activation of bladder mast cells and their association with nerve processes in interstitial cystitis. Br J Urol 77:41–54.

64. Lowe EM, Anand P, Terenghi G, Williams-Chestnut RE, Sinicropi DV, Osborne JL (1997) Increased nerve growth factor levels in the urinary bladder of women with idiopathic sensory urgency and interstitial cystitis. Br J Urol 79:572–577.

65. Dupont MC, Spitsbergen JM, Kim KB, Tuttle JB, Steers WD (2001) Histological and neurotrophic changes triggered by varying models of bladder inflammation. J Urol 166:1111–1118.

66. Dmitrieva N, Shelton D, Rice ASC, McMahon SB (1997) The role of nerve growth factor in a model of visceral inflammation. Neuroscience 78:449–459.

67. Tuttle JB, Steers WD (1992) Nerve growth factor responsiveness of cultured major pelvic ganglion neurons from the adult rat. Brain Res 588:29–40.

68. Dupont MC, Persson K, Spitsbergen J, Tuttle JB, Steers WD (1995) The neuronal response to bladder outlet obstruction, a role for NGF. Adv Exp Med Biol 385:41–54.

69. Bjorling DE, Jerde TJ, Zine MJ, Busser BW, Saban MR, Saban R (1999) Mast cells mediate the severity of experimental cystitis in mice. J Urol 162:231–236.

70. Spanos C, Pang X, Ligris K, Letourneau R, Alferes L, Alexacos N, Sant GR, Theoharides TC (1997) Stress-induced bladder mast cell activation: implications for interstitial cystitis. J Urol 157:669–672.

71. Chancellor MB, de Groat WC (1999) Intravesical capsaicin and resiniferatoxin therapy: spicing up the ways to treat the overactive bladder. J Urol 162:3–11.

72. Suzuki H, Miura S, Liu YY, Tsuchiya M, Ishii H (1995) Substance P induces degranulation of mast cells and leukocyte adhesion to venular endothelium. Peptides 16:1447–1452.

73. Figini M, Emanueli C, Grady EF, Kirkwood K, Payan DG, Ansel J, Gerard C, Geppetti P, Bunnett N (1997) Substance P and bradykinin stimulate plasma extravasation in the mouse gastrointestinal tract and pancreas. Am J Physiol 272:G785–G793.

74. Moussaoui SM, Montier F, Carruette A, Blanchard PM, Laduron PM, Garret C (1993) A non-peptide NK_1- receptor antagonist, RP 67580, inhibits neurogenic inflammation postsynaptically. Br J Pharmacol 109:259–264.

75. Lembeck F, Donnerer J, Tsuchiya M, Nagahisa A (1992) The non-peptide tachykinin antagonist, CP-96, 345, is a potent inhibitor of neurogenic inflammation. Br J Pharmacol 105:527–530.

76. Kumar V, Chapple CC, Chess-Williams R (2004) Characteristics of adenosine triphosphate release from porcine and human normal bladder. J Urol 172: 744–747.

77. Sun Y, Keay S, De Deyne PG, Chai TC (2001) Augmented stretch activated adenosine triphosphate release from bladder uroepithelial cells in patients with interstitial cystitis. J Urol 166:1951–1956.

78. Burnstock G (1999) Release of vasoactive substances from endothelial cells by shear stress and purinergic mechanosensory transduction. J Anat 194:335–342.

79. Sun Y, Chai TC (2006) Augmented extracellular ATP signaling in bladder urothelial cells from patients with interstitial cystitis. Am J Physiol Cell Physiol 290: C27–C34.

80. Keay S, Zhang C-O, Trifillis AL, Hise MK, Hebel JR, Jacobs SC, Warren JW (1996) Decreased ^{3}H-thymidine incorporation by human bladder epithelial cells following exposure to urine from interstitial cystitis patients. J Urol 156:2073–2078.

81. Keay S, Zhang C-O, Hise MK, Hebel JR, Jacobs SC, Gordon D, Whitmore K, Bodison S, Gordon N, Warren JW (1998) A diagnostic in vitro urine assay for interstitial cystitis. Urology 52:974–978.

82. Keay S, Kleinberg M, Zhang C-O, Hise MK, Warren JW (2000) Bladder epithelial cells from patients with interstitial cystitis produce an inhibitor of heparin-binding epidermal growth factor-like growth factor production. J Urol 164:2112–2118.

Question 7

What are the treatment options for patients with interstitial cystitis?

Answer

Because the etiology of interstitial cystitis remains unknown and the pathogenesis has not been clarified, the current treatment focuses on decreasing symptoms and achieving remission. Various types of pharmacotherapy and surgical manipulations have been tried with varying degrees of success. Among the latter, cystoscopic hydrodistention may provide only temporary relief, and cystectomy and urinary diversion have an unacceptable high failure rate for pain control. Standard pharmacotherapy with a tricyclic antidepressant (amitriptyline), intravesical dimethylsulfoxide, anticholinergics, antihistamines, cyclosporin A, and pentosan polysulfate sodium has been tested with some effects but also often with significant side effects. Although at this time all encouraging data are limited to animal studies, antineuropeptide therapy appears to offer the best hope. According to recent studies, neuromodulation via direct stimulation of the sacral nerves is another approach with lasting favorable results.

Comments

Treatment methods that have demonstrated some effects in human and animal studies are described below.

Intravesical Dimethyl Sulfoxide

Intravesical dimethyl sulfoxide (DMSO) is the first drug approved in 1978 by the U.S. Food and Drug Administration (FDA) for the treatment of interstitial cystitis (IC) [1]. Although the pharmacologic mechanism of action is unclear, it is thought to act as an anti-inflammatory, analgesic agent and muscle relaxant [1]. Alleviation of the symptoms is reported in 50%–90% of patients [1–3]. DMSO has an acceptable morbidity rate and an excellent safety profile [1]. It is probably the most widely used intravesical treatment for IC [4, 5]. Its favorable action is not related to mast cell release of histamine [3]. A significant side effect is a garlic-like breath odor and taste in the mouth due to the metabolite dimethyl sulfide [6].

Tricyclic Antidepressant (Amitriptyline)

Hanno and Wein [7] were the first to report the efficacy of amitriptyline in the treatment of IC. Recently, a prospective randomized placebo-controlled, double-blind study was conducted [8]. Pain and urgency intensity was significantly alleviated in the amitriptyline group compared with the placebo group ($P < 0.001$). The frequency and functional bladder capacity improved to a much greater degree in the amitriptyline group ($P = 0.063$, $P = 0.083$, respectively). Mouth dryness was the most frequent side effect in the treated group (79%). The authors concluded that amitriptyline therapy for 4 months was safe and effective in treating IC.

Oral Pentosan Polysulfate Sodium

The rationale behind using oral pentosan polysulfate sodium (PPS) is based on the proposal that defective barrier function is responsible for the voiding symptoms, as described under Question 6. This is another agent approved by the FDA. After the initial apparently favorable clinical data with either oral [9, 10] or intravesical [11] PPS or intravesical heparin [12] therapy, several subsequent double-blind placebo-controlled studies demonstrated variable results; two of them reported positive results, and two others demonstrated negative results. A double-blind controlled study by Holm-Bentzen from Denmark [13] observed no difference between the pretrial and posttrial values in the drug-treated and placebo-treated groups in regard to diminished symptoms or improved urodynamics, cystoscopic appearance, or mast cell counts. In the study reported by the Parsons' group [14] in 1990, a total of 110 patients were enrolled and treated for 3 months with PPS. Overall improvement was observed in 28% of patients assigned to PPS and in 13% of the controls ($P = 0.03$). Sant and others [15] in 2003 reported a study from the Interstitial Cystitis Clinical Trials Group. It was a multicenter, randomized trial testing oral PPS and hydroxyzine (antihistamine), either alone or in combination, and placebo. The response rate for hydroxyzine was 31% for those treated and 20% for those not treated ($P = 0.26$). A nonsignificant trend of effect was seen in the PPS treatment group (34%) compared to the no-PPS group (18%, $P = 0.064$). The response rates were low, and there was no significant difference among the PPS, hydroxyzine, and placebo groups. A fourth study, reported by Nickel et al. [16] in 2005, consisted of 380 patients and evaluated three dosages of PPS. For all three dosages, a clinically significant but similar response was demonstrated, and the duration of therapy appeared to be more important than the dosage. Hwang et al. [17], after a data search using MEDLINE, Excerpta Medica, and International Pharmaceutical Abstracts databases, came to the conclusion that PPS is more efficient than placebo in the treatment of pain, urgency, and frequency but not significantly different from placebo in treating nocturia. In summary, PPS may be marginally effective in a small fraction of patients. If one accepts the report by Elbadawi and Light, who demonstrated severe urothelial damage in all cases of nonulcer-type IC [18], glycosaminoglycan administration is unlikely to repair barrier function.

Immunosuppressant

An immunosuppressant has been tested based on the rationale that an immunologic mechanism may be involved in the pathogenesis of IC. In a randomized prospective study reported from Finland [19], a total of 64 patients were divided into a group receiving cyclosporin A (CyA) 1.5 mg/kg twice daily and another group receiving 100 mg PPS three times daily for 6 months. At 6 months, the CyA was superior to PPS in all clinical outcome parameters evaluated. This study did not have a placebo group. There were more adverse effects with CyA than with PPS.

Intravesical BCG Therapy

Intravesical bacillus Calmette-Guerin (BCG) therapy was initiated because of an anecdotal observation that BCG therapy was effective in ameliorating the symptoms of IC [20]. In a subsequent study by Peters et al. [21], 15 patients were assigned to a BCG group and 12 to a placebo group in an open-label study. Results showed a 60% response rate in the BCG group compared to a 27% rate in the placebo group. With a minimum 2-year follow-up, 89% of the original responders (8/9) continued to experience an improved clinical course with no additional treatment. Encouraged by the data, a double-blind randomized placebo-controlled study was conducted [22]. A total of 265 patients were randomized. Patient-reported global response assessment at 34 weeks was 21% for the BCG group and 12% for the placebo ($P = 0.062$). In contrast to the initial promising data, the results were disappointing. In the Peters group study, those who did not respond to BCG had more severe baseline symptoms. Mayer et al. [22] expressed a similar impression that those presenting with severe symptoms were unlikely to respond as their participants represented a relatively severe and chronic type of IC.

Antineuropeptide Therapy

The rationale behind antineuropeptide therapy is the hypothesis that IC is associated with sensory nerve hyperactivity–mast cell activation (refer to Question 6). Excessive release of sensory nerve neurotransmitters (substance P [SP], galanin, calcitonin gene-related peptide [CGRP], nitric oxide synthase) [23] and subsequently activated mast cell-released cytokines are responsible for increased vascular permeability and inflammation. At this time, all available data are limited to studies with animal models. However, because of the encouraging data, it is hoped that clinical data will become available in the near future. In a mouse model with *Escherichia coli* lipopolysaccharide (LPS)-induced acute cystitis, Gonzalez et al. [24] demonstrated that the anti-inflammatory peptide RDP58 (NH_2-arg-norleucine (nle)-nle-arg-nle-nle-nle-gly-tyr-$CONH_2$) significantly decreased the inflammatory response compared with that of controls ($P < 0.05$). This was associated with a reduced level of tumor necrosis factor-α (TNFα), SP, and NGF production. The anti-inflammatory effect of RDP58 was previously demonstrated in a mouse model of chronic colitis as well [25]. In humans, oral RDP58 has been shown to be highly effective in reducing chemotherapeutic agent-associated gastrointestinal toxicity due to the production of proinflammatory cytokines such as TNFα produced by epithelial cells and infiltrating leukocytes [26].

Another approach based on the same theme is the intravesical use of the neurotoxin capsaicin, the main pungent ingredient in hot peppers. Also used is resiniferatoxin, an ultra-potent analogue of capsaicin that has similar efficacy but less-acute side effects. These agents are specific neurotoxins that desensitize C nerve fibers of the sensory afferent neurons [27] (also refer to Question 6).

L-Arginine has been shown to be effective in reducing voiding symptoms and pelvic and vaginal/urethral pains [28, 29]. Its use is based on the observation that nitric oxide synthase is reduced in urine of IC patients and the assumption that nitric oxide may be an important determinant of the symptoms.

Neurokinin-1 (NK1) receptor antagonist has potential to be used in IC patients. Release of tachykinins, including SP, from afferent C nerve fibers is thought to be responsible for vasodilatation and plasma protein extravasation. Experimentally, the NK1 receptor antagonist RP67580 is effective in modulating inflammatory edema induced by SP [30]. The anti-NK1 approach should be considered as an option for treating IC.

Sacral Nerve Modulation

Direct neuromodulation via sacral nerve stimulation was introduced during the 1980s as a novel treatment for chronic voiding dysfunction [31]. The approach was theorized to cause afferent inhibition of sensory processing in the spinal cord via the spinobulbospinal pathways to the pontine micturition center [32, 33]. Although sacral root neuromodulation is gaining popularity for managing refractory detrusor instability and nonobstructive voiding dysfunction [34, 35], it was also shown to be effective for treating IC [36]. Lately, a number of groups have reported sustained significant alleviation of the voiding symptoms [32,

34, 37, 38] with the use of permanent sacral nerve stimulator implantation [32, 37].

References

1. Parkin J, Shea C, Sant GR (1997) Intravesical dimethyl sulfoxide (DMSO) for interstitial cystitis: a practical approach. Urology 49(suppl):105–107.
2. Perez-Marrero R, Emmerson LE, Feltis JT (1988) A controlled study of dimethyl sulfoxide in interstitial cystitis. J Urol 140:36–39.
3. Stout L, Gerspach JM, Levy SM, Yun SK, Lad PM, Leach GE, Zimmern PE (1995) Dimethyl sulfoxide does not trigger urine histamine release in interstitial cystitis. Urology 46:653–656.
4. Sant GR (1987) Intravesical 50% dimethyl sulfoxide (RIMSO-50) in treatment of interstitial cystitis. Urology 29(suppl):17–21.
5. Selo-Ojeme DO, Onwude JL (2004) Interstitial cystitis. J Obstet Gynecol 24:216–225.
6. Jacob SW, Hershler R (1975) Biological actions of dimethyl sulfoxide. Ann N Y Acad Sci 243:497–503.
7. Hanno PM, Wein AJ (1987) Medical treatment of interstitial cystitis (other than Rimso-50/Elmiron). Urology 29 (suppl):22–26.
8. Van Ophoven A, Pokupic S, Heinecke A, Hertle L (2004) A prospective, randomized, placebo controlled, double-blind study of amitriptyline for the treatment of interstitial cystitis. J Urol 172:533–536.
9. Parsons CL, Schmidt JD, Pollen JJ (1983) Successful treatment of interstitial cystitis with sodium pentosanpolysulfate. J Urol 130:51–53.
10. Parsons CL, Mulholland SG (1987) Successful therapy of interstitial cystitis with pentosanpolysulfate. J Urol 138:513–516.
11. Bade JJ, Mensink HJA, Laseur M (1995) Intravesical treatment of interstitial cystitis with a heparin analogue. Br J Urol 75:260.
12. Parsons CL, Housley JD, Schmidt JD, Lebow D (1994) Treatment of interstitial cystitis with intravesical heparin. Br J Urol 73:504–507.
13. Holm-Bentzen M, Jacobsen F, Nerstrom B, Lose G, Kristensen JK, Pedersen RH, Krarup T, Feggetter J, Bates P, Barnard R, Larsen S, Hald T (1987) A prospective double blind clinically controlled multicenter trial of sodium pentosan polysulfate in the treatment of interstitial cystitis and related painful bladder disease. J Urol 138:503–507.
14. Mulholland SG, Hanno P, Parsons CL, Sant GR, Staskin DR (1990) Pentosan polysulfate sodium for therapy of interstitial cystitis: a double-blind placebo-controlled clinical study. Urology 35:552–558.
15. Sant GR, Propert KJ, Hanno PM, Burks D, Culkin D, Diokno AC, Hardy C, Landis JR, Mayer R, Madugan R, Messing EM, Peters K, Theoharides TC, Warren J, Wein AJ, Steers W, Kusek JW, Nyberg LM: the

Interstitial Cystitis Clinical Trials Group (2003) A pilot clinical trial of oral pentosan polysulfate and oral hydroxyzine in patients with interstitial cystitis. J Urol 170:810–815.

16. Nickel JC, Barkin J, Forrest J, Mosbaugh PG, Hernandez-Graulau J, Kaufman D, Lloyd K, Evans RJ, Parsons CL, Atkinson LE (2005) Randomized, double-blind, dose-ranging study of pentosan polysulfate sodium for interstitial cystitis. Urology 65:654–658.

17. Hwang P, Auclair B, Beechinor D, Diment M, Einarson TR (1997) Efficacy of pentosan polysulfate in the treatment of interstitial cystitis: a meta-analysis. Urology 50:39–43.

18. Elbadawi AE, Light JK (1996) Distinctive ultrastructural pathology of nonulcerative interstitial cystitis: new observations and their potential significance in pathogenesis. Urol Int 56:137–162.

19. Sairanen J, Tammela TLJ, Leppilahti M, Multanen M, Paananen I, Lehtoranta K, Ruutu M (2005) Cyclosporine A and pentosan polysulfate sodium for the treatment of interstitial cystitis: a randomized comparative study. J Urol 174:2235–2238.

20. Zeidman EJ, Helfrick B, Pollard C, Thompson IM (1994) Bacillus Calmette-Guerin immunotherapy for refractory interstitial cystitis. Urology 43:121–124.

21. Peters KM, Diokno AC, Steinert BW, Gonzalez JA (1998) The efficacy of intravesical bacillus Calmette-Guerin in the treatment of interstitial cystitis: long-term followup. J Urol 159:1483–1486.

22. Mayer R, Propert KJ, Peters KM, Payne CK, Zhang Y, Burks D, Culkin DJ, Diokno A, Hanno P, Landis JR, Madigan R, Messing EM, Nickel JC, Sant GR, Warren J, Wein AJ, Kusek JW, Nyberg LM, Foster HE: the Interstitial Cystitis Clinical Trials Group (2005) A randomized controlled trial of intravesical bacillus Calmette-Guerin for treatment refractory interstitial cystitis. J Urol 173:1186–1191.

23. Callsen-Cancic P, Mense S (1997) Expression of neuropeptides and nitric acid synthase in neurones innervating the inflamed rat bladder. J Auton Nerv Syst 65:33–44.

24. Gonzalez RR, Fong T, Belmar N, Saban M, Felsen D, Te A (2005) Modulating bladder neuro-inflammation: RDP58, a novel anti-inflammatory peptide, decreases inflammation and nerve growth factor production in experimental cystitis. J Urol 173:630–634.

25. Murthy S, Flannigan A, Coppola D, Buelow R (2002) RDP58, a locally active TNF inhibitor, is effective in the dextran sulfate mouse model of chronic colitis. Inflamm Res 51:522–531.

26. Zhao J, Huang L, Belmar N, Buelow R, Fong T (2004) Oral RDP58 allows CPT-11 dose intensification for enhanced tumor response by decreasing gastrointestinal toxicity. Clin Cancer Res 10:2851–2859.

27. Chancellor MB, De Groat WC (1999) Intravesical capsaicin and resiniferatoxin therapy: spicing up the ways to treat the overactive bladder. J Urol 162:3–11.

28. Smith SD, Wheeler MA, Foster HE Jr, Weiss RM (1997) Improvement in interstitial cystitis symptom scores during treatment with oral L-arginine. J Urol 158:703–708.

29. Korting GE, Smith SD, Wheeler MA, Weiss RM, Foster HE Jr (1999) A randomized double-blind trial of oral L-arginine for treatment of interstitial cystitis. J Urol 161:558–565.

30. Wilsoncroft P, Euzger H, Brain SD (1994) Effect of a neurokinin-1 (NK1) receptor antagonist on oedema formation induced by tachykinins, carrageenin and an allergic response in guinea-pig skin. Neuropeptides 26:405–411.

31. Schmidt RA, Senn E, Tanagho EA (1990) Functional evaluation of sacral nerve root integrity: report of a technique. Urology 35:388–392.

32. Comiter CV (2003) Sacral neuromodulation for the symptomatic treatment of refractory interstitial cystitis: a prospective study. J Urol 169:1369–1373.

33. de Groat WC (1996) Neuroanatomy and neurophysiology: innervation of the lower urinary tract. In: Raz S (ed) Female urology. Saunders, Philadelphia, pp 28–42.

34. Maher CF, Carey MP, Dwyer PL, Schulter PL (2001) Percutaneous sacral nerve root neuromodulation for intractable interstitial cystitis. J Urol 165:884–886.

35. Yokozuka M, Namima T, Nakagawa H, Ichie M, Handa Y (2004) Effects and indications of sacral surface therapeutic electrical stimulation in refractory urinary incontinence. Clin Rehabil 18:899–907.

36. Fall M (1985) Conservative management of chronic interstitial cystitis: transcutaneous electrical nerve stimulation and transurethral resection. J Urol 133:774–778.

37. Peters KM, Konstandt D (2004) Sacral neuromodulation decreases narcotic requirements in refractory interstitial cystitis. BJU Int 93:777–779.

38. Chai TC, Zhang C-O, Warren JW, Keay S (2004) Percutaneous sacral third nerve root neurostimulation improves symptoms and normalizes urinary HB-EFG levels and antiproliferative activity in patients with interstitial cystitis. BJU Int 93:777–779.

Question 8

Is there a difference in clinical behavior between urothelial carcinoma of the upper urinary tract and that of the lower urinary tract? What is the risk of developing tumors in the contralateral and lower urinary tracts in patients presenting initially with an upper urinary tract cancer? Conversely, what is the risk of developing an upper urinary tract tumor in patients who initially present with a lower urinary tract tumor?

Answer

Urothelial neoplasms involving the upper urinary tract are uncommon, accounting for about 5% of primary urothelial neoplasms. Unlike tumors involving the lower urinary tract (mostly urinary bladder), more than 50% of them are of high grade and high stage (pT2 or higher) and typically require radical surgery such as nephrectomy or ureterectomy with or without nephrectomy. The risk of developing carcinoma in the contralateral kidney is 1%–3%. The projected incidence of a tumor in the contralateral kidney rises progressively from 2.7% to 6.5% during a follow-up from 5 years to 15 years, respectively. The incidence of bladder carcinoma subsequent to an upper tract carcinoma ranges from 9% to 48%. Bladder cancer is also significantly more common among patients with bilateral upper tract cancer. This high risk is probably due to both spreading of the original cancer and field changes (new cancer). For patients presenting with bladder cancer, the risk for developing upper tract cancer is 1%–4%. Several mechanisms have been proposed to account for this event. Among these, multiplicity of tumors and the presence of widely spreading carcinoma in situ in the urinary bladder are distinctive risk factors for the development of upper urinary tract cancer.

Comments

Urothelial neoplasms of the renal pelvis are uncommon, accounting for approximately 5% of all primary urothelial neoplasms [1–5]. The incidence of ureteral cancer is far less, about 1% of the entire urothelial neoplasms [6].

Are there significant differences in pathologic and clinical characteristics between tumors of the lower urinary tract (primarily urinary bladder) and those of the upper urinary tract?

Although the renal pelvis and ureter have anatomic structure similar to that of the urinary bladder, the lamina propria is absent to quite thin in the upper urinary tract (UUT), and the muscularis propria is considerably thinner than that in the urinary bladder [7]. These differences may be important in regard to tumor progression (invasion). According to the latest American Joint Committee on Cancer Staging System, pTa is defined as "papillary noninvasive carcinoma"; pT1, "tumor invades subepithelial connective tissue"; pT2, "tumor invades the muscularis"; pT3 for the renal pelvis. "tumor invades beyond the muscularis propria into peripelvic fat or renal parenchyma"; pT3 for the ureter only, "tumor invades beyond muscularis into periureteral fat"; and pT4, "tumor invades adjacent organs, or through the kidney into the perinephric fat" [8]. The TNM system combines renal pelvic and ureteral carcinomas into one classification. Although histologically similar, the renal pelvis and ureter are anatomically and biologically different, as transmural invasion of the tumor is

TABLE 3-8-1. Pathologic stage of urothelial neoplasms at renal pelvis

Study	No.	Noninvasive pTa, pTis	pT1	pT2	PT3	PT4	Noninvasive / invasive	Superficial (≤ pT1)/ Deeply invasive (≥ pT2)
Johansson [55], (1976)	94	21		17		56	0.29	—
Davis [56], (1987)	46	8	8	9		21	0.21	0.53
Huben [57], (1988)	54	10	18	14	12	—	0.23	1.07
Krogh [23], (1991)	197	92		105[a]			0.88	—
Guinan [3], (1992)	607	21	285[b]		176	125	0.03	—
Solsona [40], (1997)	100	48	8		20	24	0.92	1.27
Hall [15], (1998)	247	38	101	35	53	20	0.18	1.28
Kang [27], (2003)	223	77[c]		37	54	55	—	0.52
Olgac [7], (2004)	123	42	23	14	39	5	0.52	1.12
Genega (2005)	102	50	20	4	19	9	0.96	2.18
Holmang [25], (2006)[d]	201	89	35	19	51	7	0.79	1.45
Perez-Montiel (2006)	42	8	4	4	23	3	0.2	0.40

[a] All invasive tumors combined.
[b] pT_1 and pT_2 tumors combined.
[c] Noninvasive and pT_1 tumors combined.
[d] This study includes contralateral upper urinary tract cancers that developed after the initial nephroureterectomy.

associated with a poorer prognosis for a ureteral cancer than a renal pelvis cancer [9–11]. Keeping this definition in mind, we look at the frequency of tumors by stage and grade.

In the bladder, most urothelial tumors (approximately 75%–80%) are superficial (pTa, pTis, pT1) and of low grade (including both papillary urothelial neoplasm of low malignant potential (PUNLMP) and low-grade carcinoma[1]). These are papillary and are characterized by frequent recurrences over the course of many years. Muscle-invasive carcinomas eventually develop in 10%–20% of low-grade tumors. In contrast, the remaining 20% and 5% of the entire bladder cancer population presents with invasive disease (pT2) and metastatic disease, respectively [12]. Most of the patients with invasive high-grade tumors do not have a known history of papillary tumors, and the lesions are commonly associated with carcinoma in situ elsewhere in the bladder [13]. Papillary superficial tumors are typically treated with organ-sparing transurethral resection (TUR), with radical cystectomy being saved for those who present with locally advanced-stage cancer. Ureteroscopic treatment of upper tract tumors has been tried for apparently localized low-grade tumors; it met, however, with a high recurrence rate (15%–53%) [14]. Therefore, this strategy is not recommended as standard treatment of upper tract tumors, particularly because of its close association with a high-stage presentation. Thus, nephroureterectomy with the distal ureter-bladder cuff removal has been the standard treatment.

Several reports have classified primary urothelial tumors of the renal pelvis by grade and pathologic stage (Table 3-8-1). The frequency ratio of superficial tumors (pTa, pTis, pT1) to muscle-invasive tumors (pT2 or higher) ranges from 1:0.5 to 1:2.1. These ratios are apparently lower than the commonly accepted ratio of 3:1 in the urinary bladder. In two recent studies reporting renal pelvis urothelial neoplasms using the WHO/ISUP classification, PUNLMPs were not recorded; of 87 cases in the Genega et al. series [2], 30 cases (34%) and the remaining 57 cases (66%) were classified as low-grade and high-grade carcinomas, respectively. It is not clear that the lack of PUNLMP in the UUT was due to a true difference in biologic behavior or difference in interpretation. In the Olgac series [7] of 130 cases, the frequencies of low-grade and high-grade carcinomas were 29% and 71%, respectively. Thus, in these studies most of the cases were classified as high-grade carcinoma. However, using the 1973 WHO classification, Hall et al. [15] reported a 9% frequency of grade 1 carcinoma (which would be comparable with PUNLMP) in the UUT.

Despite some reported variations, it is safe to conclude that UUT tumors at presentation are more frequently of higher grades and at more advanced stages (Figs. 3-8-1, 3-8-2).

What are possible reasons for more high-grade and high-stage urothelial carcinomas in the upper urinary tract?

Although the incidence of UUT urothelial tumors is far less common than that in the bladder, it is significant that most of them are more aggressive. Many, in

[1] Some authors keep pTis with the superficial tumor group, but one should realize that their biologic potential is different from that of superficial tumors.

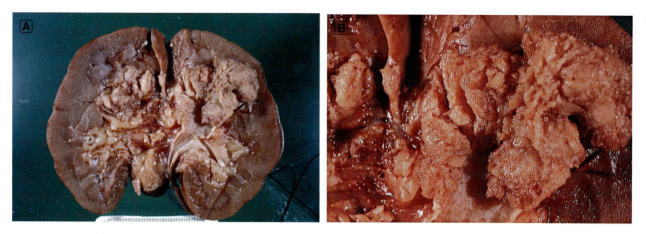

FIG. 3-8-1. **A, B** Bisected nephrectomy specimen showing a papillary urothelial carcinoma which has invaded the renal sinus fat tissue. In **B**, a shaggy surface indicative of papillary configuration is demonstrated

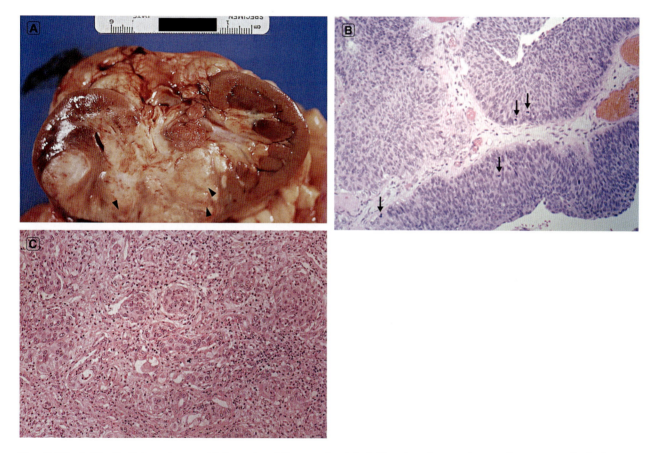

FIG. 3-8-2. **A** Urothelial carcinoma, high grade of the renal pelvis infiltrating the renal parenchyma extensively (*arrowheads*). **B** High-grade urothelial carcinoma replacing the renal pelvic lining. Note the frequent mitotic figures (*arrows*) **C** In this field, the renal parenchyma has been replaced by infiltrating urothelial carcinoma

fact, are already invading the muscularis propria or beyond when detected.

Multiple risk factors have been linked to bladder cancer both epidemiologically and experimentally [16]. The urogenous hypothesis of urinary tract carcinogenesis was firmly supported by a number of investigators during the late 20th century. The well-known bladder carcinogens 2-naphthylamine and 4-aminobiphenyl [17] have been found in tobacco smoke [18]. Hepatic *N*-hydroxylation of aromatic carcinogens is the initial step in urinary tract carcinogenesis. *N*-Hydroxy derivatives of bladder carcinogens are then conjugated to glucuronic acid in the liver and are transported to the bladder via kidney [19]. Hydrolysis of these conjugates and liberation of the *N*-hydroxyl arylamines are acid-dependent and occur in urine [20]. After hydrolysis, the proximate carcinogen is absorbed by the urothelium and undergoes final metabolic activation to a DNA-binding form to induce neoplastic transformation.

The much higher incidence of tumors in the urinary bladder than in the prostatic urethra or the UUT can be attributed to constant contact of the bladder urothelium to urine-borne carcinogens. The risk is a function of the concentration of, and duration of exposure to, carcinogens in urine. Therefore, it is higher in the bladder than in the remaining urinary tract. In the urinary bladder of rodents, tumors are more frequent in the ventral wall than the dorsal surface, a fact attributed to longer contact with urine [21]. In humans, although the entire mucosal surface should be equally susceptible to neoplasia, posterolateral areas around the ureteral orifices are the common sites of tumor development.

Several factors may contribute to the aggressive nature of the UUT tumors. (1) In the urinary bladder, tumors tend to be detected at an early stage of neoplasia because most of these tumors are papillary in configuration and the delicate papillary fronds with a vascular core may be susceptible to trauma induced by micturition-associated bladder contractions. Thus, the earliest manifestation of tumors is either gross hematuria or microscopic hematuria, more commonly the former. (2) The less confinement of the UUT tumors may be due to the much thinner wall than that of the bladder. (3) It is difficult to detect UUT tumors by imaging or endoscopic studies. (4) There are some suggestions that UUT tumors have molecular genetic characteristics different from the lower tract (bladder) tumors, although the studies are preliminary and need more study. The difference, if any, could reflect detection of the tumors at a more advanced stage and thus with more accumulated genetic changes.

Although most bladder tumors, when discovered, are at a low grade and low stage, it is not uncommon to observe more than one histologic grade in a given tumor sample. This suggests that continuous carcinogenic insult leads to the development of a more aggressive subclone. Heterogeneity was well documented in a recent study by Cheng et al. [22]; 52 of 164 Ta urothelial cell tumors consisted of two grades, and the prognosis was worse in the presence of a worse secondary grade.

What is the risk of developing a tumor in the contralateral kidney in patients with an upper urinary tract cancer?

Metachronous bilateral UUT tumors are rare, with an estimated incidence of 1%–3% [23, 24]. Of 768 patients from the Swedish Cancer Registry [25], a contralateral UUT cancer developed in 24 (3.1%) after a median of 46 months. The projected incidences after the initial diagnosis of UUT tumor were 2.7%, 5.8%, and 6.5% at 5, 10, and 15 years, respectively. An important observation was that bladder cancer was significantly more common among patients with bilateral UUT cancers than among those with a unilateral UUT cancer (83% vs. 30%, $P < 0.0001$). The authors proposed several possibilities to account for the difference: retrograde urinary bladder tumor implantation through the defective ureteral orifice; a field effect of urothelial carcinogens acting at multiple sites; and a risk of developing UUT cancer in patients with hereditary nonpolyposis colon cancer syndrome (HNPCC), or so-called Lynch syndrome [26]. For more discussion on this subject, readers are referred to Question 9.

What is the risk of developing a urinary bladder tumor in patients who present with an upper urinary tract tumor?

Inasmuch as the urinary bladder is the major site of urothelial cancer development, it is not surprising that high incidences are reported for patients in whom the initial manifestation of a urothelial tumor involved the UUT. The reported incidences range from 9% to 48% [23, 24, 27, 28]. There is a high frequency of developing bladder cancer in UUT tumors involving both the renal pelvis and ureter [28]. Data from the Habuchi group [29] indicate that approximately one-half of the bladder tumors in these patients were new cancers, and the other half were from intraureteral spread (i.e., monoclonal origin). This is in contrast to the fact that most recurrent or multiple tumors confined to the bladder are monoclonal [30].

What is the risk for developing an upper urinary tract tumor in patients with a history of bladder cancer?

It is well known that patients with bladder cancer have a significant risk of developing tumors elsewhere in the urinary tract, including the prostatic urethra. The reported incidence of subsequent UUT tumors is 0.7%–4.0% based on a large series [31]. Proposed risk factors are vesicoureteral reflux [32–35], previous BCG treatment [36, 37], pathologic characteristics of the primary bladder tumor that include multiplicity including so-called recurrences [38–42], high-grade tumors, presence of carcinoma in situ [36, 37, 40, 41, 43], and a history of occupational exposure to bladder carcinogens (e.g., bladder cancer in dye factory employees) [39].

Vesicoureteral Reflux

Repeat TUR for bladder cancer can damage the anti-reflux function of the ureteral ostia [25]. Whether vesicoureteral reflux is associated with an increased risk for UUT tumors is controversial. The proposed mechanism is implantation of bladder tumor cells via incompetent ureteral orifices. If this hypothesis is correct, the incidence of UUT cancer should be higher at the refluxing UUT unit.

Palou et al. [34] reported a 1.5% incidence of metachronous UUT tumors among bladder tumor patients (30/1962). Of the 30 patients, 18 had retrograde cystography-confirmed vesicoureteral reflux. Of eight patients with right-sided UUT tumors, five had right-sided reflux, one had left-sided reflux, and two had bilateral reflux. Of seven patients with left-sided UUT tumors, five presented with bilateral reflux and two with left-sided reflux. Among three patients with bilateral UUT tumors, two presented with bilateral reflux. Thus, the reflux/tumor-site correlation was good. However, it must be noted that in those 30 patients who developed a UUT tumor, 21 (70%) had multiple bladder tumors, and 21 (93%) experienced recurrences (see the discussion to follow for the significance of multiplicity on the subsequent development of UUT tumor). Amar and Das [32] reported that only 1 patient developed a UUT tumor among 222 without reflux, whereas 3 of 47 patients with reflux developed a UUT tumor. The authors thus concluded that reflux was associated with a 15-fold increase in the risk of UUT tumor development. Statistical comparison was not provided; but by our cal-culation, the difference is significant ($P < 0.002$, χ^2 test). Each of the three patients, however, experienced multiple recurrences of a bladder tumor before UTT tumors developed (see the discussion to follow for the significance of multiple recurrences). According to De Torres Mateos et al. [33], of 288 patients with superficial bladder tumors, vesicoureteral reflux developed in 26% after TUR (The incidence was higher [77%] among those whose tumors were located near the ureteral orifices). The incidence of UUT tumors was significantly higher in patients with reflux than those without it (20% vs. 0.9%, $P < 0.001$). On the other hand, Mukamel et al. [35] did not observe a single case of UUT tumor during a follow-up of up to 18 years among 27 patients who had unilateral or bilateral reflux and recurrent low-grade, low-stage bladder carcinoma. Solsona et al. [40], in their interim analysis of 172 patients with a mean follow-up of 78.3 months, saw no significant difference in the UUT tumor incidence with or without reflux.

Those articles reporting a positive effect of reflux are relatively old, and the data were not subjected to critical statistical analysis (i.e., with multivariate analysis), possibly due to a small number of cases to provide enough statistical power. It is to be concluded that vesicoureteral reflux may be associated with an increased risk of UUT tumor, but it cannot be stated with certainty that reflux is causally related to UUT tumor development.

BCG Treatment

Bacillus Calmette-Guerin (BCG) is an effective therapy for superficial papillary tumors and carcinoma in situ of the bladder [44]. As a result, many patients live longer with a functioning bladder, but they must be monitored regularly for a recurrent urothelial tumor [37]. Several groups have reported a high incidence of UUT tumors after intravesical BCG therapy for superficial bladder tumors. The incidence ranges from 13% to 15% [36, 45]. Miller et al. [36] reported a 13.4% incidence among 82 patients who received BCG therapy for recurrent superficial bladder tumors. The median interval between initiation of BCG therapy and the diagnosis of a UUT tumor was 38 months (range 7–124 months). The indication for BCG treatment was the presence of a high-grade tumor, T1 tumors, multiplicity, associated carcinoma in situ, and failure of prior intravesical therapy. According to the Memorial Sloan-Kettering

Cancer Center series reported by Schwalb et al. [45], there was a 14.6% incidence of UUT cancer among 219 patients treated with BCG. The mean interval was 44 months.

Thus, BCG therapy appears to be associated with an apparently higher incidence of UUT tumors. It is to be noted, however, that in both series cited patients treated with BCG had high-grade lesions and/or Tis. In the Miller series [36], all UUT tumors developed were of high grade (grade 2 or 3) with or without Tis. These high-grade bladder cancers can possibly influence the development of urothelial neoplasms outside the bladder. It is pertinent to point out that the success of BCG therapy depends on direct contact with the urothelium. Thus, the UUT and urethra are potential areas of BCG failure [46]. Unless vesicoureteral reflux is present, the urothelium of the UUT is never in contact with BCG instilled intravesically [36].

To assess the prevalence and significance of carcinoma in situ, Herr et al. made a detailed pathology examination on 105 cystectomy specimens removed for invasive carcinomas plus diffuse carcinoma in situ. Among the 105 patients, 37 (35%) had evidence of carcinoma in situ involving some or all portions of the distal 8- to 10-cm segment of the ureter including the vesical intramural portion. BCG treatment, when administered to patients with carcinoma in situ, may achieve a complete response in the bladder and possibly also the prostatic urethra. In the Herr series, 66 patients with diffuse carcinoma in situ of the bladder received BCG therapy and achieved a complete response as evidenced by negative cystoscopy, biopsy, and urine cytology study. After more than 1 year of being free of bladder or urethral carcinoma in situ, 29% of the patients had clinical evidence of distal ureteral carcinoma in situ with no evidence of carcinoma in situ in the bladder or prostatic urethra. Foci of carcinoma in situ were a potential source of development of a high-grade urothelial cell carcinoma (see next section for further discussion).

Pathologic Characteristics of Bladder Cancers

Many investigators have pointed out that the risk of UUT tumors is closely related to the pathologic characteristics of the primary bladder cancer. Factors considered as risk are grade, stage, and recurrence (multiplicity) of tumors, and the presence of carcinoma in situ. Hurle et al. [41] divided bladder tumors into three risk groups. The low-risk group consisted of 216 patients with primary, solitary, low-grade (grade1 and 2), and low-stage (Ta, T1) tumors. They were treated with TUR alone. The intermediate-risk group consisted of 182 patients with recurrent or multifocal superficial tumors, which were treated with chemotherapy after TUR. The high-risk group consisted of 193 patients, including those with carcinoma in situ, grade 3 superficial tumors, and failed intravesical-chemotherapy or intravesical BCG treatment. After a median follow-up of 86 months, UUT tumors developed in 0.9%, 2.2%, and 9.8%, respectively, of the three risk groups. The risk was significantly higher in the high-risk group compared with the low-risk group [$P = 0.0004$; odds ratio (OR) 11.6, 95% confidence interval (CI) 2.5–40.7) or with the intermediate risk group ($P = 0.004$; OR 4.8, 95%CI 1.5–17.2), or both ($P = 0.000006$, OR 7.3, 95%CI 2.6–20.3).

Several reports have emphasized the history of multiplicity (primarily metachronous tumors but also simultaneous multiple tumors) as a significant risk factor. Millan-Rodriguez et al. [38] evaluated the prognostic factors of primary superficial bladder tumors based on 1529 patients. The overall incidence of UUT tumors was 2.6%. Independent variables considered for statistical analysis were pT stage, multiplicity, tumor size, Tis association, previous or synchronous UUT tumor, and intravesical BCG therapy. Risk groups were divided into a low-risk group consisting of patients with a Ta, grade 1 tumor or a single-stage T1 grade 1 tumor; the intermediate group consisted of multiple stage T1 grade 1 or stage Ta grade 2 tumors, or a single T2 grade 2 tumor; and the high-risk group consisted of multiple T1 grade 2, Ta grade 3, or T1 grade 3 tumors, or association with carcinoma in situ. The frequency of UUT tumor development was 0.6% in the low-risk group, 1.8% in the intermediate-risk group, and 4.1% in the high-risk group ($P = 0.007$). By multivariate analysis, the only factor significant for UUT tumor development was multiplicity of bladder tumors ($P < 0.04$, relative risk 2.7, 95%CI 1.06–6.84).

Canales et al. [42] reviewed a database of 375 patients who underwent resection of Ta urothelial carcinomas with a median follow-up of 6 years. Patients with T1 tumors and carcinoma in situ were not included. Upper urinary tract tumors developed in 13 patients (3.4%) at an average of 22 months after an initial bladder tumor. Both time to recurrence and the number of bladder tumor recurrences were statistically significant predictors of a UUT tumor ($P <$

0.04 and 0.01, respectively, by multivariate analysis). Patients with two or more recurrences within 12 months of each other were at a 4.5-fold risk for a UUT tumor.

Data to suggest an association of tumor multiplicity (both synchronous and metachronous) with UUT tumor development were also presented by Palou et al. [34] but were not analyzed statistically.

Many investigators have proposed the importance of carcinoma in situ as a risk factor. Solsona et al. [40] had four groups of patients. The first group consisted of 789 patients with superficial bladder tumor(s) but without associated carcinoma in situ. A second group consisted of 132 patients with either primary carcinoma in situ or carcinoma in situ associated with superficial tumors. A third group was made up of 179 patients who underwent cystectomy for invasive carcinoma. The fourth group consisted of 46 patients who had cystectomy for carcinoma in situ. The subsequent incidence of UUT cancer was 2.3% for group 1, 21.2% for group 2, 3.9% for group 3, and 17.4% for group 4. The difference between the group with superficial bladder cancer without associated carcinoma in situ (group 1) and with carcinoma in situ (group 2) was significant ($P < 0.001$), and the difference between the group who underwent cystectomy because of invasive cancer (group 3) and the group who had cystectomy because of carcinoma in situ (group 4) was also significant ($P < 0.01$). Among patients with bladder carcinoma in situ (group 2), 34 developed cytologic evidence of carcinoma in situ involving the UUT. Of these 34 patients, 23 developed UUT tumors, most of them located in the distal ureter. This was in sharp contrast to the predominantly pyelocaliceal location (69%) of UUT tumors as an initial manifestation of urothelial carcinoma (Table 3-8-1). Among patients with bladder carcinoma in situ, development of a UUT tumor did not affect the prognosis. In the multivariate analysis, however, only the presence of carcinoma in situ in the prostatic urethra had a negative impact on the prognosis; thus, bladder carcinoma in situ with panurothelial involvement (i.e., renal pelvis, ureter, prostatic urethra) ($P = 0.0001$) and bladder carcinoma in situ with prostatic urethral involvement ($P = 0.007$) had a negative impact on prognosis. Based on these findings, they concluded that (1) carcinoma in situ in the bladder is associated with a high propensity of developing carcinoma in situ in the UUT and urothelial carcinoma in the ureters, primarily in the distal segment; and (2) the presence of carcinoma in situ in the prostatic urethra has a significant negative impact on prognosis. They believed that the multicentricity and diffuseness of carcinoma in situ (including pagetoid spread) is the important etiologic factor for the development of urothelial carcinomas at multiple sites. This conclusion is supported by the observation that cystectomy performed because of carcinoma in situ does not reduce the incidence of subsequent UUT tumor development (group 3 vs. group 4) (see next section). Herr and Whitmore [37] also observed that UUT tumors in patients with bladder carcinoma in situ were predominantly in the distal ureter, suggesting pagetoid spread as an etiologic factor.

Does cystectomy lower the incidence of upper urinary tract tumors?

The reported incidence of UUT tumors after cystectomy ranges widely, from 2.0% to 8.5% [47–53]. Thus, there is no difference from the reported incidence among patients with an intact bladder. In general, tumors developing in the upper urinary tract after cystectomy tend to be multifocal and are at an advanced stage and high grade and thus are associated with a poor prognosis [47, 51, 53]. Reported risks present in the bladder associated with the development of UUT tumors are multiplicity/recurrences [47, 50, 54], the presence of carcinoma in situ [48, 51, 52], and involvement of an intramural portion and/or distal end of the resected ureters with invasive tumor or carcinoma in situ [47, 50, 51, 53, 54]. As a result, more tumors develop at the distal portion of the ureter in comparison to the incidence of ureteral tumors in patients who present with a UUT tumor as an initial manifestation of urothelial cancer.

In the study by Huguet-Perez et al. [50], the overall incidence after cystectomy was 4.5% (26/568). However, the incidence varied among several subgroups; it was significantly higher among patients who had a history of repeated recurrence of superficial tumors before development of invasive carcinoma than among those without a history of prior superficial tumors ($P < 0.0005$). Tumors of the bladder in patients who subsequently developed UUT tumors were of high grade in 84%, multifocal in 80%, and associated with carcinoma in situ in the bladder in 65%, in the prostatic urethra in 52%, and in the distal ureter in 57%.

In summary, carcinoma in the UUT is more aggressive than carcinoma in the lower urinary tract although its incidence is lower. Patients with UUT carcinoma carry a much higher risk of developing lower urinary tract carcinoma probably through both spreading and a field effect. Patients who undergo cystectomy for bladder cancer carry all sorts of risk factors that are known for the development of UUT tumor. Nevertheless, the incidence of UUT tumor is no higher than that among patients with an intact bladder. When it does occur, though, it tends to be in the distal ureter and multifocal and at an advanced stage.

References

1. Murphy WM, Beckwith JB, Farrow GM (1994) Tumors of the kidney, bladder, and related urinary structures. Fascicle 11, 3rd series. In: Rosai J, Sobin LH (eds) Atlas of tumor pathology. Armed Forces Institute of Pathology, Washington, DC, pp 313–321.
2. Genega P, Vogelzang NJ, Randazzo R, Sener S, Chmiel J, Fremgen A, Sylvester J (1992) Renal pelvic cancer: a review of 611 patients treated in Illinois 1975–1985, 1992. Urology 40:393–399.
3. Guinan P, Chmiel J, Vogelzang NJ, Fremgen A, Randazzo R, Sylvester J, Sener S (1992) Renal pelvic cancer: a review of 611 patients treated in Illinois 1975–1985. Urology 40:393–399.
4. Melamed MR, Reuter VE (1993) Pathology and staging of urothelial tumors of the kidney and ureter. Urol Clin North Am 20:333–347.
5. Nocks BN, Heney NM, Daly JJ, Perrone TA, Groffin PP, Prout GR Jr (1982) Transitional cell carcinoma of renal pelvis. Urology 19:472–477.
6. Dudak SC, Soloway MS, Neulander EZ (2000) Management of upper tract transitional cell carcinoma: surgical management. In: Vogelzang NJ, Scardino PT, Shipley WU, Coffey DS (eds) Comprehensive textbook of genitourinary oncology. Lippincott Williams & Wilkins, Philadelphia, pp 367–376.
7. Olgac S, Mazmdar M, Dalbagni G, Reuter VE (2004) Urothelial carcinoma of the renal pelvis: a clinicopathologic study of 130 cases. Am J Surg Pathol 28:1545–1552.
8. Anonymous (2002) Renal pelvis and ureter. In: Greene FL, Page DL, Fleming ID, Fritz AG, Blech CM, Haller DG, Morrow M (eds) AJCC cancer staging manual. Springer-Verlag, New York, pp 329–331.
9. Bloom NA, Vidone RA, Lytton B (1970) Primary carcinoma of the ureter: a report of 102 new cases. J Urol 103:590–598.
10. Batata MA, Whitmore WF, Hilaris BS, Tokita N, Grabstald H (1975) Primary carcinoma of the ureter: a prognostic study. Cancer 35:1626–1632.
11. Heney NM, Nocks BN, Daly JJ, Blitzer PH, Parkhurst EC (1981) Prognostic factors in carcinoma of the ureter. J Urol 125:632–636.
12. Reuter VE (2004) The urothelial tract: renal pelvis, ureter, urinary bladder, and urethra. In: Mills SE (ed) Sternberg's Diagnostic Surgical Pathology. Lippincott Williams & Wilkins, Philadelphia, pp 2035–2081.
13. Knowles MA (2001) What we could do now: molecular pathology of bladder cancer. Mol Pathol 54:215–221.
14. Huffman JL (2000) Management of upper tract transitional cell carcinomas: endoscopic management In: Vogelzang NJ, Scardino PT, Shipley WU, Coffey DS (eds) Comprehensive textbook of genitourinary oncology. Lippincott Williams & Wilkins, Philadelphia, pp 367–376.
15. Hall MC, Womack S, Sagalowsky AI, Carmody T, Erickstad MD, Roehrborn CG (1998) Prognostic factors, recurrence, and survival in transitional cell carcinoma of the upper urinary tract: a 30-year experience in 252 patients. Urology 52:594–601.
16. Kroft SH, Oyasu R (1994) Biology of disease—urinary bladder cancer: mechanisms of development and progression. Lab Invest 71:158–174.
17. IARC (1979) IARC Monographs on the evaluation of the carcinogenic risk of chemicals to humans. Supplement 1. Chemicals and industrial processes associated with cancer in humans. International Agency for Research on Cancer, Lyon.
18. US DHEW (1979) Smoking and health: a report of the Surgeon General. PHS Publ 79-50066. Department of Health, Education and Welfare, Washington, DC.
19. Kadlubar FF, Miller JA, Miller EC (1977) Hepatic microsomal N-glucuronidation and nucleic acid binding of N-hydroxyarylamines in relation to urinary bladder carcinogenesis. Cancer Res 37:805–814.
20. Bladder Cancer (1981) In: Skrabanek P, Walsh, A (eds) UICC technical report series, vol 60. UICC, Geneva, pp 118–143.
21. Dominick MA, White MR, Sanderson TP, Van Fleet T, Cohen SM, Arnold LE, Cano M, Tannehill-Gregg S, Moehlenkamp JD, Waites CR, Schilling BE (2006) Urothelial carcinogenesis in the urinary bladder of male rats treated with muraglitazar, a PPAR alpha/gamma agonist: evidence for urolithiasis as the inciting event in the mode of action. Toxicol Pathol 34:903–920.
22. Cheng L, Neumann RM, Nehra A, Spotts BE, Weaver AL, Bostwick BG (2000) Cancer heterogeneity and its biologic implications in the grading of urothelial carcinoma. Cancer 88:1663–1670.
23. Krogh J, Kvist E, Rye B (1991) Transitional cell carcinoma of the upper urinary tract: prognostic variables and post-operative recurrences. Br J Urol 67:32–36.
24. Charbit L, Gendreau MC, Mee S, Cukier J (1991) Tumors of the upper urinary tract: 10 years of experience. J Urol 146:1243–1246.
25. Holmang S, Johansson SL (2006) Bilateral metachronous ureteral and renal pelvic carcinomas: incidence, clinical presentation, histopathology, treatment and outcome. J Urol 175:69–73.
26. Lynch HT, Taylor RJ, Lynch JF, Knezetic JA, Barrows A, Fodde R, Wijnen J, Wagner A (2003) Multiple primary cancer, including transitional cell carcinoma of the upper uroepithelial tract in a multigeneration HNPCC family: molecular genetic, diagnostic, and

management implications. Am J Gastroenterol 98: 664–670.

27. Kang C-H, Yu T-J, Hsieh H-H, Yang JW, Shu K, Huang C-C, Chiang P-H, Shiue Y-L (2003) The development of bladder tumors and contralateral upper urinary tract tumors after primary transitional cell carcinoma of the upper urinary tract. Cancer 98:1620–1626.

28. Kakizoe T, Fujita J, Murase T, Matsumoto K, Kishi K (1980) Transitional cell carcinoma of the bladder in patients with renal pelvic and ureteral cancer. J Urol 124:17–19.

29. Takahashi T, Kakehi Y, Mitsumori K, Akao T, Terachi T, Kato T, Ogawa O, Habuchi T (2001) Distinct microsatellite alterations in upper urinary tract tumors and subsequent bladder tumors. J Urol 165:672–677.

30. Takahashi T, Habuchi T, Kakehi Y, Mitsumori K, Akao T, Terachi T, Yoshida O (1998) Clonal and chronologic genetic analysis of multifocal cancers of the bladder and upper urinary tract. Cancer Res 58: 5835–5841.

31. Kirkali Z, Tuzel E (2003) Transitional cell carcinoma of the ureter and renal pelvis. Crit Rev Oncol Hematol 47:155–169.

32. Amar AD, Das S (1985) Upper urinary tract transitional cell carcinoma in patients with bladder carcinoma and associated vesicoureteral reflux. J Urol 133:468–471.

33. De Torres Mateos JA, Banus Gassol JM, Palou Redorta J, Morote Robles J (1987) Vesicorenal reflux and upper urinary tract transitional cell carcinoma after transurethral resection of recurrent superficial bladder carcinoma. J Urol 138:49–51.

34. Palou J, Farina LA, Villavicencio H, Vicente J (1992) Upper tract urothelial tumor after transurethral resection for bladder tumor. Eur Urol 21:110–114.

35. Mukamel E, Nissenkorn I, Glanz I, Vilcovsky E, Servadio C (1985) Upper tract tumours in patients with vesico-ureteral reflux and recurrent bladder tumours. Eur Urol 11:6–8.

36. Miller EB, Eure GR, Schellhammer PF (1993) Upper tract transitional cell carcinoma following treatment of superficial bladder cancer with BCG. Urology 42:26–30.

37. Herr HW, Whitmore WF Jr (1987) Ureteral carcinoma in situ after successful intravesical therapy for superficial bladder tumors: incidence, possible pathogenesis and management. J Urol 138:292–294.

38. Millan-Rodriguez F, Chechile-Toniolo G, Salvador-Bayarri J, Huguet-Perez J, Vicente-Rodriguez J (2000) Upper urinary tract tumors after primary superficial bladder tumors; prognostic factors and risk group. J Urol 164:1183–1187.

39. Shinka T, Uekado Y, Aoshi H, Hirano A, Ohkawa T (1988) Occurrence of uroepithelial tumors of the upper urinary tract after the initial diagnosis of bladder cancer. J Urol 140:745–748.

40. Solsona E, Iborra I, Ricos JV, Dumont R, Casanova JL, Calabuig C (1997) Upper urinary tract involvement in patients with bladder carcinoma in situ (Tis): its impact on management. Urology 49:347–352.

41. Hurle R, Losa A, Manzetti A, Lembo A (1999) Upper urinary tract tumors developing after treatment of superficial bladder cancer: 7-year follow-up of 591 consecutive patients. Urology 53:1144–1148.

42. Canales BK, Anderson JK, Premoli J, Slaton JW (2006) Risk factors for upper tract recurrence in patients undergoing long-term surveillance for stage Ta bladder cancer. J Urol 175:74–77.

43. Schwartz CB, Bekirov H, Melman A (1992) Urothelial tumors of upper tract following treatment of primary bladder transitional cell carcinoma. Urology 40:509–511.

44. Han RF, Pan JG (2006) Can intravesical bacillus Calmette-Guerin reduce recurrence in patients with superficial bladder cancer? A meta-analysis of randomized trials. Urology 67:1216–1223.

45. Schwalb DA, Herr HW, Sogani PC, Russo P, Sheinfeld J, Fair WR (1992) Upper tract disease following intravesical BCG for superficial bladder cancer: five year follow-up. J Urol 147(suppl):273A.

46. Ratliff TL (1991) Bacillus Calmette-Guerin (BCG): mechanism of action in superficial bladder cancer. Urology 37(suppl 5):8–11.

47. Malkowicz SB, Skinner DG (1990) Development of upper tract carcinoma after cystectomy for bladder carcinoma. Urology 35:20–22.

48. Hastie KJ, Hamdy FC, Collins MC, Williams JL (1991) Upper tract tumours following cystectomy for bladder cancer: is routine intravenous urography worthwhile? Br J Urol 67:29–31.

49. Mufti GR, Gove JRW, Riddle PR (1988) Nephroureterectomy after radical cystectomy. J Urol 139:588–589.

50. Huguet-Perez J, Palou J, Millan-Rodriguez F, Salvador-Bayarri J, Villavicencio-Mavrich H, Vicente-Rodriguez J (2001) Upper tract transitional cell carcinoma following cystectomy for bladder cancer. Eur Urol 40:318–323.

51. Zincke H, Garbeff PJ, Beahrs JR (1984) Upper urinary tract transitional cell cancer after radical cystectomy for bladder cancer. J Urol 131:50–52.

52. Schellhammer PF, Whitmore WF Jr (1976) Transitional cell carcinoma of the urethra in men having cystectomy for bladder cancer. J Urol 115:56–60.

53. Balaji KC, McGuire M, Grotas J, Grimaldi G, Russo P (1999) Upper tract recurrences following radical cystectomy: an analysis of prognostic factors, recurrence pattern and stage at presentation. J Urol 162:1603–1606.

54. Kenworthy P, Tanguay S, Simon T, Dinney CP (1996) The risk of upper tract recurrence following cystectomy in patients with transitional cell carcinoma involving the distal ureter. J Urol 155:501–503.

55. Johansson S, Angervall L, Bengtsson U, Wahlqvist L (1976) A clinicopathologic and prognostic study of epithelial tumors of the renal pelvis. Cancer 37:1376–1383.

56. Davis BW, Hough AJ, Gardner WA (1987) Renal pelvic carcinoma: morphological correlates of metastatic behavior. J Urol 137:857–861.

57. Huben RP, Mounzer AM, Murphy GP (1988) Tumor grade and stage as prognostic variables in upper tract urothelial tumors. Cancer 62:2016–2020.

Question 9

Do multifocal or recurrent urothelial carcinomas originate from a single transformed cell or from multiple transformed cells? What is the clinical significance of this argument?

Answer

Currently two hypotheses are being considered for the origin of multifocal or recurrent urothelial carcinomas. The clonogenic hypothesis (hypothesis 1) describes tumors as descendants of a single transformed cell that undergoes further multiple genetic alterations, proliferates, and spreads through the urothelial tract either by intraepithelial migration or intraluminal seeding. The "field changes" hypothesis (hypothesis 2) states that urothelial cells undergo malignant transformation at multiple sites and become the source of multifocal tumors. Based on reports with several available techniques, both hypotheses are viable to account for human bladder carcinogenesis. Hypothesis 1 may apply most of the urothelial carcinomas that result from exposure to the conventional carcinogen source (cigarette smoking). The underlying mechanism responsible for oligoclonal tumor development (hypothesis 2) remains unknown. It would be intriguing to suggest that heavy carcinogen exposure (e.g., aromatic amines, irradiation, heavy smoking) may cause the "field changes."

Comments

One characteristic of urothelial tumors is multiple synchronous and metachronous development. To explain this phenomenon, two hypotheses have been proposed. The first is a "field changes" hypothesis in which multiple cells undergo initial transformation as a first step in carcinogenesis. This hypothesis makes sense because every day millions of urothelial cells (in particular, of the bladder) are uniformly exposed to the carcinogens present in urine. Therefore, multiple tumors of independent origin could develop either simultaneously or metachronously. A second hypothesis postulates that a single transformed cell is the source of multiple tumors (clonal derivatives[1]), either simultaneous or metachronous, although they may appear heterogeneous in microscopic, genetic, and clinical characteristics. Monoclonal tumors should exhibit identical initial genetic alterations that are responsible for tumor development. As transformed cells continue to accumulate genetic changes, proliferating cells would spread by the intraepithelial route or by intraluminal seeding. Multifocal development of tumors from new sources ensues with variable genetic and epigenetic differences.

There have been considerable debates on this subject, and data supporting both hypotheses have been published. Studies based on molecular evidence indicate, however, that most urothelial tumors are of monoclonal origin. Those readers who are keenly interested in this subject, are encouraged to read the review articles by Duggan et al. [1], Habuchi [2], Hafner et al. [3], and Garcia et al. [4]. In the Garcia article, the discussion is not limited to urothelial tumors.

Why is it important to determine whether urothelial tumors originate in a single clone or multiple clones? The knowledge could be used to establish a new strategy for the prevention of urothelial tumors and an individual treatment strategy against molecular targets of the tumor [1, 2, 5].

---

[1] Clone is defined as a family of cells that derive from a common progenitor.

What are the methods commonly used for clonality studies?

Several techniques are available. They are based on two principles: (1) whether every cell in all multiple tumors exhibits the same type of X-chromosome inactivation; and (2) if all tumors share the same genetic (allelic) changes that have been accepted as early-stage alterations (i.e., fingerprints). Several techniques are available for studying the latter type. Understandably, the more markers utilized, the more reliable is the conclusion.

X-Chromosome Inactivation

The X-chromosome inactivation technique is based on the principle that one of the two X chromosomes in females is inactivated in individual cells during early embryonic development as a result of methylation of cytosine residues in the promoter region [6]. Thus, normal tissue in females is a closely knit mosaic of cells with one active X chromosome of either maternal or paternal origin. If a tumor is of monoclonal origin, all cells should express the same type of X chromosome of either paternal or maternal origin, and this can be determined by digesting DNA with a methylation-sensitive enzyme (commonly HpaII or HhaI) and amplifying the remaining allele via the polymerase chain reaction (PCR) at a polymorphic X-chromosome-linked marker, such as the human androgen receptor gene. A drawback of this method is that only tumors from female patients can be studied. Additional caveats are the possibility of unstable DNA methylation in tumors [7] and the possible preferential inactivation of the maternal or paternal allele [8]. Another potential problem is that each tissue type, including the urothelium, contains "patches" of varying size derived from a single cell, thus exhibiting an identical regional inactivation pattern [4]. Should two independent tumors happen to arise in patches of identical X-chromosome inactivation, the tumors would be identified as of monoclonal origin. In urothelium, these patches are estimated to be about 120 mm^2 in size and contain approximately 2×10^6 cells; and 200–300 founder cells participate in the formation of a urinary bladder [9]. Furthermore, different patches may possess a different predisposition to tumorigenesis (for further discussion see below).

Using the X-chromosome inactivation method, Sidransky et al. [10] demonstrated for the first time that the same allele (of either paternal or maternal origin) was inactivated in all tumors in each patient, strongly indicating that multiple tumors were clonal. Reports of similar findings followed [11, 12].

Loss of Heterozygosity

The Knudson's "two-hit" hypothesis [13] has provided the rationale for studies that aim to identify tumor suppressor genes by mapping regions of allelic loss (loss of heterozygosity, or LOH). Gene loss in a cancer cell often occurs by deletion of a relatively large segment of a chromosome. As a result, one copy of tumor suppressor gene in a cancer cell may undergo an inactivating point mutation, whereas a gross deletion eliminates the other copy along with some neighboring genes [14]. Because certain chromosomal regions in bladder cancer cells (e.g., 9q) are known to have been lost at an early stage and at high frequency, LOH has been used as a tool for the clonality assay.

Microsatellite analysis has been used to detect LOH in tumor cells [15]. Two types of alteration can be detected; one is LOH as a result of allelic deletion, and a second is due to alteration in the microsatellite repeats either by shortening or expansion (which indicates microsatellite instability) [2]. Identical LOH patterns suggest a monoclonal origin of the tumors. LOH on chromosome 9 is the most frequent genetic alteration identified in bladder tumors and has been accepted as an early event in urothelial tumorigenesis [16]. Chromosome 9 is the site of multiple important cyclin-dependent kinase inhibitors with tumor suppressor activity related to cell cycle regulation. Approximately 60%–70% of bladder tumors show LOH of at least one locus on either arm of this chromosome [16–18]. A discrepant LOH pattern among tumors can be due to polyclonality but could still be due to omission of a right marker locus in an LOH analysis. In the case of partial chromosomal arm loss, if an identical chromosomal breakpoint is demonstrated on 9q with the use of multiple probes, it gives strong support for monoclonality of the tumors [19].

As was discussed under Question 8, urothelial cancer can be divided into two types—superficial low-grade papillary and nodular high-grade invasive—and a distinctly different mode of development has been proposed for each [20]. Regions commonly showing deletion and predicted to contain tumor suppressor genes have been identified by LOH [21, 22].

Some of the changes are linked to special tumor properties: tumor initiation, 9p–,[2] 9q–, Y–, 1q+, 17+; papillary growth, –9q [23]; T1 tumor (in addition to the Ta changes) 2q–, 4p–, 4q–, 5q–, 6p–, 8p–, 10q–, 11p–, 11q–, 13q–, 17p–, 18q–, 3p+, 5p+, 6p+, 8q+, 10p+, 10q+[3], 17q+, 20q+; and deeply invasive phenotype (T2-4) (in addition to the above) 15q–, 7p+, Xq+ [21–30].

Comparative Genomic Hybridization

The comparative genomic hybridization technique detects gains and losses at each chromosome [23, 24, 30–32]. The advantage is that DNA from either fresh tissue or paraffin-embedded tumor can be used, and a hybridization kit is commercially available [28]. Complex changes (deletion, addition, amplification) affecting numerous chromosomal loci can be visualized. They vary by the bladder tumor grade [23–25, 32]. By comparing the pattern changes, one can suggest a clonal origin of multiple tumors [32].

Fluorescence in Situ Hybridization

The fluorescence in situ hybridization (FISH) technique has been found extremely useful in cytogenetics and oncology studies [33]. To demonstrate certain chromosome or chromosomal loci, a probe (e.g., CDK12 for 9p21) is hybridized with the chromosome. Copy numbers for centromeres and a specific gene locus are counted in all cells available on the slides. Although sensitive, intact nuclei and a significant number of analyzable cells are required [5], and a subchromosomal location cannot be determined unless multiple markers are used.

Mutational Analysis of Suppressor Genes

Mutational analysis of suppressor genes is most commonly used for the studying the p53 gene. The mutation site and pattern of changes of this gene vary. The p53 mutations occur in 65% of carcinomas in situ and only 3% of papillary Ta tumors [20]. Because in the urinary bladder the p53 mutation does not show significant carcinogen-specific hot spots, identical mutation among multiple tumors is interpreted as evidence for monoclonal derivation [34–36]. However, Yasunaga et al. [37] found specific mutations among

patients who were exposed to aromatic amine dye carcinogens at work. Mutations occurred in exon 5 (at codons 151 and 152) in 70% of neoplastic lesions.

Identical alteration in tumors at late stages could reflect monoclonal occurrence of multiple tumors [34] but could also indicate dominant overgrowth of the most malignant tumor cell clone. Conversely, tumors showing diverse p53 mutations can still be monoclonal because p53 mutations tend to occur late in carcinogenesis, especially in papillary tumors [20, 38–40]. There are no convincing data that confirm their role in clonality, but p53 status appears to be involved in the evolution of urothelial tumors.

What have investigators found on clonality and molecular basis of bladder tumors? How reliable is the reported frequency?

The results and conclusions are tabulated in Table 3-9-1. A comprehensive and persuasive report comes from Habuchi's group. Multiple markers (ranging from two to four) representing subchromosomal loci of several chromosomes were used [19]. Three groups of patients were found. Group 1 consisted of 16 patients whose tumors demonstrated identical LOH patterns. Thus, all tumors in these patients were considered clonal. Group 2 consisted of 9 patients showing discordant alterations, of which multiple tumors in 4 patients were judged to be of clonal origin because they exhibited identical alterations in the fingerprint chromosome loci (i.e., 9p/9q), and discordances were interpreted as subsequent genetic changes. In the remaining 5 cases, clonality could not be established (although the tumors could still be found to be clonal if more early genetic change markers had been used). Group 3 consisted of 4 patients whose tumors did not show detectable microsatellite alterations; thus, the data were not informative. The authors concluded that at least 80% of 25 evaluated patients had multiple tumors of monoclonal origin. Their study provided an additional piece of useful information: the genetic alterations detected were fairly stable for at least 3 years in 5 patients. The findings are consistent with the clinical observation that low-grade superficial tumors progress to invasive tumors in only 10% of patients after a long follow-up [41].

Multifocal cancers involving the upper urinary tract and lower urinary tract were discussed under

---

[2] – indicates loss, and + indicates gain.
[3] 10q– and 10q+ indicate that both types of changes may be associated with invasive growth.

TABLE 3-9-1. Clonal analysis of urothelial tumors

Investigator (year)	Method used	Type of tumors			Results	Conclusions and comments
		Superficial	Deeply invasive tumors	All types		
Sidransky [10], (1992)	X-chromosome inactivation		Yes		Inactivation of same chromosome in all (13) tumors in 4 patients	Monoclonal origin
Miyao [38], (1993)	LOH (9p, 9q, 17p), p53 mutation			Yes	Multiple tumors (13) judged to be clonal in each of 5 patients	Concordance in clonality also observed in all 13 patients between bladder tumor and lymph node metastasis
Habuchi [35], (1993)	p53 mutation		Yes		Identical mutations in all tumors in each of 4 patients	Monoclonal origin
Xu [34], (1996)	p53 mutation	Yes (pTa, pT1, grades 2 and 3)			Identical mutation in 21 of 22 tumors from 5 patients	All but 1 of 22 are clonal
Goto [36], (1997)	p53 mutation			Yes	Nine patients had identical mutation in multiple tumors, 11 had tumors with discordant mutations, and 2 had a mutation in one tumor and no mutation in another	Both monoclonal and polyclonal origins of multiple tumors
Takahashi [19], (1998)	LOH and microsatellite alteration	Yes			Judged monoclonal in 20 of 25 patients (65 tumors)	At least 80% of 25 evaluable patients considered to have monoclonal tumors
Li [11], (1999)	X-chromosome inactivation	Yes			Inactivation of same chromosome in all (35) tumors in 10 patients	Monoclonal origin. In 4 of the 10 patients, bladder and upper urinary tract tumors analyzed
Diaz-Cano [12], (2000)	X-chromosome inactivation androgen receptor gene		Yes		Identical mutation in 37 of 39 patients	All but 2 of 39 are monoclonal. This study compares tumor cells located above and below musularis mucosa to look for intratumoral heterogeneity (one sample from each compartment studied)
Hartmann [50], (2000)	FISH (chromosomes 9, 17) LOH (9q22, 9p21, 17p13)	Yes			Judged monoclonal in 8 of 9 patients (44 tumors), oligoclonal in 1 (5 tumors)	Most multiple bladder tumors are monoclonal, but recurrent tumors show additional genetic alterations
Hafner [24], (2001)	LOH (9p, 9q, p53), p53 mutation	Yes			Overall, 9 of 14 patients (64%) judged to have tumors of clonal origin	Clonal (64%) and oligoclonal (36%). Every patients had at least one tumor in the upper (renal pelvis ureter) and one lower (bladder, urethra) tumor. In all, 4 of 5 oligoclonal cases involved both upper and lower urinary tract
Denzinger [5], (2006)	FISH, LOH, p53 mutation			Yes	Overall, 4 of 6 carcinoma in situ samples showed LOH of 9p and 17p 13.1. All 9 tumor samples with deletion of identical alleles on 9p and 17p 13.1. All 7 analyzable tumor samples with deletion of 9p, 9q, and 17p 13.1 by FISH. Identical p53 mutation (in codon 281) in all 7 analyzable tumor samples	Samples from a single bladder with multiple tumors demonstrate changes indicative of monoclonality. FISH analysis is sensitive in detecting LOH

Question 8. Patients presenting initially with an upper tract cancer carry a risk as high as 48% of developing a bladder tumor after nephrectomy [42]. The Habuchi group addressed the genetic correlation of these two types of urothelial tumor [43]. Confirming the earlier finding [19], they found that recurrent bladder tumors affecting the bladder only were judged to be clonal in 16 of 19 evaluated cases (84%), whereas bladder tumors developing subsequent to an upper tract cancer were clonal in only 7 of the 13 evaluable cases (47%). Furthermore, compared with recurrent carcinomas confined to the bladder, additional genetic alterations were found in six of the seven bladder tumors developing after nephrectomy ($P < 0.005$). These findings indicate that bladder tumors developing in patients initially presenting with a upper urinary tract carcinoma are due to both "field changes" and spread from the original tumor and that upper urinary tract carcinomas are genetically more unstable than bladder-specific tumors.

X-chromosome inactivation, if performed properly, should provide a decisive conclusion on clonality. Monoclonal origin was reported in all tumors studied [10–12].

Chimeric animals may be a useful model for studying clonality of multiple tumors. In their study with chimeric mice (C3H/BALB/c) exposed to a powerful bladder carcinogen, N-butyl-N-(4-hydroxybutyl)nitrosamine, Yamamoto et al. [44] observed that multiple tumors were of different strain origin, but individual tumors were monoclonal. Although the data favor the multiclonal hypothesis, one must recognize that an identical genetic background of tumors does not necessarily indicate monoclonality. Another potential problem that was recognized was that animals were exposed to a potent bladder carcinogen at high levels. There has been no human study that directly addresses carcinogen dosage effect on polyclonal tumor development. It is possible that exposure to carcinogens at high levels increases the number of oligoclonal tumors. In this regard, a clonality study would be of value on tumors of dye industry workers or Chernobyl irradiation victims [45].

Recently, two groups [46, 47] claimed a high frequency of polyclonality of bladder tumors. In the Paiss study [46], 27 female patients who were heterozygous for androgen receptor polymorphism were studied. Both fresh and formalin-fixed paraffin-embedded tissues were used as a DNA source. Altogether, 16 of 45 tumors revealed a polyclonal pattern.

The tumors studied ranged from Ta to T3. There was no correlation between clonality status and tumor stage. Cheng's group [47] used the same technique. Unlike the Paiss group, this group examined intratumoral clonality of a muscle-invasive tumor derived from cystectomy specimens from 18 female patients; multiple tumor samples representing different parts of the same tumor were microdissected from 5-μm histologic sections under direct light microscopy visualization. Seven of nine informative patients showed different patterns of nonrandom X-chromosome inactivation; thus, only two patients showed the same pattern of nonrandom X-chromosome inactivation. In both studies the investigators were fully cognizant of possible technical problems that could have led to their unexpected results, but they were reportedly ruled out. In one patient of the Paiss study, four samples taken from different parts of one tumor demonstrated a polyclonal pattern.

Several possibilities may be offered to reconcile these discrepant reports on clonality. First, in support of monoclonal development (hypothesis 1), multiple clones with initial genetic alterations erupt at multiple sites in the urinary tract, especially in the bladder. With accumulated mutational events, one of the clones emerges as dominant over the others. The progeny of this clone spread to the surrounding mucosa or discontinuously to other sites as intraluminal transplants. With additional genetic and epigenetic changes (e.g., hypermethylation), papillary neoplasms or dysplastic epithelium ensue (Fig. 3-9-1A). A second possibility (hypothesis 2), which supports the "field change" hypothesis, is that multiple clones that have undergone heavy mutational events occur in the bladder (Fig. 3-9-1B). This situation might apply to individuals who have developed urothelial neoplasms as a consequence of heavy exposure to carcinogens for an extended period of time. The observation by Paiss et al. and Yamamoto et al. obtained with the use of a chimeric mouse model may fall into this category. A third possibility (hypothesis 3), which may be considered a variant of hypothesis 2, is that two closely spaced clones develop into a single (collision) tumor (Fig. 3-9-1C1). This hypothesis can account for the intratumoral polyclonality reported by Cheng et al. For this event to become a realistic possibility, numerous cells need to be "hit hard" by carcinogens. Data from the chimeric mouse study cited above (Yamamoto, 1998), however, do not support this hypothesis because separate tumors

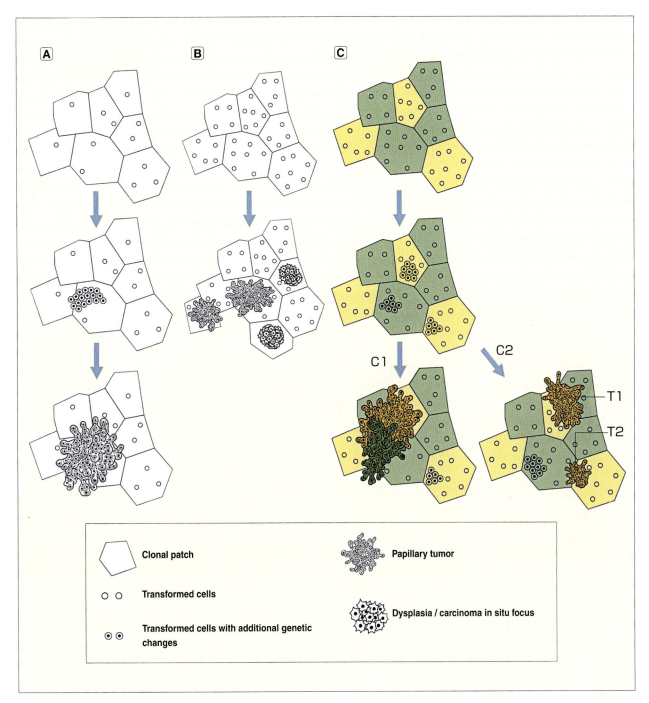

FIG. 3-9-1. Proposed mechanisms of monoclonal and oligoclonal development of urothelial tumors. **A** Hypothesis 1. Urothelial mucosa consists of two types of "patches" arranged in a mosaic pattern. Initial neoplastic changes have occurred involving a few cells at random distribution (*open circles, top figure*). Additional genetic alterations involve one of them and its clonal expansion (*circles with central dot, middle figure*). Further accumulation of genetic changes has resulted in a papillary neoplasm (*lower figure*). **B** Hypothesis 2. In this model, several cells have undergone genetic alterations independently (*top figure*) and progressed to a papillary neoplasm and foci of dysplasia/carcinoma in situ (*bottom figure*). **C** Hypothesis 3. **C1** In this model, two clones from different patches have undergone progressive genetic alterations (*middle figure*), continue to proliferate, and ultimately collide and fuse to form a single tumor mass (*lower figure*). **C2** In this model, two clones of the same genetic background (*yellow-colored patches*) have grown into two independent tumors (pseudomonoclonal phenomenon)

were polyclonal but none of tumors demonstrated intratumoral polyclonality. However, another theoretical possibility exists: By chance, two cells within a patch or one cell of each of adjoining patches of the same genetic background have undergone neoplastic transformation, and subsequently each clone gives rise to a separate tumor. These two (T1 and T2 in Fig. 3-9-1C2) would be indistinguishable when studied by the X-chromosome inactivation assay. Hence, they would be interpreted as being of monoclonal origin despite their independent development (pseudo-monoclonal phenomenon).

In summary, based on reports using several available techniques, we conclude that both hypothesis 1 (clonogenic) and hypothesis 2 (field changes) are viable to explain human bladder carcinogenesis. Hypothesis 1 may apply to many of the papillary carcinomas that develop following exposure to a conventional carcinogen source (cigarette smoking). The underlying mechanism responsible for oligoclonal tumor development (hypothesis 2) remains unknown. It would be intriguing to suggest that heavy carcinogen exposure (e.g., aromatic amines, irradiation, and heavy smoking) causes the "field changes." A puzzling question is whether intratumoral oligoclonality is as frequent an event as a recent publication cited above suggests.

The LOH assay and the X-chromosome inactivation method are not without potential technical faults [8, 48, 49]. To improve the quality of studies, future investigations should use fresh samples (if feasible) or a substantial amount of tumor DNA if paraffin-embedded tissue to be used [49] as well as multiple methods including the FISH analysis with multiple microsatellite probes and the X-chromosome assay, if applicable.

References

1. Duggan BJ, Gray SB, McKnight JJ, Watson CJ, Johnston SR, Williamson KE (2004) Oligoclonality in bladder cancer: the implication for molecular therapies. J Urol 171:419–425.
2. Habuchi T (2005) Origin of multifocal carcinomas of the bladder and upper urinary tract: molecular analysis and clinical implication. Int J Urol 12:709–716.
3. Hafner C, Knuechel R, Stoehr R, Hartmann A (2002) Clonality of multifocal urothelial carcinomas: 10 years of molecular genetic studies. Int J Cancer 101:1–6.
4. Garcia SB, Park HS, Novelli M, Wright NA (1999) Field cancerization, clonality, and epithelial stem cells: the spread of mutated clones in epithelial sheets. J Pathol 187:61–81.
5. Denzinger S, Mohren K, Knuechel R, Wild PJ, Burger M, Wieland WF, Hartmann A, Stoehr R (2006) Improved clonality analysis of multifocal bladder tumors by combination of histopathologic organ mapping, loss of heterozygosity, fluorescence in situ hybridization, and p53 analysis. Hum Pathol 37:143–151.
6. Lyon MF (1972) X-chromosome inactivation and developmental patterns in mammals. Biol Rev Camb Philos Soc 47:1–35.
7. Jones PA, Buckley JD (1990) The role of DNA methylation in cancer. Adv Cancer Res 54:1–23.
8. Mutter GL, Boynton KA (1995) PCR bias in amplification of androgen receptor alleles, trinucleotide repeat marker used in clonality studies. Nucleic Acids Res 23:1411–1418.
9. Tsai YC, Simoneau AR, Spruck CH III, Nichols PW, Steven K, Buckley JD, Jones PA (1995) Mosaicism in human epithelium: macroscopic monoclonal patches cover the urothelium. J Urol 153:1697–1700.
10. Sidransky D, Frost P, Von Eschenbach A, Oyasu R, Preisinger AC, Vogelstein B (1992) Clonal origin bladder cancer. N Engl J Med 326:737–740.
11. Li M, Cannizzaro LA (1999) Identical clonal origin of synchronous and metachronous low-grade, noninvasive papillary transitional cell carcinomas of the urinary tract. Hum Pathol 30:1197–1200.
12. Diaz-Cano SJ, Blanes A, Rubio J, Matilla A, Wolfe HJ (2000) Molecular evolution and intratumor heterogeneity by topographic compartments in muscle invasive transitional cell carcinoma of the urinary bladder. Lab Invest 80:279–289.
13. Knudson AG (1996) Hereditary cancer: two hits revisited. J Cancer Res Clin Oncol 122:135–140.
14. Alberts B, Johnson A, Lewis J, Raff M, Roberts K, Walter P (2002) Molecular biology of the cell. Garland Science, New York, pp 1313–1362.
15. Mao L, Lee DJ, Tockman MS, Erozan YS, Askin F, Sidransky D (1994) Microsatellite alterations as clonal markers for the detection of human cancer. Proc Natl Acad Sci USA 91:9871–9875.
16. Simoneau AR, Spruck CH III, Gonzalez-Zulueta M, Gonzalgo ML, Chan MF, Tsai YC, Dean M, Steven K, Horn T, Jones PA (1996) Evidence for two tumor suppressor loci associated with proximal chromosome 9p to q and distal chromosome 9q in bladder cancer and the initial screening for GAS1 and PTC mutations. Cancer Res 56:5039–5043.
17. Keen AJ, Knowles MA (1994) Definition of two regions of deletion on chromosome 9 in carcinoma of the bladder. Oncogene 9:2083–2088.
18. Stadler WM, Sherman J, Bohlander SK, Roulston D, Dreyling M, Rukstalis D, Olopade OI (1994) Homozygous deletions within chromosomal bands 9p21–22 in bladder cancer. Cancer Res 54:2060–2063.
19. Takahashi T, Habuchi T, Kakehi Y, Mitsumori K, Akao T, Terachi T, Yoshida O (1998) Clonal and

chronological genetic analysis of multifocal cancers of the bladder and upper urinary tract. Cancer Res 58:5835–5841.

20. Spruck CH, Ohneseit PF, Gonzalez-Zulueta M, Esrig D, Miyao N, Tsai YC, Lerner SP, Schmutte C, Yang AS, Cote R, Dubeau L, Nichols PW, Hermann GG, Steven K, Horn T, Skinner DG, Jones PA (1994) Two molecular pathways to transitional cell carcinoma of the bladder. Cancer Res 54:784–788.

21. Knowles MA, Elder PA, Williamson M, Cairns JP, Shaw ME, Law MG (1994) Allelotype of human bladder cancer. Cancer Res 54:531–538.

22. Knowles MA (2001) What we could now: molecular pathology of bladder cancer. Mol Pathol 54:215–221.

23. Richter J, Beffa L, Wagner U, Schraml P, Gasser TC, Moch H, Mihatsch MJ, Sauter G (1998) Patterns of chromosomal imbalances in advanced urinary bladder cancer detected by comparative genomic hybridization. Am J Pathol 153:1615–1621.

24. Simon R, Burger H, Brinkschmidt C, Bocker W, Hertle L, Terpe HJ (1998) Chromosomal aberrations associated with invasion of papillary superficial bladder cancer. J Pathol 185:345–351.

25. Richter J, Jiang F, Gorog JP, Sartorius G, Egenter C, Gasser TC, Moch H, Mihatsch MJ, Sauter G (1997) Marked genetic differences between stage pTa and stage pT1 papillary bladder cancer detected by comparative genomic hybridization. Cancer Res 57:2860–2864.

26. Hafner C, Knuechel R, Zanardo L, Dietmaier W, Blaszyk H, Cheville J, Hofstaedter F, Hartmann A (2001) Evidence for oligoclonality and tumor spread by intraluminal seeding in multifocal urothelial carcinomas of the upper and lower urinary tract. Oncogene 20:4910–4915.

27. Orlow I, Lianes P, Lacombe L, Dalbagni G, Reuter VE, Cordon-Cardo C (1994) Chromosome 9 allelic losses and microsatellite alterations in human bladder tumors. Cancer Res 54:2848–2851.

28. Zhao J, Richter J, Wagner U, Roth B, Schraml P, Zellweger T, Ackermann D, Schmidt U, Moch H, Mihatsch MJ, Gasser TC, Sauter G (1999) Chromosomal imbalances in noninvasive papillary bladder neoplasms (pTa). Cancer Res 59:4658–4661.

29. Presti JC Jr, Reuter VE, Galan T, Fair WR, Gordon-Cardo C (1991) Molecular genetic alterations in superficial and locally advanced human bladder cancer. Cancer Res 51:5405–5409.

30. Hovey RM, Chu L, Balasz M, DeVries S, Moore D, Sauter G, Carroll PR, Waldman FM (1999) Genetic alterations in primary bladder cancers and their metastases. Cancer Res 58:3555–3560.

31. Brinkschmidt C, Christiansen H, Terpe HJ, Simon R, Boecker W, Lampert F, Stoerkel S (1997) Comparative genomic hybridization (GCH) analysis of neuroblastomas: an important methodological approach in paediatric tumour pathology. J Pathol 181:394–400.

32. Simon R, Eltze E, Schafer K-L (2001) Cytogenetic analysis of multifocal bladder cancer supports a monoclonal origin and intraepithelial spread of tumor cells. Cancer Res 61:355–362.

33. Jain KK (2004) Current status of fluorescent in-situ hybridisation. Med Device Technol 15:14–17.

34. Xu X, Stower MJ, Reid IN, Garner RC, Burns PA (1996) Molecular screening of multifocal transitional cell carcinoma of the bladder using p53 mutations as biomarkers. Clin Cancer Res 2:1795–1800.

35. Habuchi T, Takahashi R, Yamada H, Kakehi Y, Sugiyama T, Yoshida O (1993) Metachronous multifocal development of urothelial cancers by intraluminal seeding. Lancet 342:1087–1088.

36. Goto K, Konomoto T, Hayashi K, Kinukawa N, Naito S, Kumazawa J, Tsuneyoshi M (1997) p53 mutation in multiple urothelial carcinomas: a molecular analysis of the development of multiple carcinomas. Mod Pathol 10:428–437.

37. Yasunaga Y, Nakanishi H, Naka N, Miki T, Tsujimura T, Itatani H, Okuyama A, Aozasa K (1997) Alterations of the p53 gene in occupational bladder cancer in workers exposed to aromatic amines. Lab Invest 77:677–684.

38. Miyao N, Tsai YC, Lerner SP, Olumi AF, Spruck C III, Gonzalez-Zulueta M, Nichols PW, Skinner DG, Jones PA (1993) Role of chromosome 9 in human bladder cancer. Cancer Res 53:4066–4070.

39. Habuchi T, Ogawa O, Kakehi Y, Ogura K, Koshiba M, Sugiyama T, Yoshida O (1992) Allelic loss of chromosome 17p in urothelial cancer: strong association with invasive phenotype. J Urol 148:1595–1599.

40. Fujimoto K, Yamada Y, Okajima E, Kakizoe T, Sasaki H, Sugimura T, Terada M (1992) Frequent association of p53 gene mutation in invasive bladder cancer. Cancer Res 52:1393–1398.

41. Greene LF, Hanash KA, Farrow GM (1973) Benign papilloma or papillary carcinoma of the bladder? J Urol 110:205–207.

42. Kakizoe T, Fujita J, Murase T, Matsumoto K, Kishi K (1980) Transitional cell carcinoma of the bladder in patients with renal pelvic and ureteral cancer. Cancer Res 124:17–19.

43. Takahashi T, Kakehi Y, Mitsumori K, Akao T, Terachi T, Kato T, Ogawa O, Habuchi T (2001) Distinct microsatellite alterations in upper urinary tract tumors and subsequent bladder tumors. J Urol 165:672–677.

44. Yamamoto S, Tatematsu M, Yamamoto M, Fukami H, Fukushima S (1998) Clonal analysis of urothelial carcinomas in C3H/HeN-BALB/c chimeric mice treated with N-butyl-N-(4-hydroxybutyl)nitrosamine. Carcinogenesis 19:855–860.

45. Yamamoto S, Romanenko A, Wei M, Masuda C, Zaparin W, Vinnichenko W, Vozianov A, Lee CCR, Morimura K, Wanibuchi H, Tada M, Fukushima S (1999) Specific p53 gene mutations in urinary bladder epithelium after the Chernobyl accident. Cancer Res 59:3606–3609.

46. Paiss T, Wohr G, Hautmann RE, Mattfeldt T, Muller M, Haeussler J, Vogel W (2002) Some tumors of the bladder are polyclonal in origin. J Urol 167:718–723.

47. Cheng L, Gu J, Ulbright TM, MacLennan GT, Sweeney CJ, Zhang S, Sanchez K, Koch MO, Eble JN (2002) Precise microdissection of human bladder tumor carcinomas reveals divergent tumor subclones in the same tumor. Cancer 94:104–110.

48. Tomlinson IP, Lambros MB, Roylance RR (2002) Loss of heterozygosity analysis: practically and conceptually flawed? Genes Chromosomes Cancer 34:349–353.

49. Sieben NLG, Ter Haar NT, Cornelisse CJ, Fleuren GJ, Cleton-Jansen A-M (2000) PCR artifacts in LOH and MSI analysis of microdissected tumor cells. Hum Pathol 31:1414–1419.

50. Hartmann A, Moser K, Kriegmair M, Hofstetter A, Hofstaedter F, Knuechel R (1999) Frequent genetic alterations in simple urothelial hyperpasias of the bladder in patients with papillary urothelial carcinoma. Am J Pathol 154:721–727.

Part 4. Testis

Question 1

What is the latest classification of male germ cell tumors? How do the pathology subtypes relate to their biologic behavior and malignant potential?

Answer

Histologically, germ cell tumors (GCTs) mimic early embryogenesis. They consist of a heterogeneous group of tumors. All GCTs in postpubertal males are malignant except for epidermoid cysts. Most GCTs originate in dormant neoplastic cells located inside seminiferous tubules. They are identified as intratubular germ cell neoplasia of unclassified type (IGCNU). Seminoma, the prototype of invasive GCTs, is the most common and accounts for approximately 50% of all GCTs. Nonseminomatous tumors can occur in a pure form, but more commonly they are seen in combination with several types including seminoma.

There are two GCTs that typically occur in children and infants. Teratoma is benign; and yolk sac tumor, more common than teratoma, is malignant. Both develop by an unknown mechanism different from those in adult GCTs. They are not associated with IGCNU. For detailed discussion on histogenetic mechanisms of adult GCTs and prepubertal GCTs, readers are referred to Questions 2 and 3, respectively.

Comments

Based on the histologic and biochemical features and the clinical behavior, the male germ cell tumors (GCTs) are divided into the groups shown in Table 4-1-1 [1].

An important message is that GCTs consist of a heterogeneous group of tumors and that their biologic behavior differs greatly depending on the sex and age at which tumors develop. Only two types of GCT are observed in infants and young children. Teratoma in this age group is benign, whereas yolk sac tumor (YST) is malignant. In adults, virtually all GCTs are malignant regardless of the direction or degree of differentiation—undifferentiated (seminoma and spermatocytic seminoma), zygotic (embryonal carcinoma and teratoma), or extraembryonic (YST and choriocarcinoma). The only exception is the epidermoid cyst. It is distinctly different from the rest of the testicular GCTs in terms of its histogenesis and behaves in a benign fashion. The presence of a "benign" dermoid cyst is questionable as most of these cysts represent a mature-looking portion of malignant teratomas.

Pathologic Features of Testicular Germ Cell Tumors

Because the gross and microscopic appearance of GCTs has been described in detail in many textbooks, readers are referred to the latest publications for a detailed discussion [1, 4, 5]. Here, essential pathologic features are described in brief.

The histogenetic model for the development of GCTs in prepubertal and postpubertal males is depicted in Fig. 4-1-1. The currently widely accepted view states that intratubular germ cell neoplasia of unclassified type (IGCNU) is the precursor to all types of GCT in the adult testis except the spermatocytic seminoma. It is speculated, although not definitively proven, that seminoma may progress to embryonal carcinoma, which then is believed to give rise to other types of nonseminomatous GCTs, including yolk sac tumor (YST), teratoma, and choriocarcinoma. Evidence for development of embryonal carcinoma (EC) from seminoma is supported by chromosome analysis data as well as histologic/immunohistochemical study [6–8]. It does not imply that the sequential order depicted in Fig. 4-1-1 is the only route of development of GCTs. YST derivation from seminoma has been demonstrated [9]. At presentation, approximately 50% of GCTs are pure seminomas, and the remaining 50% consist of nonseminomatous types, either in pure form or in various combinations of all types (mixed nonseminomatous GCT). Embryonal carcinomas may occur in pure form in only 2%–10% of cases and far more commonly as a mixed type [10]. Teratoma more commonly than not occurs as a mixed type with either seminoma, EC, YST, or choriocarcinoma, or in combination of more than two elements [4]. According

TABLE 4-1-1. Classification of male germ cell tumors: effect of age on clinical behavior

Postpubertal testis	Prepubertal testis
Malignant tumors	
Seminoma	Yolk sac tumor
Nonseminomatous GCTs	
Embryonal carcinoma	
Yolk sac tumor	
Teratoma, mature and immature	
Choriocarcinoma	
Secondary malignant transformation	
Spermatocytic seminoma[1]	
Benign tumors	
Epidermoid cyst	Teratoma

GCTs, germ cell tumors.
[1] Although spermatocytic seminomas reportedly behave benignly, an authentic case of retroperitoneal lymph note metastasis has been reported [2]. In addition, rarely, the neoplasm may be accompanied by sarcomatous components [3].

to Mosharafa et al. [11], the closest association was teratoma with YST in a review of 2589 orchiectomy specimens.

Intratubular Germ Cell Neoplasia of Unclassified Type

Skakkebaek [12] was the first to describe the presence of atypical cells in the testes of two infertile men. He speculated that these cells represented the preinvasive phase of testicular cancer. He and his associates used the term "carcinoma in situ." Because these cells do not demonstrate epithelial characteristics, "carcinoma in situ" is inappropriate. The currently widely accepted term is intratubular germ cell neoplasia of unclassified type (IGCNU). Among 812 consecutive testicular biopsies from 555 infertile men, IGCNU was found in 6 oligospermic men (1.1%); and 4 of 6 developed an invasive GCT within 1.3–4.5 years [13]. IGCNU is also found in men with a history of cryptorchidism (2%–8%) [14–17] or dysgenetic testes and in the contralateral testis of men with a prior history of testicular GCT (5%) [18–20].

IGCNU consists of large clear (glycogen-rich) cells that are located along the basal portion of seminiferous tubules (Fig. 4-1-2A,B). The nuclei are round, significantly larger than those of spermatogonia (Fig. 4-1-2C), and hyperchromatic; and they have one prominent nucleolus. The tubules, in general, are atrophic with a thickened hyalinized basement membrane, and they lack germ cells. Often the only remaining cells are Sertoli cells, which are displaced off the basal portion of the tubule (Fig. 4-1-2A,B). Leydig cells may be prominent (Fig. 4-1-2A). Immunohisto-

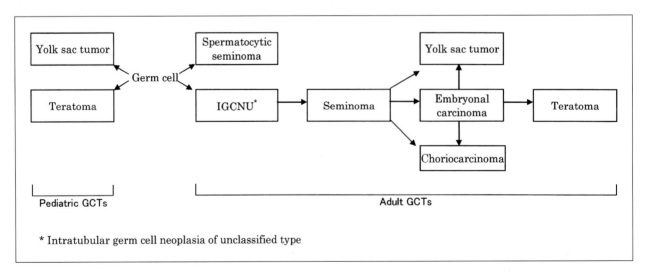

* Intratubular germ cell neoplasia of unclassified type

FIG. 4-1-1. Histogenesis of male germ cell tumors (GCTs)

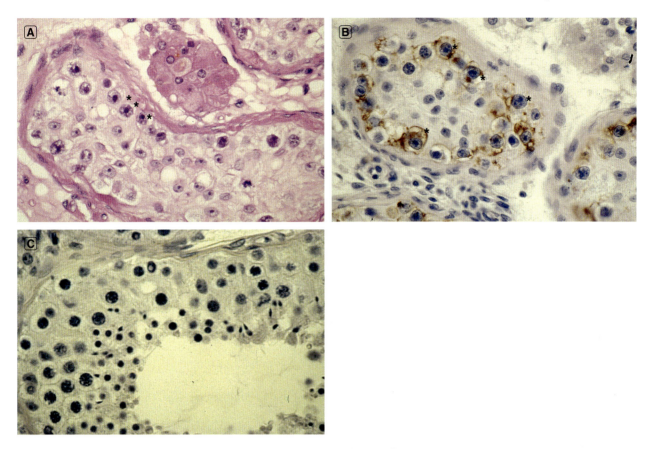

FIG. 4-1-2. Intratubular germ cell neoplasia of unclassified type (IGCNU). This 25-year old man underwent bilateral testicular biopsy because of infertility. The biopsies demonstrate atrophic tubules containing atypical large cells (*) with clear cytoplasm and a prominent large nucleolus. Sertoli cells are located just inside the atypical cells. Gonadal cells are absent. A cluster of Leydic cells is between tubules (**A**). Antibodies against placenta-like alkaline phosphatase stain the cell membrane of the atypical cells (*) (**B**), whereas none of the germ cells in normal tubules (from a normal testis biopsy) are stained (**C**)

chemically, IGCNU cells are highlighted by distinct membrane staining for placental-like alkaline phosphatase (Fig. 4-1-2B), whereas Sertoli cells and nonneoplastic germ cells are nonreactive to this enzyme (Fig. 4-1-2C). Recently, OCT4 has been advocated to be a highly specific marker for IGCNU, seminoma, and embryonal carcinoma but not for other types of GCTs, including adult YST and teratoma, spermatocytic seminoma, and infantile teratoma and YST [21, 22]. OCT4 is a transcription factor expressed in pluripotent mouse and human embryonic stem cells and germ cells including primordial germ cells. Its expression is downregulated during differentiation [21].

Seminoma

Seminoma forms a discrete mass that on sectioning reveals a gray to pale tan homogeneous or nodular cut surface (Fig. 4-1-3). Microscopically, it typically consists of uniform round cells arranged in sheets or in clusters divided by delicate fibrous trabeculae that contain a varying number of lymphocytes and plasma cells (Fig. 4-1-4A). A granulomatous reaction and fibrosis are common (Fig. 4-1-4B); and as a result, tumor cells may be dispersed as small clusters or in delicate cords (Fig. 4-1-4C). Rarely, seminoma cells grow in the intertubular space without forming a discrete tumor mass (Fig. 4-1-4B). This lesion, termed intertubular seminoma, may escape clinical recognition and be indistinguishable from IGCNU on a gross morphologic basis alone [23]. Seminoma cells have a clear to pale cytoplasm (rich in glycogen or lipid), and mitosis is readily recognized.

Seminoma with cellular pleomorphism, large nuclei, a high mitotic rate, and a paucity of

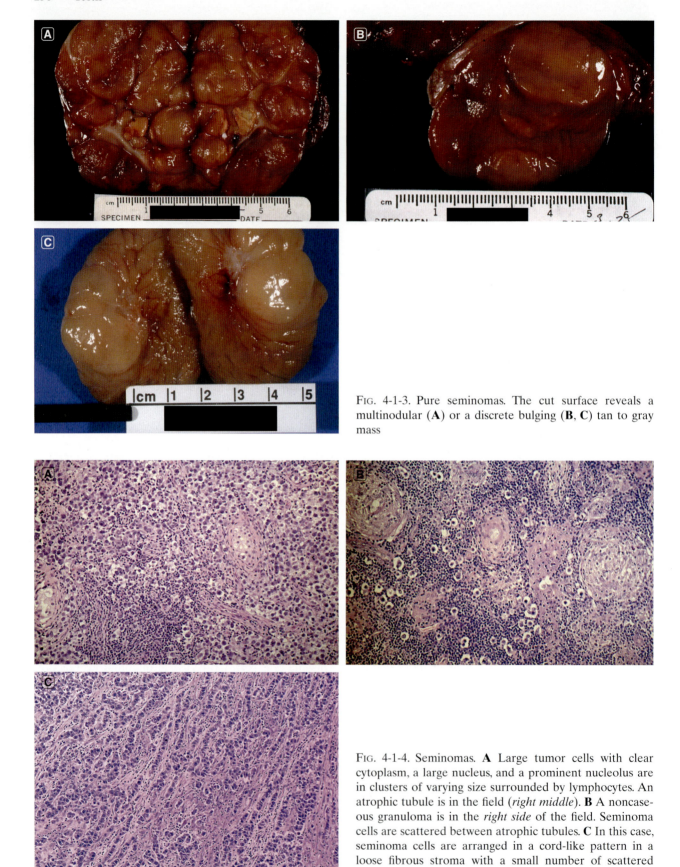

FIG. 4-1-3. Pure seminomas. The cut surface reveals a multinodular (**A**) or a discrete bulging (**B**, **C**) tan to gray mass

FIG. 4-1-4. Seminomas. **A** Large tumor cells with clear cytoplasm, a large nucleus, and a prominent nucleolus are in clusters of varying size surrounded by lymphocytes. An atrophic tubule is in the field (*right middle*). **B** A noncaseous granuloma is in the *right side* of the field. Seminoma cells are scattered between atrophic tubules. **C** In this case, seminoma cells are arranged in a cord-like pattern in a loose fibrous stroma with a small number of scattered lymphocytes

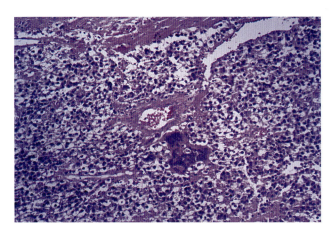

FIG. 4-1-5. Seminoma with a syncytiotrophoblastic giant cell

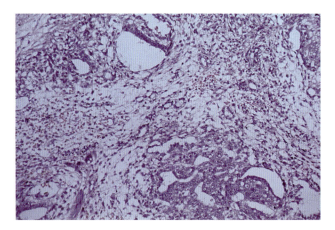

FIG. 4-1-6. Polyembryoma. A cystic structure (*top middle*) resembles the embryonic disk observed in an embryo about 2 weeks old

lymphocytes has been called anaplastic seminoma or atypical seminoma. The prognostic significance is controversial. According to a recent study, patients with atypical seminoma are at a higher stage, and the tumors possibly represent an early step toward a more aggressive phenotype (i.e., embryonal carcinoma) [8]. This study may have a selection bias as most of the cases included were from a major cancer center treating a selected group of patients with advanced-stage testicular cancer.

Three immunohistochemical markers that are diffusely positive in seminoma are placental-like alkaline phosphatase in 85%–100% of cases with membrane stain [4, 24], c-kit (CD117) in 90%–95% of cases with membrane stain [8, 25], and OCT4 in 100% of cases with nuclear stain [21].

Syncytiotrophoblastic cells can be seen in 4%–7% of seminomas (Fig. 4-1-5) [4]. These syncytiotrophoblastic cells are immunoreactive to human chorionic gonadotrophin beta chain (HCGβ). Their presence does not qualify the diagnosis of nonseminomatous GCT nor alter the clinical behavior of seminoma. Caution is advised not to call them choriocarcinomas unless syncytiotrophoblastic cells are accompanied by additional features for choriocarcinoma differentiation (i.e., rich vascular proliferation and areas showing cytotrophoblastic differentiation).

Embryonal Carcinoma

Embryonal carcinoma (EC) in its pure form occurs in only 2%–10% of cases and far more commonly as mixed tumors with other types [10]. It has acquired

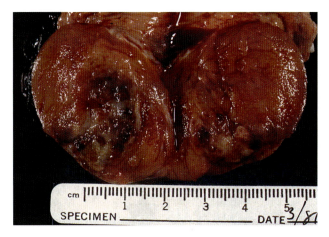

FIG. 4-1-7. Embryonal carcinoma, pure. The tumor occupies the central half of the cut surface, which in the left half of the testis reveals central necrosis

epithelial characters. Tumor cells express cytokeratin markers that can be detected in most cases (94%–100%) [24, 26]. The tumor cell differentiation in EC is similar to that of a 2-week-old embryo with the embryonic disc. An extremely rare variant of EC, polyembryoma, consists of an EC portion arranged in a pattern resembling the embryonic disc admixed with a yolk sac component (Fig. 4-1-6). EC occurred as a pure form in only 2.3% in the Mostofi series [27]. According to the Indiana University series, the EC component was observed in 84% of mixed GCTs, and association with YST was the most common [11].

Grossly, EC is generally smaller than seminoma, and the cut surface exhibits a bulging gray to pink to tan color (Fig. 4-1-7). Foci of necrosis may be

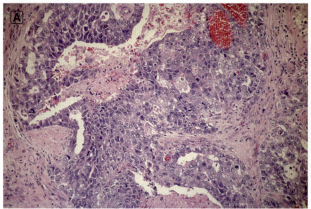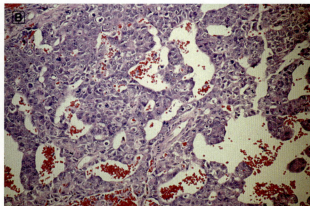

Fɪɢ. 4-1-8. Embryonal carcinoma. **A** Large amphophilic epithelioid tumor cells are arranged, in large part, in solid sheets surrounded by scanty fibrous stroma. An area of necrosis is in the *left upper corner*. **B** In the same case, tumor cells form an incomplete papilloglandular pattern. Several mitotic figures can be recognized

present. Microscopically, the tumor cells are large, appear undifferentiated but with some epithelial appearance, and have basophilic, amphophilic to eosinophilic cytoplasm. The nuclei are large and irregular and have one or more prominent nucleoli. Mitotic figures are easily found. The cells are arranged in two major patterns: as cohesive solid nests (Fig. 4-1-8A) and in a papillary/tubular pattern (Fig. 4-1-8B). The stroma consists of undifferentiated oval to spindle cells (Fig. 4-1-8A). A lymphocytic infiltrate and a granulomatous reaction may be found but not as frequently as in seminomas. Immunohistochemically, most ECs stain for the pancytokeratins (AE1/AE3) and CAM5.2 but do not react with epithelial membrane antigen (EMA) [28]. Useful immunohistochemical markers to distinguish them from seminomas are CD30 and CD 117. CD30 is positive in most ECs (86-100%) and negative in most seminomas (94%) [22, 24, 25]; and CD 117 (c-kit) is positive in 91% of seminomas and negative in 93% of ECs [25].

Yolk Sac Tumor (Endodermal Sinus Tumor)

A second type of nonseminomatous GCT is yolk sac tumor (YST). It shows differentiation comparable to that of extraembryonic membranes such as the allantois, the yolk sac, and extraembryonic mesenchyme [29]. Teilum observed that one of the typical morphologic subtypes, "glomerulous-like" structures (Schiller-Duval body) of YST closely resembled that of the endodermal sinus of the rat placenta[2] [30] and therefore were thought that this type of tumor in the human ovary and testis should be regarded as an extraembryonic membrane tumor or endodermal sinus tumor. Currently, the term YST has been accepted rather than endodermal sinus tumor. YST is the most common type of testicular GCT of children and is four times as common as testicular teratomas [4]. GCTs in children are discussed under Question 3.

In adults, a pure YST is rare in the testis. Most occur as a component of the mixed germ cell tumors [34]. YSTs may demonstrate one or more of the following 11 microscopic patterns [4]: (1) reticular (microcytic); (2) macrocytic; (3) endodermal sinus (perivascular, festoon); (4) papillary; (5) solid; (6) glandular-alveolar (including intestinal and endometrioid-like); (7) myxomatous; (8) sarcomatoid; (9)

---

[2] It must be pointed out that the endodermal sinus, a term coined by Duval, is a structure unique to the rat and mouse placenta. It is formed by the reflection of the visceral endoderm to the pariental endoderm in a 9-day-old placenta [30]. The glomeruloid structure, a hallmark of YST, is formed by ingrowth of advancing allantoic vessels surrounded by mesoderm, which lift the overlying endodermal epithelium and result in a festoon-like structure. In elaborating the concept of an endodermal sinus tumor, Teilum's idea was not to extrapolate directly from the rodent's placenta and apply it to human tumors but, rather, to choose the endodermal sinus as a model [30]. The parietal portion of the endodermal lining is supported by a thick basement membrane also called Reichert membrane, which contains laminin and type IV collagen [31–33].

polyvesicular vitelline; (10) hepatoid; and (11) parietal. These patterns often occur as admixtures in varying combinations. There is no known difference in the biologic potential among the different histologic patterns. The importance lies in recognizing these histologic variants as manifestations of YST. The microcystic (reticular) pattern (Fig. 4-1-9A) is the most common and consists of a meshwork of vacuolated cells. Hyaline globules are often found. Macrocystic patterns are created as microcysts fuse to form large cysts. The endodermal sinus pattern (Fig. 4-1-9B) is the most characteristic with a distinct histologic appearance; it consists of a papillary core with a central small vascular space surrounded by a layer of cuboidal or columnar cells with large nuclei (glomeruloid body or Schiller-Duval body). The papillary pattern (Fig. 4-1-9C) exhibits fine papillae lined by cuboidal cells around delicate fibrovascular cores projecting into cystic spaces. The solid pattern (Fig. 4-1-9D) consists of polygonal tumor cells arranged in sheets (Note that Figs. 4-1-9A and D are from the same tumor). In glandular and alveolar patterns, the glandular structure is arranged in tubules and the alveolar pattern scattered in myxomatous stroma. These glands represent more differentiated embryonal tissues of endodermal origin such as enteric-type glands and islands of hepatoid cells. The hepatoid pattern (Fig. 4-1-9E) occurs in approximately 20% of YSTs [35] as small clusters of eosinophilic cells. These cells are usually immunoreactive to α-fetoprotein (AFP). The glands resemble enteric glands but lack a peripheral smooth muscle layer [4]. Glands resembling endometrioid carcinoma were first described in ovarian YSTs [36] (Fig. 4-1-9F). These glands, reported by Clement et al., were immunoreactive to AFP in five of seven cases and also positive to carcinoembryonic antigen (CEA) in all six cases studied. Despite considerable resemblance to endometrial glands or endometrioid carcinoma, the presence of AFP and CEA indicates an enteric differentiation of these glands. The polyvesicular vitelline type (Fig. 4-1-9G) consists of round to oval cysts scattered in a myxomatous background. The cysts have cuboidal to low columnar lining cells. Occasionally, the cysts demonstrate constriction in the middle, thereby creating the pattern resembling the primary and secondary yolk sacs observed in a 2-week-old embryo. The parietal yolk sac differentiation (Fig. 4-1-9H,I) is characterized by eosinophilic membranes of basement membrane material

(Reichert membrane—see footnote 2). In the Ulbright series, it was found in 92% of YSTs. It occurs most often as anastomosing bands between tumor cells of either reticular or solid type and also as globules. The membranes are immunoreactive to laminin and type IV collagen, and this reaction is highly specific for YST with parietal yolk sac differentiation [4] (see footnote 2).

The stroma of YST of any histologic pattern, but particularly the reticular/microcystic type, consists of spindle cells embedded within a myxoid stroma (Fig. 4-1-9J). Teilum considered that the myxoid stroma with spindle cells recapitulated the extraembryonic mesenchyme (magma reticulare). Transition from the spindle cells to epithelial cell components is demonstrated, and these spindle cells express cytokeratins [37]. This observation led Michael et al. to propose that they are derived from epithelial elements. Furthermore, they believed that the mesenchyme-like component represents a chemotherapy-resistant pluripotential cell population and may give rise to sarcoma in patients with treated GCTs. (See the discussion on somatic type tumor development [malignant transformation of GCT] under Question 4.)

α-Fetoprotein is demonstrated in high frequency in YSTs, but its cytoplasmic staining may be patchy. The staining is more intense in hepatoid cells [35]. Another characteristic finding is the presence of eosinophilic hyaline globules in the cytoplasm of tumor cells. They are periodic acid-Schiff (PAS)-positive and diastase-resistant, and they are negative for AFP [4].

Teratoma

Teratomas are made up of cells of somatic differentiation from two or more germ layers (ectoderm, mesoderm, and endoderm). The component cells may be mature (adult type) or immature (fetal or embryonic type). As has been emphasized repeatedly, all adult male teratomas are malignant regardless of the degree of cellular maturation. Similar to seminomas and nonseminomatous GCTs, which are associated with IGCNU in high frequency, teratomas in postpubertal testes are also associated with IGCNU in 80%–88% of the cases [38, 39]. This is in a sharp contrast to its lack of association with prepubertal teratomas. In the ovarian teratomas, on the other hand, immaturity is an important determinant of

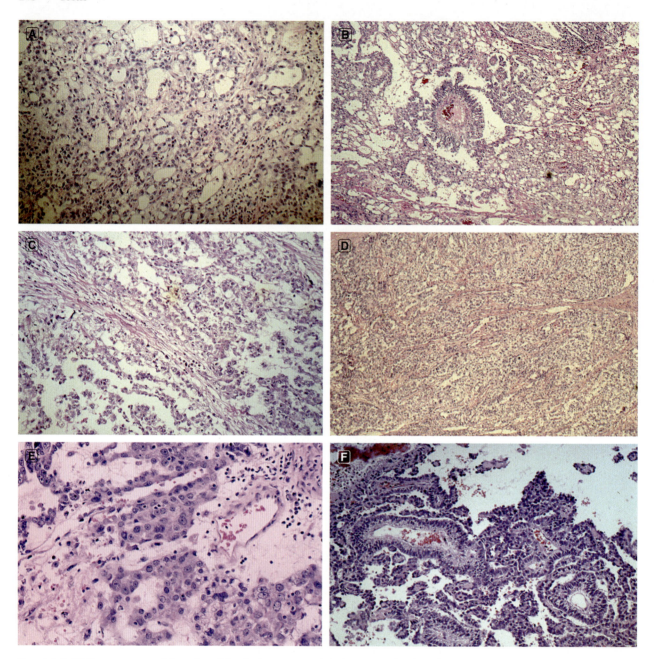

FIG. 4-1-9. Yolk sac tumor with various histologic patterns. **A** Microcystic (reticular) pattern, the most common type. Thin cords of vacuolated neoplastic cells create microcysts. **B** Endodermal sinus pattern. An endodermal sinus-like structure with a central vessel (Schiller-Duval body) is surrounded by thin anastomosing cords of pale tumor cells in a microcystic pattern. Focally, tumor cells form solid sheets. **C** Papillary pattern. **D** Solid pattern. **E** Hepatoid pattern. Eosinophilic cells with a round nucleus and a large nucleolus represent hepatoid differentiation. **F** Endometrioid pattern. Tall columnar cells are arranged in tubulopapillary structures. Subnuclear vacuoles resemble those of early secretor-phase endometrial glands

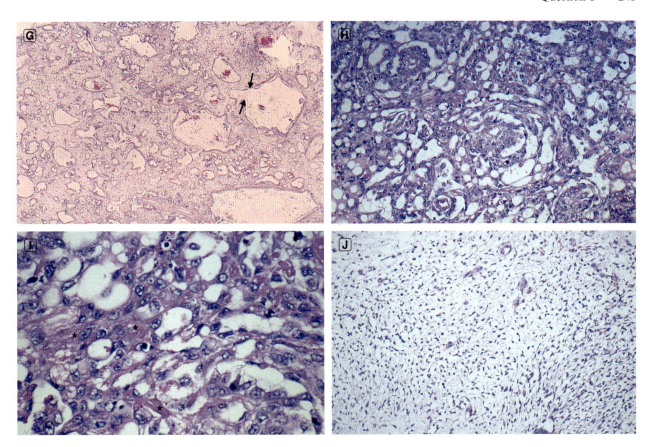

Fig. 4-1-9. (*Continued*) **G** Polyvesicular vitelline pattern. Cysts of varying size are in myxomatous stroma. Some of the cysts show an eccentric constriction (*arrows*) resembling the formation of primary and secondary yolk sacs of around 2-week-old human embryos. **H, I** Parietal differentiation. Eosinophilic bands of basement membrane material (*) (Reichert membrane) are distributed between cells. The bands contain laminin and type IV collagen and are equated to parietal yolk sac differentiation in a rodent placenta. **H** Several Schiller-Duval bodies are recognized. **J** Magma reticulare. Spindle cells are diffusely scattered within myxomatous stroma. These cells are considered to be a chemotherapy-resistant pluripotential cell population that may give rise to sarcomatous cells

prognosis in postpubertal patients. Mature ovarian teratomas are benign, whereas mature testicular teratomas are malignant in postpubertal males [40].

Mature teratomas consist of differentiated somatic tissues that resemble adult structures, such as intestinal glandular elements with underlying smooth muscle arranged in organoid structure, cartilage, nerve, brain, and epidermis and its adnexae, among others (Fig. 4-1-10A, B). However, unlike the ovarian counterpart or prepubertal teratomas, a fair degree of cytologic atypia and mitotic activity may be demonstrated (Fig. 4-1-10B). The immaturity involving the testicular teratoma in the adult as well as the ovary requires the presence of tissues with embryonal appearance; they are almost always neuroepithelium (Fig. 4-1-10C). Fetal type tissues should not be considered elements of an immature teratoma [4].

Immature elements, when they show overgrowth, constitute a "malignant transformation of GCT" (secondary malignancy of somatic cell components on top of the already malignant tumor). When not resectable surgically, they worsen the prognosis because of their resistance to chemotherapy [41]. This subject is discussed under Question 4.

Dermoid Cyst and Epidermoid Cyst

A dermoid cyst contains skin appendages, whereas an epidermoid cyst lacks them. Strictly speaking, these lesions are tumors composed only of tissues of ectodermal origin. Unlike teratomas, epidermoid cysts are mostly benign [42]. Most patients with epidermoid cyst are in the third decade, and the lesion is detected as an incidentally discovered nodule by the

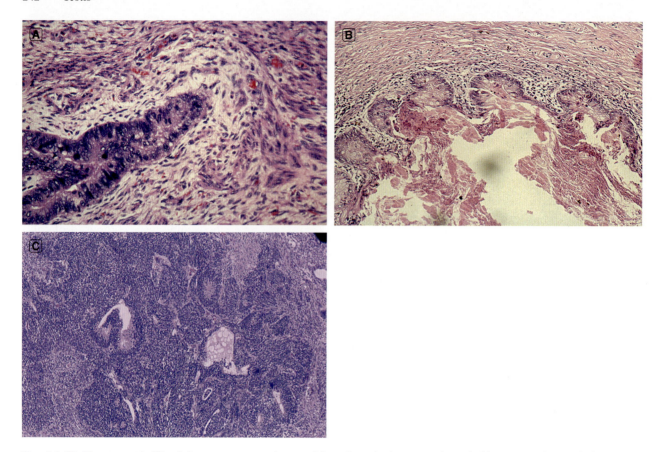

FIG. 4-1-10. Teratoma. **A** Glandular structure consistent with an intestinal crypt surrounded by a smooth muscle layer. The lining cells are cytologically atypical in that the nuclei are large and hyperchromatic. Several cells are in mitosis. **B** Cystically dilated gland contains eosinophilic secretion from the columnar lining cells. This lesion represents a supraclavicular lymph node metastasis of a testicular teratoma. **C** Primitive neuroepithelium (primitive neuroectodermal tumor) in an immature teratoma from a 47-year-old man. Tubular structures are lined by pseudostratified epithelium surrounded by undifferentiated cells (medulloepithelioma). This represents a focus of immature teratoma

patients or on physical examination [42]. The nature of dermoid cysts is controversial. Recently, Ulbright and Srigley [43] reported a few cases of dermoid cysts that contained ciliated epithelium, respiratory-type epithelium with goblet cells, and even intestinal-type columnar epithelium with goblet cells and an underlying layer of smooth muscle (thus, all three germ layers were represented). There was no cytologic atypia or apparent mitotic figures. However, to distinguish it from the conventional adult testis teratoma, the term "dermoid cyst" was retained by Ulbright and Srigley. Although these cases may be benign, a study with a small number of cases may have a selection bias. Second, a low-grade malignant tumor may not reveal malignant potential in a small cohort. In fact, the cases appearing to be dermoid cysts may actually represent an undersampled mature teratoma. One of the present authors has seen a patient with a testicular "dermoid' cyst" who had elevated serum markers and developed lymph node metastasis. Therefore, a diagnosis of benign testicular dermoid cyst in an adult male should be made with caution. These lesions, which they regarded as dermoid cysts, can no longer be designated dermoid cysts in our opinion but should be classified as cystic teratomas. Dermoid cysts should not be associated with IGCNU; there should not be elevated serum markers; and the lesion must be adequately sampled, preferably totally submitted. Finally, these patients should be closely followed [38, 39, 43].

Ulbright and Srigley [43] proposed that there might be two ways for the development of testicular teratomas in the postpubertal testis. The more common pathway is the development from the IGCNU, and the less common pathway is from a nonmalignant germ cell [42].

A bisected testis through an epidermoid cyst reveals a cyst containing cheesy material (Fig. 4-1-11A, B). Microscopically, the cyst is filled with layered keratin, and the wall is covered with welldifferentiated squamous epithelium (Fig. 4-1-11C). Skin adnexae, such as sebaceous glands and hair follicles, are not seen, in contrast to that in the dermoid cyst.

If the concept of the dermoid cysts is expanded, how are these neoplasms differentiated from teratoma of the adult testis? Because at present there is no marker characteristic of dermoid cysts, the absence of IGCNU in the surrounding tubules is the only objective criterion. Adequate sampling of the surrounding parenchyma to look for IGCNU is mandatory for the surgical pathologist. With the diagnosis of dermoid cyst, the urologist would perform local resection instead of orchiectomy. Unfortunately, however, IGCNU is not detectable in all cases of teratomas in the adult testis (88%) [38]. Failure to detect IGCNU does not guarantee a benign nature of the lesion. The presence of or absence of cytologic atypia would be an important ancillary finding (Fig. 4-1-11c).

Choriocarcinoma

Choriocarcinoma is the least common type of testicular GCT. It is, by definition, composed of an intimate admixture of syncytiotrophoblastic and cytotrophoblastic cells. The pure form is extremely rare (0.3%) [44]. Mixed GCT with areas of choriocarcinoma is found in only 8% of GCTs [4]. The most common manifestations of pure choriocarcinoma are the symptoms of metastasis [4]. The primary site may be quite small or even undetectable owing to regression. Microscopically, the lesion consists of sheets of pale polygonal cytotrophoblastic cells surrounded by an outer rim of eosinophilic multinucleated syncytiotrophoblastic cells (Fig. 4-1-12). Foci of hemorrhage and necrosis are common.

Spermatocytic Seminoma

Spermatocytic seminoma is a distinct entity of testicular neoplasms. It differs from other GCTs in many respects. First, it affects patients older (mean age 54 years) than those with seminoma. Second, it occurs exclusively in the testis. Third, it is not associated with other types of GCTs or IGCNU [45]. Fourth,

none of the cases has arisen in a cryptorchid testis. Fifth, AFP and human choriogonadotropin-β are not produced by spermatocytic seminoma cells [45]. Finally, it is a very low-grade neoplasm. Only one case of retroperitoneal lymph node metastasis has been reported [2]. Orchiectomy is curative.

Spermatocytic seminoma was first reported by Masson in 1946 [46]. He thought that it was composed of cells similar to primary spermatocytes. Grossly, spermatocytic seminoma presents as a sharply demarcated mass that on sectioning has a tan-gray mucoid surface (Fig. 4-1-13A). Microscopically, spermatocytic seminoma is composed of solid sheets of tumor cells with little or no intervening stroma. The diagnostic feature is the marked difference in tumor cell size. Three types of cells are recognized: (1) small cells with a small dark nucleus, resembling lymphocytes; (2) medium-sized cells with a round nucleus and finely granular chromatin surrounded by a rim of lightly eosinophilic cytoplasm; (3) large mononucleated or multinucleated cells with abundant eosinophilic cytoplasm. The chromatin has a unique pattern, being arranged in a filamentous fashion that Masson likened to the "spiremes" formed during the meiotic division phase of normal spermatocytes (Fig. 4-1-13B). Mitoses are abundant. Intratubular growth is a regular feature, but IGCNU is not present. Takahashi et al. [47] measured the DNA content of each type of cell by fluorescence cytometry. The small cells exhibited diploidy (2C) or near 2C, the intermediate cells, 2C to 6C and the large cells, 3C to 18C. No cases showed haploid DNA content. The authors concluded that these cells were not involved in meiosis and that small cells created large cells by continuous sequential polyploidization.

Immunohistochemical reactions of spermatocytic seminoma are distinctly different from those of seminoma; spermatocytic seminoma cells were negative for placental-like alkaline phosphatase except for a few scattered cells [45, 48].

As stated earlier, it is a low-grade tumor with an excellent prognosis after orchiectomy. However, rare secondary malignant transformation analogous to that of other types of GCT has been reported. A sarcomatous component coexisted with the typical spermatocytic seminoma. Rhabdomyosarcoma was one of the sarcomas reported. Distant metastases were all due to the sarcomatous elements [3].

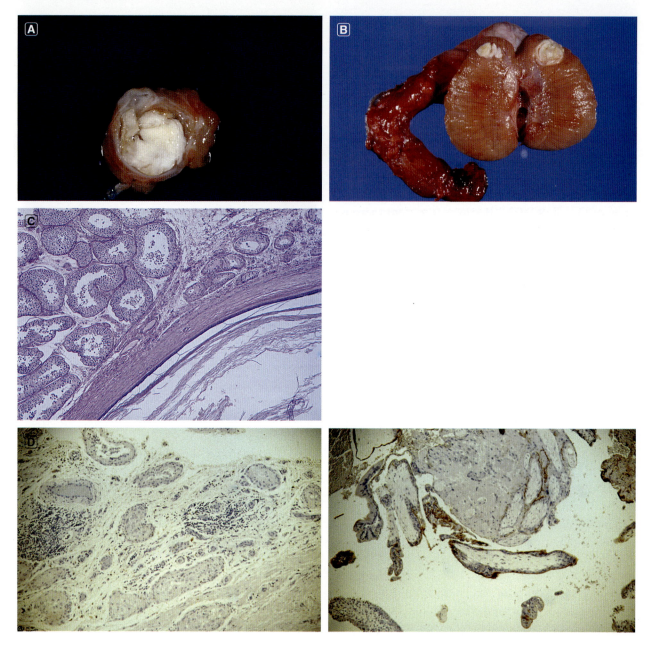

FIG. 4-1-11. Epidermoid cyst. **A** This 17-year-old boy had a testicular nodule. The cut surface reveals an encapsulated cyst filled with keratin material. **B** Another epidermoid cyst filled with cheesy material. **C** Epidermoid cyst. The lining of the cyst is well-differentiated squamous epithelium. The cyst lumen contains laminated keratin material. There are no skin appendages such as hair follicles or a sweat gland. Hence it is an epidermoid cyst. Note that seminiferous tubules around the cyst show normal spermatogenesis without atypical germ cells. **D** Another case of an epidermoid cyst (not shown). The adjacent seminiferous tubules (*left half*) are completely atrophic but do not contain IGCNU, as evidenced by negative staining reaction to placenta-like alkaline phosphatase. Positive control (placental villi) is shown in the *right half*

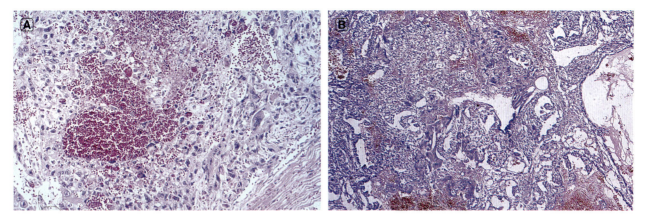

FIG. 4-1-12. Choriocarcinoma. **A** Disseminated GCT in a 52 year-old man. A biopsy demonstrated choriocarcinoma. Note the mononuclear (cytotrophoblastic) cells (*center*) of photograph. There are a few multinucleated syncytiotrophoblastic giant cells (*right side*). The latter cells were reactive to human chorionic gonadotropin-beta (HCGβ) antibodies (not shown). It is presumed to be of testicular origin. **B** Focus of choriocarcinoma in a testicular GCT in a different case

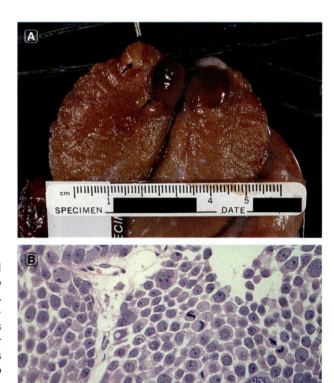

FIG. 4-1-13. Spermatocytic seminoma from a 24-year-old man (unusual for this age). **A** Cross section reveals two nodules (*arrows*), one of which reveals a mucoid cut surface. **B** Microscopic examination reveals typical features of spermatocytic seminoma; solid sheets of medium-sized cells with little cytoplasm, round nuclei, and a finely granular chromatin. In two nuclei (*arrowheads*), the chromatin is arranged in a filamentous structure that Masson likened to spiremes formed during the meiosis of normal spermatocytes. A large multinucleated cell is on the right side. Mitotic activity is brisk. There is minimal intervening stroma. Mucoid material demonstrated in the gross photograph is not shown in this field

References

1. Anonymous (2006) Tumours of the urinary system and genital organs. In: Eble JN, Sauter G, Epstein JI, Sesterhenn IA (eds) World Health Organization classification of tumours. IARC Press, Lyon, p 218.
2. Matoska J, Ondrus D, Hornak M (1988) Metastatic spermatocytic seminoma: a case report with light microscopic, ultrastructural, and immunohistochemical findings. Cancer 62:1197–1201.
3. True LD, Otis CN, Delprado W, Scully RE, Rosai J (1988) Spermaticytic seminoma of testis with sarcomatous transformation. Am J Surg Pathol 12:75–82.
4. Ulbright TM, Amin MB, Young RH (1999) Tumors of the testis, adnexa, spermatic cord, and scrotum. In: Atlas of tumor pathology. Armed Forces Institute of Pathology, Washington, DC, pp 41–191.
5. Ulbright TM (2005) Germ cell tumors of the gonads: a selective review emphasizing problems in differential diagnosis, newly appreciated, and controversial issues. Mod Pathol 18:S61–S79.
6. Oosterhuis JW, Castedo SMMJ, de Long Cornelisse CJ, Dam A, Slewijfer DT (1989) Ploidy of primary germ cell tumors of the testis: pathologic and clinical relevance. Lab Invest 60:14–21.
7. Faulkner SW, Leigh DA, Oosterhuis JW, Roelofs H, Loojienga LHL, Friedlander ML (2000) Allelic loss in carcinoma in situ and testicular germ cell tumors of adolescents and adults: evidence in support of the linear progression model. Br J Cancer 83:729–736.
8. Tickoo SK, Hutchinson B, Bacik J, Mazumdar M, Motzer RJ, Bajorin DF, Bosl GJ, Reuter VE (2002) Testicular seminoma: a clinicopathologic and immunohistochemical study of 105 cases with special reference to seminomas with atypical features. Int J Surg Pathol 10:23–32.
9. Czaja JT, Ulbright TM (1992) Evidence for the transformation of seminoma to yolk sac tumor, with histogenetic considerations. Am J Clin Pathol 97:468–477.
10. Anonymous (2004) Tumours of the urinary system and male genital organs. In: Eble JN, Sauter G, Epstein JI, Sesterhenn IA (eds) World Health Organization classification of tumours. IARC Press, Lyon, p 236.
11. Mosharafa AA, Foster RS, Leibovich BC, Ulbright TM, Bihrle R, Einhorn LH, Donohue JP (2004) Histology in mixed germ cell tumors: is there a favorable pairing? J Urol 171:1471–1473.
12. Skakkebaek NE (1972) Abnormal morphology of germ cells in two infertile men. Acta Pathol Microbiol Scand (A) 80:374–378.
13. Skakkebaek NE (1978) Carcinoma in situ of the testis: frequency and relationship to invasive germ cell tumours in infertile men. Histopathology 2:157–170.
14. Giwercman A, Bruun E, Frimodt-Moller C, Skakkebaek NE (1989) Prevalence of carcinoma-in-situ and other histopathologic abnormalities in testes of men with a history of cryptorchidism. J Urol 142:998–1002.
15. Gondos B, Migliozzi JA (1987) Intratubular germ cell neoplasia. Semin Diagn Pathol 4:292–303.
16. Krabbe S, Skakkebaek NE, Berthelsen JG, Eyben FV, Volsted P, Mauritzen K, Nielsen AH (1979) High incidence of undetected neoplasia in maldescended testes. Lancet 1:999–1000.
17. Pedersen KV, Boiesen P, Zetterlund CG (1987) Experience of screening for carcinoma-in-situ of the testis among young men with surgically corrected maldescended testes. Int J Androl 10:181–185.
18. Mumperow E, Lauke H, Holstein AF, Hartmann M (1992) Further practical experiences in the recognition of carcinoma in situ of the testis. Urol Int 48:162–166.
19. Von der Masse H, Rorth M, Walbom-Jorgensen S (1986) Carcinoma in situ of contralateral testis in patients with testicular germ cell cancer: study of 27 cases in 500 patients. BMJ 293:1398–1401.
20. Berthelsen JG, Skakkebaek NE, von der Masse H, Sorensen BL, Morgensen P (1982) Screening for carcinoma in situ of the contralateral testis in patients with germinal testicular cancer. BMJ 285:1683–1686.
21. Looijenga LHJ, Stoop H, de Leeuw HPJC, de Gouveia Brazao C, Gillis AJM, van Roozendaal KEP, van Zoelen EJJ, Weber RFA, Wolffenbuttel KP, van Dekken H, Honecker F, Bokemeyer C, Perlman EJ, Scneider DT, Kononen J, Sauter G, Oosterhuis JW (2003) POU5F1 (OCT3/4) identifies cells with pluripotent potential in human germ cell tumors. Cancer Res 63:2244–2250.
22. Jones TD, Ulbright TM, Eble JN, Baldridge LA, Cheng L (2004) OCT4 staining inn testicular tumors: a sensitive and specific marker for seminoma and embryonal carcinoma. Am J Surg Pathol 28:935–940.
23. Henley JD, Young RH, Wade CL, Ulbright TM (2004) Seminomas with exclusive intertubular growth: a report of 12 clinically and grossly inconspicuous tumors. Am J Surg Pathol 28:1163–1168.
24. Cheville JC, Rao S, Iczkowski KA, Lohse CM, Pankratz VS (2000) Cytokeratin expression in seminoma of the human testis. Am J Clin Pathol 113:583–588.
25. Leroy X, Augusto D, Leteurtre E, Gosselin B (2002) CD30 and CD117 (c-kit) used in combination are useful for distinguishing embryonal carcinoma from seminoma. J Histochem Cytochem 50:283–285.
26. Ferreiro JA (1994) Ber-H2 expression in testicular germ cell tumors. Hum Pathol 25:522–524.
27. Mostofi FK, Sesterhenn IA, Davis CJ Jr (1998) Developments in histopathology of testicular germ cell tumors. Semin Urol 6:171–188.
28. Niehans GA, Manivel JC, Copeland GT, Scheithauer BW, Wick MR (1998) Immunohistochemistry of germ cell and trophoblastic neoplasms. Cancer 62:1113–1123.
29. Teilum G (1959) Endodermal sinus tumors of the ovary and testis: comparative morphogenesis of the so-called mesonephroma ovarii (Schiller) and extraembryonic (yolk sac-allantoic) structures of the rat's placenta. Cancer 12:1092–1105.

30. Gonzalez-Crussi F (1979) The human yolk sac and yolk sac (endodermal sinus) tumors. In: Rosenberg HS, Bolande RP (eds) Perspectives in pediatric pathology, vol 5. Year Book, Chicago, pp 179–214.

31. Laurie GW, Leblond CP (1982) Intracellular localization of basement membrane precursors in the endodermal cells of the rat parietal yolk sac. I. Ultrastructure and phosphatase activity of endodermal cells. J Histochem Cytochem 10:973–982.

32. Laurie GW, Leblond CP, Martin GR, Silver MH (1982) Intracellular localization of basement membrane precursors in the endodermal cells of the rat parietal yolk sac. II. Immunostaining for type IV collagen and its precursors. J Histochem Cytochem 10:983–990.

33. Laurie GW, Leblond CP, Martin GR (1982) Intracellular localization of basement membrane precursors in the endodermal cells of the rat parietal yolk sac. III. Immunostaining for laminin and its precursors. J Histochem Cytochem 10:991–998.

34. Talerman A (1975) The incidence of yolk sac tumor (endodermal sinus tumor) elements in germ cell tumors of the testis in adults. Cancer 36:211–215.

35. Ulbright TM, Roth LM, Brodhecker CA (1986) Yolk sac differentiation on germ cell tumors: a morphologic study of 50 cases with emphasis on hepatic, enteric, and parietal yolk sac features. Am J Surg Pathol 10:151–164.

36. Clement PB, Young RH, Scully RE (1987) Endometrioid-like variant of ovarian yolk sac tumor: a clinicopathological analysis of eight cases. Am J Surg Pathol 11:767–778.

37. Michael H, Ulbright TM, Brodhecker CA (1989) The pluripotential nature of the mesenchyme-like component of yolk sac tumor. Arch Pathol Lab Med 113:1115–1119.

38. Manivel JC, Reinberg Y, Niehans GA, Fraley EE (1989) Intratubular germ cell neoplasia in testicular teratomas and epidermoid cysts. Cancer 64:715–720.

39. Simmonds PD, Lee AH, Theaker JM, Tung K, Smart CJ, Mead GM (1996) Primary pure teratoma of the testis. J Urol 155:939–942.

40. Leibovich H, Foster RS, Ulbright TM, Donohue JP (1995) Adult primary pure teratoma of the testis: the Indiana experience. Cancer 75:2244–2250.

41. Michael H, Hull MT, Ulbright TM, Foster RS, Miller KD (1997) Primitive neuroectodermal tumors arising in testicular germ cell neoplasms. Am J Surg Pathol 21:896–904.

42. Price EB (1969) Epidermoid cysts of the testis: a clinical and pathological analysis of 69 cases from the testicular tumor registry. J Urol 102:708–713.

43. Ulbright TM, Srigley JR (2001) Dermoid cyst of the testis: a study of five cases, including a pilomatrixoma-like variant, with evidence supporting its separate classification from mature testicular teratoma. Am J Surg Pathol 25:788–793.

44. Mostofi FK, Price EB Jr (1973) Tumors of the male genital system. In: Atlas of tumor pathology, 2nd series. Armed Forces Institute of Pathology, Washington, DC.

45. Eble JN (1994) Spermatocytic seminoma. Hum Pathol 25:1035–1042.

46. Masson P (1946) Etude sur le seminome. Rev Cancer Biol 5:361–387.

47. Takahashi H, Aizawa S, Konishi E, Furusato M, Kato, H, Ashihara T (1993) Cytofluorometric analysis of spermatocytic seminoma. Cancer 72:549–552.

48. Dekker I, Rozeboom T, Delemarre J, Dam A, Oosterhuis JW (1992) Placental-like alkaline phosphatase and DNA flow cytometry in spermatocytic seminoma. Cancer 69:993–996.

Question 2

What is the pathogenesis of testicular germ cell tumors? Are there specific changes that characterize the development of germ cell tumors?

Answer

The germ cell tumors (GCTs) can be divided into three major groups based on the presumed differences in oncogenesis and clinical behavior.

- *Group 1*. Yolk sac tumors (YST) and teratomas in the pediatric population are believed to arise in primordial cells at an earlier stage of embryonal development than the cells that give rise to adult GCTs. Infantile teratoma is benign and exhibits no aberration in chromosomal constitution, but YST is malignant and shows aneuploidy.
- *Group 2*. Adult seminomas and nonseminomatous GCTs originate in the intratubular germ cell neoplasm of unclassified type (IGCNU). These cells are near tetraploid in karyotype. Invasive GCTs follow with sequential stepwise net loss of chromosomes, leading to seminoma (hypertriploid) and then nonseminomas (hypotriploid). A characteristic alteration associated with invasive growth is acquisition of isochromosome 12p or amplification of the 12 p11.2-p12.1 region. It is a distinct marker specific for adult GCTs including extragonadal and certain ovarian GCTs. This abnormal chromosome and its specific amplified portion provide GCTs with invasive potential. The isochrome 12p is so specific to adult GCTs that it may be used to identify tumors of unknown origin as GCTs.

- *Group 3*. Spermatocytic seminoma is thought to originate in a spermatogonia/spermatocytic cell type. Gain of chromosome 9 is a constant finding, and neither IGCNU nor isochromosome 12p is identified. Thus, difference in oncogenesis is suggested.

Comments

The GCTs of the testis are a heterogeneous group of neoplasms. Based on the patient's age at clinical presentation and the histologic differences, GCTs are divided to three major groups: group 1, YSTs and teratomas in neonates, infants, and children; group 2, seminomas and nonseminomas of adolescents and adults; group 3, spermatocytic seminomas that appear later in adult life. The GCTs of the first two groups may occur at extragonadal sites along the midline of the body, including the hypothalamus/pineal gland, neck, mediastinal, and retroperitoneal and sacrococcygeal regions. This distribution has been related to the migration path of primordial germ cells from the yolk sac to the genital ridge [1]. Spermatocytic seminoma has not been found at extratesticular sites.

Origin of Testicular GCT

Gonadal and extragonadal GCTs of prepubertal age (group 1 GCTs) share a common origin and appear to derive from primordial germ cells that are in an earlier developmental stage in embryogenesis than the primordial germ cells (PGCs) that give rise to adult GCTs (group 2 GCTs) [2, 3]. Studying the imprinting patterns is one way to assess the origin of the primordial germ cells that generate GCTs. This conclusion is based on the premise that during their development primordial germ cells erase their inherited imprint and establish a new sex-specific imprinting[1] pattern and that the imprinting status alters during the stage of their migration to the gonadal ridges [3]. Incomplete erasure of the marker genes *H19* and *IGF-2* (in contrast to complete erasure in adult GCTs) suggest that the initiation of childhood GCTs may occur during germ cell migration, whereas the initiation of testicular GCTs in adults occurs at a later stage of PGC development [3]. Infantile teratomas, which are benign, exhibit no aberrations in chromosomal constitution as studied by comparative genomic hybridization, whereas YSTs, which are malignant, show aneuploidy [4].

The origin of spermatocytic seminoma is distinct in that it is neither associated with i(12p) (vide infra) [5] nor intratubular germ cell neoplasia of unclassified type (IGCNU) [6, 7], the characteristic features of the seminoma/nonseminoma group. The origin has been proposed to be spermatogonial/spermatocytic cell type, cells in a much later stage of gonadal cell maturation than those for group 1 and 2 tumors. This conclusion is based on a comparison of the stage-specific expression of marker genes synaptonemal complex protein 1 (*SCP1*) and synovial sarcoma on X chromosome (*SSX*) between spermatocytic seminoma and normal spermatogenesis [8]. Spermastocytic seminomas show the paternal pattern of genomic imprinting, indicating they have striking morphologic features characteristic of spermatogonia stage B

[9, 10], without expression of placental-like alkaline phosphatase [6], the marker of seminomas and embryonal carcinomas, or c-kit, a marker of seminoma [11]. Comparative genomic hybridization together with cytogenetic analysis demonstrated numerical chromosomal aberrations; a consistent finding was gain of chromosome 9 in spermatocytic seminoma [12].

The best studied is the genetics of the seminoma/non-seminoma group. It has been firmly established that they develop from precursor cells called IGCNU (referred to as carcinoma in situ by the Skakkebaeck group [13]). The cells are believed to originate from diploid PGCs that migrated to the seminiferous tubules during fetal life. Currently, the prevailing model is that of Oosterhuis and colleagues [14, 15]. In their seminal investigation on ploidy of GCTs, Oosterhuis et al. proposed that oncogenesis of GCTs is initiated by polyploidization of "dysplastic" precursors to tetraploid, followed by a sequential stepwise net loss leading to the development of seminoma (hypertriploid) and then to other type GCTs (hypotriploid). Their findings gave strong support to the earlier model proposed by Friedman [16] in which all GCTs (with the exception of spermatocytic seminoma) pass through a seminoma stage as part of their evolution. However, the strong evidence inconsistent with this seminoma common pathway is that most nonseminomatous GCTs developed in younger males, whereas seminomas develop in males 10 years older than those with nonseminomatous GCTs. Particularly in young children, pure YST develops without any evidence of seminoma. That the frequency of *c-kit* mutations is higher in seminomas than in nonseminomatous GCTs [17] is likewise not supportive of the hypothesis of a common seminoma pathway unless these *c-kit* mutations could be fixed after transforming to nonseminomatous GCTs.

Subsequent studies demonstrated that IGCNU, the microscopically recognizable earliest neoplastic stage, already has the same hypertriploidy as seminoma [18–21]. In agreement with the data from DNA flow cytometry, seminomas have chromosome numbers in the hypertriploid range and nonseminomas in the hypotriploid range [4, 22]. Karyotyping demonstrated over- and underrepresentation of (parts of) chromosomes; chromosomes 7, 8, 12, 21, and X are overrepresented, whereas chromosomes 11, 13, 18, and Y are underrepresented [23].

---

[1] Genomic imprinting refers to the phenomenon that in somatic cells the two alleles of some genes are expressed in an asymmetrical pattern depending on the inheritance of the allele from either paternal or maternal origin. DNA methylation of CpG dinucleotides represents the most significant biochemical marker of imprinting and allows the distinction between the paternal and maternal alleles. The paternal genome is responsible for extraembryonic differentiation, and the maternal genome mainly supports the growth of the embryo. During a time between their migration and development to mature gametes, PGCs are characterized by the lack of imprinting. Among the imprinted genes, *H19* and *IGF-2* have been most extensively studied. They are part of an inherited gene cluster on chromosome 11p15 and share a common enhancer located downstream of the *H19* gene. During development, PGCs erase their inherited imprint and establish a new sex-specific imprinting pattern. Therefore, if GCTs preserve the original imprinting status of their cell of origin, GCTs arising from PGCs before entry to the gonadal ridge and GCTs arising from premeiotic germ cells show erased imprinting (biallelic expression of *H19* and *IGF-2*). On the other hand, GCTs arising from PGCs that have entered meiosis should display a sex-specific gametic imprinting pattern [3].

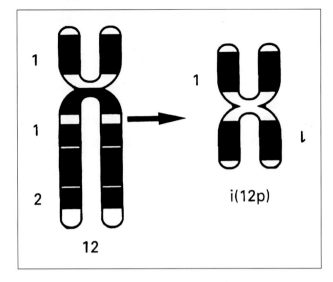

FIG. 4-2-1. Isochrome 12p, i(12p). Two identical p arms are conjugated in a mirror image

The most consistent structural abnormality is isochrome 12p (i[12p])[2] (Fig. 4-2-1), first reported by Atkin and Baker in 1983 [24]. Seminoma and non-seminomas are associated with i(12p) with a high frequency (about 80% of all GCTs). It has also been demonstrated in some ovarian GCTs (dysgerminomas, YST, and one mature teratoma) and extragonal GCTs [25, 26]. The copy number of i(12P) ranges from 1 to 4 per cell for both seminomas and nonseminomas [27]. Even in the remaining so-called i(12p)-negative testicular GCTs, overrepresentation of 12p (compared with 12q), has been demonstrated by the fluorescence in situ hybridization (FISH) technique [25, 28, 29] or comparative genomic hybridization [30]. In particular, amplification of the 12p11.2-p12.1 region has been demonstrated in 10% of GCTs, [28, 30–36], and the amplification was mainly in seminomas without an i(12p). It is of interest that the restricted amplification and i(12p) were never found in the same cell [36]. Neither gain nor amplification of 12 cases has been detected in IGCNU,[3] although many of the chromosome imbalances seen in invasive GCTs are already present [20, 38]. These results suggest that there are at least two mechanisms by which extra copies of the short arm of 12p or its restricted portion is overrepresented [36].

This frequent occurrence of i(12p) and amplification of its segment indicate that some genes located here play an important role in the development of invasive GCTs. Seminomas with 12p amplification are associated with lower levels of apoptosis than are those without it [36]. There are several candidate genes on chromosome 12p: KRAS and CCND2 (cyclin D2). A third is MYCN (N-MYC) (on chromosome 2p24.3). KRAS mutation has been demonstrated at a low frequency (11%) [39]. However, because of its location within the frequently amplified region of 12p11.1-p12.1, the amplified KRAS may be involved in invasive growth [36]. Proto-oncogenes MYCN and CCND2 are overexpressed [40]. Because a direct role for Myc in cyclin D2 amplification has been shown in plasmacytomas [41], a similar role was suggested in GCT [39]. It should be noted that upregulation of D-type cyclins and hence G_1–S phase transition in the cell cycle is a downstream event of RAS signaling. It is noteworthy that retinoblastoma (RBI) tumor suppressor gene is downregulated in virtually all IGCNU, seminomas, and embryonal carcinomas (but reexpressed in teratomas) [42]. Thus, its downstream transcription factor, E2F, is active in stimulating cell cycle-related genes [39].

What is the clinical significance of i(12p) and amplification of the chromosome 12p portion? First, invasive growth is associated with gain of 12p or amplification of the restricted 12p chromosomal region. However, the copy numbers of the restricted amplification of 12p and K-RAS mutations do not predict response to therapy or survival of patients [36]. Second, i(12p) and restricted amplification of the 12 region is specific to adult testicular and extragonadal GCTs, some ovarian GCTs [43], and secondary malignant tumors of GCT origin, such as rhabdomyosarcoma, PNET, and leukemias. Therefore, their demonstration in unclassifiable malignant tumors at extragonadal sites is diagnostic of GCT origin [35].

---

[2] i(12p) is a chromosome with two identical arms and identical genes. The arms are in a mirror image of each other.
[3] Vos et al. [37] observed two copies of i(12p) in one of three cases studied by karyotyping.

References

1. Moore KL (1977) The developing human: clinically oriented embryology. Saunders, Philadelphia, pp 220–258.
2. Ross JA, Schmidt PT, Perentesis JP, Davies SM (1999) Genomic imprinting of H19 and insulin-like growth factor-2 inn pediatric germ cell tumors. Cancer 85: 1389–1394.
3. Schneider DT, Schuster AE, Fritsch MK, Hu J, Olson T, Lauer S, Gobel U, Perlman EJ (2001) Multipotent

imprinting analysis indicates a common precursor cell for gonadal and nongonadal pediatric germ cell tumors. Cancer Res 61:7268–7276.

4. Looijenga LHJ, de Munnik H, Oosterhuis JW (1999) Molecular model for the development of germ cell cancer. Int J Cancer 83:809–814.

5. Rosenberg C, Mostert MC, Bakker T, van de Pol M, van Echten J, de Jong B, Raap MC, Tanke H, Oosterhuis JW, Looijenga LHJ (1998) Chromosomal constitution of human spermatocytic seminomas: comparative genomic hybridization supported by conventional and interphase cytogenetics. Genes Chromosom Cancer 23:286–291.

6. Soosay GN, Bobrow L, Happerfield L, Parkinson MC (1991) Morphology and immunohistochemistry of carcinoma in situ adjacent to testicular germ cell tumors in adults and children: implication for histogenesis. Histopathology 19:537–544.

7. Muller J, Skakkebaeck NE, Parkinson MC (1987) The spermatocytic seminoma: views on pathogenesis. Int J Androl 10:147–156.

8. Stoop H, van Gurp R, de Kriger R, Geurts van Kessel A, Koberle B, Oosterhuis W, Looijenga L (2001) Reactivity of germ cell maturation stage-specific markers in spermatocytic seminoma: diagnostic and etiologic implications. Lab Invest 81:919–928.

9. Verkerk AJMH, Ariel I, Dekker MC, Schneider T, van Gurp RJLM, de Groot N, Gillis AJM, Oosterhuis JW, Hochberg AA, Looijenga LHJ (1997) Unique expression patterns of the H19 in human testicular cancers of different etiology. Oncogene 14:95–107.

10. Looijenga LHJ, Oosterhuis JW (1999) Pathogenesis of testicular germ cell tumours. J Reprod Fertil 4:90–100.

11. McIntyre A, Summersgill B, Grygalewicz B, Gillis AJM, Stoop J, van Gurp RJHLM, Dennis N, Fisher C, Huddart R, Cooper C, Clark J, Oosterhuis JW, Looijenga LHJ, Shipley J (2005) Amplification and overexpression of the KIT gene is associated with progression in the seminoma subtype of testicular germ cell tumor of adolescents and adults. Cancer Res 65:8085–8089.

12. Rosenberg C, Mostert MC, Schut TB, van de Pol M, van Echten J, de Jong B, Raap AK, Tanke H, Oosrehuis JW, Looijenga LHJ (1998) Chromosomal constitution of human spermatocytic seminomas: comparative genomic hybridization supported by conventional and interphase cytogenetics. Genes Chromosom Cancer 23:286–291.

13. Skakkebaek NE (1978) Carcinoma in situ of the testis: frequency and relationship to invasive germ cell tumours in infertile men. Histopathology 2:157–170.

14. Oosterhuis JW, Castedo SMMJ, de Long B, Cornelisse CJ, Dam A, Slewijfer DT (1989) Ploidy of primary germ cell tumors of the testis: pathogenetic and clinical relevance. Lab Invest 60:14–20.

15. Oosterhuis JW, Looijenga LH (2003) Current views on the pathogenesis of testicular germ cell tumours and perspectives for further research: highlights of the 5th Copenhagen workshop on carcinoma in situ and cancer of the testis. APMIS 111:280–289.

16. Friedman NB (1951) The comparative morphogenesis of extragenital and gonadal teratoid tumors. Cancer 4:265–276.

17. Leroy X, Augusto D, Leteurtre E, Gosselin B (2002) CD30 and CD117 (c-kit) used in combination are useful for distinguishing embryonal carcinoma from seminoma. J Histochem Cytochem 50:283–285.

18. Looijernga LHJ, Rosenberg C, van Gurp RJHLM, Geelen E, van Echten-Arends J, Dejong B, Mostert MC, Oosterhuis JW (2000) Comparative genomic hybridization of microdissected samples from different stages in the development of a seminoma and nonseminoma. J Pathol 191:187–192.

19. Faulkner SW, Leigh DA, Oosterhuis JW, Roelofs H, Looijenga LHJ, Friedlander ML (2000) Allelic loss in carcinoma in situ and testicular germ cell tumors of adolescents and adults: evidence in support of the linear progression model. Br J Cancer 83:729–736.

20. Rosenberg C, van Gurp RJHLM, Geelen H, Oosterhuis JW, Looijenga LHJ (2000) Overrepresentation of the short arm of chromosome 12 is related to invasive growth of human testicular seminomas and nonseminomas. Oncogene 19:5858–5862.

21. Summersgill B, Osin P, Lu YJ, Huddart R, Shipley J (2001) Chromosome imbalances associated with carcinoma in situ and associated testicular germ cell tumors of adolescents and adults. Br J Cancer 85:213–220.

22. El-Naggar AK, Ro JY, McLemore D, Ayala AG, Batsakis JG (1992) DNA ploidy in testicular germ cell neoplasms. Am J Surg Pathol 16:611–618.

23. Van Echten-ArendsJ, Oosterhuis JW, Looijienga LHJ, Wiersma J, te Meerman G, Schraffordt Koops H, Slejifer DTH, de Jong B (1995) No recurrent structural abnormalities in germ cell tumors of the adult testis apart from i(12p). Genes Chromosom Cancer 14:133–144.

24. Atkin NB, Baker MC (1983) i(12p): specific chromosomal marker in seminoma and malignant teratoma of the testis? Cancer Genet Cytogenet 10:199–204.

25. Suijkerbuik RF, Looijenga L, de Jong B, Oosterhuis JW, Cassiman JJ, Geurts van Kessel A (1992) Verification of isochromosome 12p and identification of other chromosome 12 aberrations in human germ cell tumors by bicolor double fluorescence in situ hybridization. Cancer Genet Cytogenet 63:8–16.

26. De Bruin TW, Slater RM, Deferrari R, van Kessel AG, Suijkerbuijk RF, Jansen G, de Jong B, Oosterhuis JW (1994) Isochromosome 12p-positive pineal germ cell tumor. Cancer Res 54:1542–1544.

27. De Jong B, Oosterhuis JW, Castedo SMMJ, Vos A, te Meerman GJ (1990) Pathogenesis of adult testicular germ cell tumors: a cytogenetic model. Cancer Genet Cytogenet 48:143–167.

28. Suijkerbuik RF, Sinke RJ, Meloni AM, Parrington JM, van Echten J, De Jong BB, Oosterhuis JW, Sandberg AA, Geurts van Kessel A (1993) Overrepresentation of chromosome 12p sequences and karyotypic

evolution in i(12p)-negative testicular germ cell tumors revealed by fluorescence in situ hybridization. Cancer Genet Cytogenet 70:85–93.

29. Rodriguez E, Houldsworth J, Reuterr VE, Meltzer P, Zang J, Trent JM, Bosl GJ, Chaganti RSK (1993) Molecular cytogenetic analysis of i(12p)-negative human male germ cell tumors. Genes Chromosom Cancer 8:230–236.

30. Rodriguez S, Jafer O, Goker H, Summersgill BM, Zafarana G, Gillis AJM, van Gurp RJHLM, Ooosterhuis JW, Lu Y-J, Huddarty R, Cooper CS, Clark J, Looijenga LHJ, Shipley JM (2003) Expression profile of genes from 12p in testicular germ cell tumors of adolescent and adults associated with i(12p) and amplification at 12p11.2-p12.1. Oncogene 22:1880–1891.

31. Suijkerbuik RF, Sinke RJ, Olde Weghuis DEM, Roque L, Forus A, Stellink F, Siepman A, van de Kaa C, Soares J, Geurts van Kessel A (1994) Amplification of chromosome subregion 12p11.2–p12.1 in a metastasis of an i(12p)-negative seminoma: relationship to tumor progression? Cancer Genet Cytogenet 78:145–152.

32. Mostert MMC, van de Poll M, Olde Weghuis D, Suijkerbuik RF, Geurts van Kessel A, van Echten J, Oosterhuis JW, Looijenga LHJ (1996) Comparative genomic hybridization of germ cell tumors of the adult testis: confirmation of karyotypic findings and identification of 12p-amplicon. Cancer Genet Cytogenet 89:46–152.

33. Korn WM, Olde Weghuis DE, Suijkerbuik RK, Schmidt U, Otto T, du Manoir S, Geurts van Kessel A, Harstrick A, Seeber S, Becher R (1996) Detection of chromosomal DNA gains and losses in testicular germ cell tumors by comparative genomic hybridization. Genes Chromosom Cancer 17:78–87.

34. Rao PH, Houldsworth J, Palanisamy N, Murty VV, Reuter VE, Motzer RJ, Bosl GJ, Chaganti RS (1998) Chromosomal amplification is associated with cisplatin resistance of human male germ cell tumors. Cancer Res 58:4260–4263.

35. Summersgill B, Goker H, Osin P, Huddart R, Horwich A, Fisher C, Shipley J (1998) Establishing germ cell origin of undifferentiated tumors by identifying gain of 12p material using comparative genomic hybridization analysis of paraffin-embedded samples. Diagn Mol Pathol 7:260–266.

36. Roelofs H, Mostert MC, Pompe K, Zafarana G, van Oorschot M, van Geurp RJ, Gillis AJ, Stoop H, Beverloo B, Oosterhuis JW, Bokemeyer C, Looijernga LH (2000) Restricted 12p amplification and RAS mutation in human germ cell tumors of the adult testis. Am J Pathol 157:1155–1166.

37. Vos AM, Oosterhuis JW, de Jong B, Buist J, Koops HS (1990) Cytogenetics of carcinoma in situ of the testis. Cancer Genet Cytogenet 46:75–81.

38. Summersgill B, Osin P, Lu YJ, Huddart R, Shipley L (2001) Chromosomal imbalances associated with carcinoma in situ and associated testicular germ cell tumors of adolescents and adults. Br J Cancer 85:213–220.

39. Olie RA, Looijenga LH, Boerrigter L, Top B, Rodenhuis S, Langeveld A (1995) N- and K-RAS mutations in primary testicular germ cell tumors: incidence and possible biological implications. Genes Chromosom Cancer 12:110–116.

40. Skotheim RI, Lothe RA (2003) The testicular germ cell tumour genome. APMIS 111:136–151.

41. Mai S, Hanley-Hyde J, Rainey GJ, Kushakl TI, Paul JT, Littlewood TD, Mischak H, Stevens LM, Henderson DW, Mushinski JF (1999) Chromosomal and extrachromosomal instability of the cyclin D2 gene is induced by Myc overexpression. Neoplasia 1:241–252.

42. Strohmeyer T, Reissmann P, Cordon-Cardo C, Hartmann M, Ackermann R, Slamon D (1991) Correlation between retinoblastoma gene expression and differentiation in human testicular tumors. Proc Natl Acad Sci U S A 88:6662–6666.

43. Poulos C, Cheng L, Zhang S, Gersell DJ, Ulbright TM (2006) Analysis of ovarian teratomas for isochromosome 12p: evidence supporting a dual histogenetic pathway for teratomatous elements. Mod Pathol 19:766–771.

Question 3

How do germ cell tumors in infants and children differ from those in postpubertal males and females?

Answer

Germ cell tumors (GCTs) in the pediatric population differ significantly from adult GCTs in several respects. First, the incidence is much lower than in adults. Second, GCTs occur more commonly at extragonadal sites during the first several years. Third, except for ovarian dysgerminoma, which develops in girls after age 8, teratoma and yolk sac tumor (YST) are the only GCTs in this age group. The sacrococcygeal region is the most common extragonadal site, and teratoma is the most common type at this location. In the testis, YST is more common than teratoma, whereas in the ovary teratoma is more common than YST and there are twice as many mature teratomas as the immature type. YST is malignant. Teratoma is benign in children. Although the presence of immature elements per se does not affect prognosis, immature teratoma of high grade is significantly associated with foci of YST and higher stages of the disease. The overall prognosis is still excellent. Intratubular germ cell neoplasia of unclassified type, the precursor of adult GCTs, is not identified in tubules adjacent to teratoma or YST in the prepubertal testis. A difference in the genetic mechanism is suggested.

Comments

Germ cell tumors (GCTs) in children (prepubertal) vastly differ from those in adults (postpubertal, to be exact). The major differences are as follows: (1) GCTs occur more commonly at extragonadal sites during the first several years; (2) teratomas and yolk sac tumors (YSTs) are the only types except for a small number of dysgerminomas in the ovary; (3) YST is malignant but teratomas of the testis and extragonadal sites, and most of the ovarian teratomas are benign,[1] in contrast to the adult testicular teratoma, which is malignant regardless of the degree of differentiation. In a recent review, Ulbright proposed a reasonable (albeit provocative) histogenetic classification to account for the biologic difference of GCTs in children and adults [1, 2] (Fig. 4-3-1): The fundamental difference in the genetic makeup produces two types of gonadal teratomas, benign and malignant. The benign tumors are derived from "benign (nontransformed)" germ cells and include the usual mature ovarian teratoma, prepubertal testicular teratoma (extragonadal site teratomas included), and testicular dermoid/epidermoid cysts. The postpubertal testicular teratoma is malignant because it originates in a malignant germ cell located in atrophic tubules, recognizable as intratubular germ cell neoplasia of unclassified type (IGCNU) through the intermediate forms such as embryonal carcinoma or YST. Additionally, some gonadal teratomas become malignant because of "post-teratomatous malignant transformation"; such tumor usually occurs in the ovary of a young girl and women and exhibits a spectrum of biologic behavior ranging from grade 1 to 3 depending on the amount of immature tissues.[1] Immature teratomatous components, such as neuro-ectodermal tissue or blastema of Wilms tumor,

---

[1] The behavior of immature teratoma of the ovary is dependent on the degree of immaturity. This commonly accepted view may not apply to the immature teratomas in the pediatric patients. A recent authentic study reports that immaturity per se does not affect prognosis, but YST which develops significantly associated with the increasing degree of immaturity of teratoma affects prognosis adversely [3].

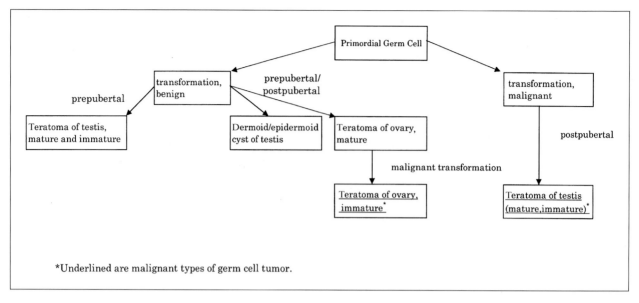

FIG. 4-3-1. Histogenesis of gonadal germ cell tumor in testis and ovary. (Adapted from Fig. 5 by Ulbright (ref. 1), with permission)

may also occur in the postpubertal testicular teratoma, but they have no established clinical significance because the adult teratoma, regardless of degree of differentiation, behaves in a malignant fashion [1].

The proposal of Ulbright seems to account for the differences in biologic behavior of teratomas by age, organ, and sex but has not addressed the genetic basis responsible for the differences. An inevitable question is what the basic genetic difference(s) between the two types of teratoma is. If the ovarian teratomas in adolescents and young women are derived from a "benign" germ cell but immature elements make the tumor more aggressive, why, then, do the immature elements in the prepubertal testicular teratoma not likewise behave aggressively? What is the genetic difference between YST and teratoma in the prepubertal age group?

Based on data reported in the world literature, the gonadal and extragonadal GCTs in prepubertal males and females can be summarized as follows.

Incidence

The incidence of the total GCTs at all sites in the prepubertal population is not available. The incidence of testicular GCTs in the prepubertal population is much lower than in postpubertal males (0.12/100 000 vs. 6.0/100 000) [4]. YST is more common than teratoma, with a reported ratio of 6:1 to 3:1 [5–7]. However, in a British registry series, more teratomas than YSTs were reported [8]. A small number of dysgerminomas occur in the ovary [8].

Tumor Sites and Type

Germ cell tumors occur more commonly at extragonadal sites [8–10]. They are, in descending order of frequency: sacrococcygeal region (42% of cases), ovary (24%), testis (9%), mediastinum (7%), central nervous system (6%), and retroperitoneum (4%) [9]. Teratoma is the most common type in the sacrococcygeal site [8, 11] and almost exclusively occurs before the age of 2 years with a fourfold predominance in girls [11], whereas in the testis the YST is far more common than teratoma [12].

Age

There is a bimodal age distribution curve for teratoma in girls: one peak at under 3 years of age and a second peak after the age of 8 years. The first peak is exclusively due to sacrococcygeal teratomas and the second to ovarian teratomas [11]. Among boys during the first 2 years of life, teratoma is more common at extragonadal sites than in the testis. After that period, the incidence remains low at any sites until after puberty [12].

Germ Cell Tumors of the Testis

Teratoma represents 14%–22% of GCTs in the testis [5, 7, 12]. YST is far more common than teratoma in the testis (59%–86%) [5, 7, 12].

Germ Cell Tumors of the Ovary

Teratomas are more common than YSTs [10], and mature teratomas are twice as common as the immature type [10]. In contrast to seminoma, which is rare to nonexistent during the prepubertal period, dysgerminoma (ovarian counterpart of seminoma) commonly accounts for about 9% of prepubertal GCTs [10] and occurs in an older age group (median age 153 months), in contrast to that of YSTs (pure) (24 months) [10].

Clinical Behavior of Yolk Sac Tumor

The yolk sac tumor is a malignant GCT. In contrast to that in postpubertal patients, it occurs mostly in a pure form. Metastases occur less frequently (9%) than in adults (61%) [7].[2] In the series of 212 patients with YSTs registered in the Prepubertal Testis Tumor Registry of the American Academy of Pediatrics, Section of Urology, 33 patients (16%) presented with metastasis [6].

Clinical Behavior of Teratoma by Site, Sex, and Age

It has been categorically accepted that childhood teratomas are benign irrespective of the sites and presence of immature elements and run a benign course provided they are excised completely. Recently, several hitherto undescribed findings were reported in a study by the Combined Pediatric Oncology Group/Children's Cancer Group [3]. Expert review of 135 immature teratoma cases revealed that 60 cases were pure immature teratomas, and 75 were mixed teratomas and YSTs but with a major component of immature teratoma. When immature teratomas were graded by their proportion of neural and blastemal components, significant correlations were detected between stage and the presence of foci of YST ($P < 0.02$) and between the presence of high-

grade teratoma and the presence of foci of YST ($P < 0.001$). The grade of immature elements per se did not affect prognosis, but the presence of YST foci did. Nevertheless, the overall 2- to 6-year survival rate was excellent (96%) and was related to the presence of YST. The adverse effects of YST components on teratomas had been pointed out earlier by Harms and Janig [10].

Congenital Teratomas

Congenital (perinatal) teratoma refers to those detected in utero and identified within 1 week of age. It is the most common perinatal tumor, comprising 37%–53% of congenital neoplasms [13]. Congenital teratomas tend to be extragonadal, and most of them are at the sacrococcygeal region. In a study of 22 fetal and neonatal tumors reported by Heerema-McKinney et al. [13], the grade of teratoma (proportion of immature elements) and foci of YST did not adversely affect the outcome. Outcome was determined predominantly by whether the tumor was completely resectable.

Intratubular Germ Cell Neoplasia of Unclassified Type and Intratubular Atypical Germ Cells in Prepubertal Testes

If the molecular mechanism of prepubertal GCTs is different from that for adult GCTs, IGCNU may not be found. Indeed, that is the case. IGCNU is extremely rare [14] to nonexistent [15, 16]. Exceptional are cryptorchid testes [17–19], male pseudohermaphroditism [20, 21], and gonadal dysgenesis [22], all of which are known to develop invasive GCTs in the later life.

The seminiferous tubules adjacent to GCTs in prepubertal children frequently contain a variable number of atypical germ cells that have abundant clear cytoplasm and enlarged nuclei. These cells may also be observed in the testes of normal boys [15]. These cells are immunohistochemically negative for placental-like alkaline phosphatase (PLAP) and are not considered by most observers to represent IGCNU [15, 23, 24]. Recently, atypical cells that were negative for PLAP but positive for p53 and proliferating cell nuclear antigen (PCNA) were described adjacent to a mature teratoma by Renedo and Trainer [25]. They equated these cells with IGCNU. Another case, described by Hu et al. [26], was a 15 month-old boy with a pure testicular YST. Located within

---

[2] The study is based on the Bonn (Germany) Registry plus their own cases totaling 799 GCT cases. Though a great majority are YST (566) and teratoma (138), a small number of other types including seminoma (37) are included. Adult male GCTs are also from the Bonn Registry.

adjacent tubules were atypical cells that were rich in glycogen, focally positive for PLAP, and triploid in DNA content. In contrast, YST cells showed modal tetraploidy. The authors concluded that these cells represented IGCNU that differed from the usual adult IGCNU in showing only minimal intratubular proliferation. The precise nature of these atypical cells and possible relation to IGCNU in adults would have become clearer if additional IGCNU markers that are now available had been used. Hawkins et al. [16] attempted to characterize the atypical clear cells with antibodies against PLAP and c-kit, another marker of IGCNU [27, 28]. In none of the 28 cases were the atypical cells found adjacent to GCTs immunoreactive to PLAP or c-kit. However, five of seven cases were positive for PCNA. Immunoreactivity to p53 was present in the two cases examined. The authors concluded that the germ cells adjacent to infantile GCT are proliferative but not neoplastic.

In summary, IGCNU as defined morphologically and immunohistochemically in adults is not identified in tubules adjacent to teratomas or YSTs in prepubertal testes. Therefore, genetic mechanisms are different from those in adults. The only exceptions are in the abnormal testes associated with cryptorchidism, male pseudohermaphroditism, and gonadal dysgenesis. The IGCNU observed in these testes is probably the precursor of adult-type GCTs.

References

1. Ulbright TM (2005) Germ cell tumors of the gonads: a selective review emphasizing problems in differential diagnosis, newly appreciated, and controversial issues. Mod Pathol 18:S61–S79.
2. Ulbright TM (2004) Gonadal terstomas. Adv Anat Pathol 11:10–23.
3. Heifetz SA, Cushing B, Giller R, Shuster JJ, Stolar CJH, Vinocur CD, Hawkins EP (1998) Immature teratomas in children: pathological considerations—a report from the Combined Pediatric Oncology Group/ Children's Cancer Group. Am J Surg Pathol 22:1115–1124.
4. Reuter VE (2005) Origins and molecular biology of testicular germ cell tumors. Mod Pathol 18:S51–S60.
5. Brosman SA (1979) Testicular tumors in prepubertal children. Urology 23:581–588.
6. Grady RW, Ross JH, Kay R (1997) Epidemiological features of testicular teratoma in a prepubertal population. J Urol 158:1191–1192.
7. Weissbach L, Altwein JE, Stiens R (1984) Germinal testicular tumors in childhood: report of observations and literature review. Eur Urol 10:73–85.
8. Marsden HB, Birch JM, Swindell R (1981) Germ cell tumours of childhood: a review of 137 cases. J Clin Pathol 34:879–883.
9. Dehner LP (1983) Gonadal and extragonadal germ cell neoplasia of childhood. Hum Pathol 14:493–511.
10. Harms D, Janig U (1986) Germ cell tumors of childhood: report of 170 cases including 59 pure and partial yolk-sac tumours. Virchows Arch Pathol Anat 409:223–239.
11. Fraumeni JF Jr, Li FP, Dalager N (1973) Teratomas in children: epidemiologic features. J Natl Cancer Inst 51:1425–1430.
12. Grady RW, Ross JH, Kay R (1995) Patterns of metastaic spread in prepubertal yolk sac tumors of the testis. J Urol 153:1259–1261.
13. Heerema-McKinney A, Harrison MR, Bratton B, Farrell J, Zaloudek C (2005) Congenital teratoma: a clinicopathologic study of 22 fetal and neonatal tumors. Am J Surg Pathol 29:29–38.
14. Stamp IM, Barlebo H, Rix M, Jacobsen GK (1993) Intratubular germ cell neoplasia in an infant testis with immature teratoma. Histopathology 23:99–100.
15. Mnanivel C, Simonton S, Wold LE, Dehner LP (1988) Absence of intratubular germ cell neoplasia in testicular yolk sac tumors in children. Arch Pathol Lab Med 112:641–645.
16. Hawkins E, Heifetz SA, Giller R, Cushing B (1997) The prepubertal testis (prenatal and postnatal): its relationship to intratubular germ cell neoplasia—a combined Pediatric Oncology Group and Children's Cancer Study Group. Hum Pathol 28:404–410.
17. Krabbe S, Skakkebaek NE, Berthelsen JG, Eyben FV, Volsted P, Mauritzen K, Eldrup J, Nielsen AH (1979) High incidence of undetected neoplasia in maldescended testes. Lancet 1:999–1000.
18. Dorman S, Trainer TD, Leeke D, Leadbetter G (1979) Incipient germ cell tumor in a cryptorchid testis. Cancer 44:1357–1362.
19. Muller J, Skakkebaek NE, Nielsen OH, Graem N (1984) Cryptorchidism and testis cancer: atypical infantile germ cells followed by carcinoma in situ and invasive carcinoma in adulthood. Cancer 54:629–634.
20. Armstrong GR, Buckley CH, Kelsey AM (1991) Germ cell expression of placental alkaline phosphatase in male pseudohermaphroditism. Histopathology 18:541–547.
21. Muller J, Skakkebaek NE (1984) Testicular carcinoma in situ in children with the androgen insensitivity (testicular feminisation) syndrome. BMJ 288:1419–1420.
22. Muller J, Skakkebaek NE, Ritzen M, Ploen L, Petersen KE (1985) Carcinoma in situ of the testis in children with 45, X/46, XY gonadal dysgenesis. J Pediatr 106:431–436.
23. Soosay GN, Bobrow L, Happerfield L, Parkinson MC (1991) Morphology and immunohistochemistry of car-

cinoma in situ adjacent to testicular germ cell tumors in adults and children: implication for histogenesis. Histopathology 19:537–544.

24. Hartwick W, Ro J, Ordonez N, Ayala A (1990) Testicular germ cell tumors under age 5: does intratubular germ cell neoplasia exist? Lab Invest 62:43A.

25. Renedo DE, Trainer TD (1994) Intratubular germ cell neoplasia (ITGCN) with p53 and PCNA expression and adjacent mature teratoma in an infant testis, an immunohistochemical and morphologic study with a review of the literature. Am J Surg Pathol 18:947–952.

26. Hu LM, Phillipson J, Barsky SH (1992) Intra tubular germ cell neoplasia in infantile yolk sac tumor: verification by tandem repeat sequence in situ hybridization. Diagn Mol Pathol 1:118–128.

27. Rajpert-de Meyts E, Skakkebaek NE (1994) Expression of c-kit protein product in carcinoma-in-situ and invasive testicular germ cell tumors. Int J Androl 17:85–92.

28. Jorgensen N, Reipert-de Meyets E, Graem N, Muller J, Giwercman A, Skakkebaek NE (1995) Expression of immunohistochemical markers for testicular carcinoma in situ by normal human fetal germ cells. Lab Invest 72:223–231.

Question 4

What is the malignant transformation (or somatic malignancy) of germ cell tumors? What is the clinical significance of this transformation?

Answer

Malignant transformation in adult germ cell tumors (GCTs) refers to the development of a new type of neoplasm of somatic cell differentiation. It can be found in the orchiectomy specimen as well as the postchemotherapy retroperitoneal lymph nodes because of its refractoriness to the cisplatin-based chemotherapy. The most frequently reported types are rhabdomyosarcoma, sarcomas not otherwise classified, primitive neuroectodermal tumor, and adenocarcinoma. Their origin from GCTs is supported by demonstrating i(12p) chromosome in the tumor cells. Clinically, occurrence of malignant transformation is suspected when there is evidence of tumor progression despite improved tumor markers. Cure or long-term survival may be expected if the tumor is removed surgically. Chemotherapy optimal against the tumor of concern should be considered for patients with advanced-stage cancer.

Comments

As was discussed under Question 1, the primordial germ cell gives rise to five basic forms of GCTs in postpubertal men; (1) seminoma, which can be equated to the neoplastic counterpart of undifferentiated early-stage embryonic cells; (2) embryonal carcinoma, which is comparable to the embryo of 10 days to 2 weeks of gestation; (3) yolk sac tumor, which resembles the developing rodent endodermal sinus structure; (4) choriocarcinoma, which is a neoplastic counterpart of the extraembryonic (placental) structures; and (5) teratoma, which represents the neoplastic counterpart of the developing fetal structure and consists of cells derived from the three germ layers (endoderm, mesoderm, ectoderm).

The organization in teratomas varies. When a teratoma is made up of well-differentiated cells arranged in a recognizable tissue or organ structure, it is referred to as a mature teratoma. For example, it consists of structures resembling intestinal mucosa and the underlining smooth muscle layer, cartilage, bone, glial cells, and/or skeletal muscle cells. Teratoma, immature type, on the other hand, consists of cells at an early stage of fetal development. For example, skeletal muscle may be at the stage of rhabdomyoblast and neural structure at the stage of primitive neuroepithelium. These immature cells still represent components of an immature teratoma coexisting with other immature or mature germ cell elements.

What is the malignant transformation in germ cell tumors?

On rare occasions, some of the mature and immature teratomatous components undergo cytologically malignant alterations and exhibit expansile or infiltrative growth. When overgrowth of somatic malignant cells occurs in the background of GCT, it is referred to as a teratoma with malignant transformation or somatic malignant transformation. Unfortunately, the term "teratoma with malignant transformation" can be misleading because it gives the impression that the underlying teratoma component is benign. Obviously, that is incorrect. All teratomas in postpubertal GCTs are malignant regardless of the degree of differentiation [1].

Malignant transformation occurs in approximately 3% of testicular tumors [2]. It also is seen at extragonadal sites including the mediastinum [3,4]. Although any teratoma components can undergo a secondary malignant alteration, the most common types involve mesenchymal cells, and the least common tumors are epithelial. The frequently reported types are rhabdomyosarcomas, sarcoma not otherwise specified (Fig. 4-4-1), primitive neuroectodermal tumor (PNET) (Figs. 4-4-2, 4-4-3), and adenocarcinoma [3–5]. Other types reported to occur at low frequency are osteosarcoma, chondrosarcoma, neuroblastoma, angiosarcoma, squamous carcinoma, lymphoma, leukemia [3, 4, 6–8], and nephroblastoma [9].

What is the genetic basis for the development of somatic type malignancy in GCTs?

Malignant transformation originates from GCTs by either malignant transformation of preexisting

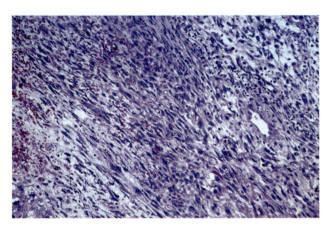

FIG. 4-4-1. Sarcoma, not otherwise specified, occurring in a testicular immature teratoma

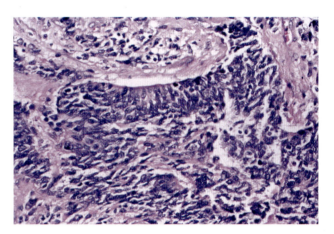

FIG. 4-4-3. Testicular immature teratoma with PNET at an advanced stage in a 26-year-old man. Shown here is an inguinal node metastasis with poorly differentiated neuroepithelioma

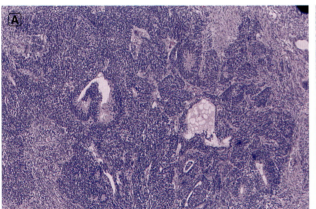
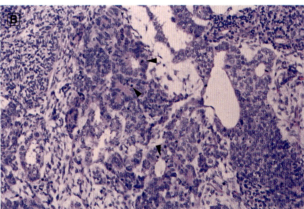

FIG. 4-4-2. Mixed germ cell tumor with immature teratoma, yolk sac tumor, and primitive neuroectodermal tumor (PNET) in a 47-year-old man. **A** Focus of PNET in the testis. Tubular structures are lined by pseudostratified epithelium surrounded by undifferentiated cells (medulloepithelioma) **B** Of 34 retroperitoneal lymph nodes tested, 1 was positive for metastasis and showed PNET. It consists of immature neuroepithelium resembling primitive neural tubes. Note the numerous cells in mitosis (*arrowheads*)

teratomatous elements or of totipotential germ cells with concomitant malignant transformation [2, 10]. Tumors' germ cell origin is supported by the almost universal coexistence of GCT elements, mainly teratoma or a yolk sac tumor [4]. The most convinc-ing evidence is the presence of i(12p) in malignant trans-formed cells including leukemia cells [11]. In Motzer's series [4], i(12p) was identified in 11 of 12 cases that included adenocarcinoma, PNET, sarcoma, and leukemia.

What is the clinical significance of somatic malignancy?

Malignant transformation may be an incidental finding in the resected specimens, including the testis and retroperitoneal lymph nodes [5], or in the tumor mass that has remained after cisplatin-based chemo-therapy [10]. Surgical resection of the residual mass is performed in patients with nonseminomatous GCTs who have attained normal serum marker levels after cisplatin-containing chemotherapy. The pres-ence of necrotic debris requires no further therapy. Enlargement of a tumor mass in the context of declin-ing or normal tumor markers represents a growing teratoma [12, 13] or a secondary somatic malignancy [4, 10]. Resected surgical specimens must be evalu-ated microscopically for the presence of somatic malignancy. In an Indiana series [10], approximately 30% of patients with disseminated GCT who received platinum-based chemotherapy had persistent radio-graphically evident disease in the retroperitoneum. Of 557 patients undergoing postchemotherapy retroperitoneal lymph node dissection, 45 (8%) had tumor tissues that were classified as somatic malignancy.

The prognosis in these patients depends on the stage when the disease is discovered. Cure or a long survival can be expected after orchiectomy and com-plete retroperitoneal lymph node dissection [4]. If the disease is already widespread, chemotherapy should be selected for the type optimal for the tumor of concern.

References

1. Leibovitch H, Foster RS, Ulbright TM, Donohue JP (1995) Adult primary pure teratoma of the testis: the Indiana experience. Cancer 75:2244–2250.
2. Ahmed T, Bosl G, Hajdu S (1985) Teratoma with malignant transformation in germ cell tumors in men. Cancer 56:860–863.
3. Manivel C, Wick MR, Abendoza P, Rosai J (1986) The occurrence of sarcomatous components in primary mediastinal germ cell tumors. Am J Surg Pathol 10:711–717.
4. Motzer RJ, Amsterdam A, Prieto V, Sheinfeld J, Murty VVVS, Mazudar M, Bosl GJ, Chaganti RSK, Reuter VE (1998) Teratoma with malignant transformation: diverse malignant histologies arising in men with germ cell tumors. J Urol 159:133–138.
5. Michael H, Hull MT, Ulbright TM, Foster RS, Miller KD (1997) Primitive neuroectodermal tumors arising in testicular germ cell neoplasms. Am J Surg Pathol 21:896–904.
6. Ahlgren AD, Simrell CR, Triche TJ, Ozols R, Bersky SH (1984) Sarcoma arising in a residual testicular tera-toma after cytoreductive chemotherapy. Cancer 54: 2015–2018.
7. Serrano-Olmo J, Tang C-K, Seidmon EJ, Ellispn NE, Elfenbein B, Ming P-M (1993) Neuroblastoma as a prominent component of a mixed germ cell tumor of testis. Cancer 72:3271–3276.
8. Fuzesi L, Rixen H, Kirschner-Hermanns R (1993) Cytogenetic findings in a metastasizing primary testicu-lar chondrosarcomma. Am J Surg Pathiol 17:738–742.
9. Emerson RE, Ulbright TM, Zhang S, Foster RS, Eble JN, Cheng L (2004) Nephroblastoma arising in a germ cell tumor of testicular origin. Am J Surg Pathol 28: 687–692.
10. Little JS Jr, Foster R, Ulbright TM, Donohue JP (1994) Unusual neoplasms detected in testis cancer patients undergoing post-chemotherapy retroperitoneal lymph-adenectomy. J Urol 152:1144–1149.
11. Ladanyi M, Samaniego F, Reuter VE, Motzer RJ, Jhanwar SC, Bosl GJ, Chaganti RS (1990) Cytogenetic and immunohistochemical evidence for the germ cell origin of a subset of acute leukemias associated with mediastinal germ cell tumors. J Natl Cancer Inst 82: 221–227.
12. Bosl G, Motzer RJ (1997) Testicular germ-cell cancer. N Engl J Med 337:242–253.
13. Logothetis CJ, Samuels ML, Tindale A (1982) The growing teratoma syndrome. Cancer 50:1629–1635.

Question 5

When a man presents with a germ cell tumor localized in the mediastinum or retroperitoneum, how can one decide whether it is a primary extragonadal tumor or a metastasis?

Answer

When the retroperitoneum or mediastinum is the initial manifestation of a germ cell tumor in an adult male, a possibility of metastasis of testicular germ cell tumors must be considered, as the retroperitoneal lymph nodes are the initial site of metastasis of testicular germ cell tumors before they spread further cranially.

During migration of the primordial germ cells from the yolk sac to the genital ridges, neoplastic transformed germ cells may remain at extragonadal sites, including the mediastinum and retroperitoneum. Thus, a primary germ cell tumor, though rare, may develop at these sites.

If a tumor is localized to the mediastinum without clinical evidence of a testicular mass and retroperitoneal lymph node involvement, it most likely represents a primary tumor. If the initial manifestation is in the retroperitoneum, it can be either a primary tumor or metastasis of a testicular tumor. If ultrasonography demonstrates a mass or a suspicious lesion in a testis, the lesional testis should be removed. If an invasive germ cell tumor is found in the testis, the retroperitoneal mass represents a metastasis. If no viable tumor tissue but a scar is found, it is reasonable to conclude that the scar represents a regressed germ cell tumor that has metastasized to the retroperitoneal lymph nodes. This conclusion is further fortified if intratubular germ cell neoplasia coexists. If intratubular germ cell neoplasia is the only finding despite exhaustive search, the retroperitoneal tumor can be either a metastasis of an unrecognized invasive testicular germ cell tumor or a primary retroperitoneal germ cell tumor.

Comments

In contrast to the prepubertal age group, primary extragonadal germ cell tumors (GCTs) are rare in adults. Nevertheless, a primary tumor may develop at the pineal gland, the anterior mediastinum, and occasionally the retroperitoneum. Autopsy studies of patients dying of testicular GCTs have disclosed several interesting findings. Among patients with an apparently pure seminoma in the testis, 32%–44% had metastases composed of nonseminomatous components; and the common sites of metastases were retroperitoneal lymph nodes (80%), lungs (73%–88%), liver (72%–73%), mediastinal lymph nodes (65%), brain (30%–31%), and bones (30%) [1, 2].

Thus, after puberty, when one presents with a GCT outside the gonads, the possibility of metastasis of a testicular GCT must be considered. Boehle et al. [3] reviewed 16 patients treated for primary extragonadal tumors whose testes were initially negative for a testicular mass by palpation. The diagnosis of GCT at the extragonadal sites was confirmed in all cases by pathology examination. Of 12 patients with a retroperitoneal GCT, a testicular primary lesion was suggested by a scar and intratubular germ cell neoplasia of unclassied type (IGCNU) in the resected testis in one patient, a scar in two cases, IGCNU in three cases, and a teratoma in one case. The remaining two had atrophy in one testis by palpation, and the other had microscopic evidence of atrophy without neoplasm. In contrast, none of the four cases presenting with a mediastinal GCT demonstrated a suspicious testicular lesion by ultrasound examination. Based on these findings, the authors concluded that the primary retroperitoneal GCT should be assumed to be of testicular origin, whereas mediastinal GCTs are extragonadal primary tumors.

A case report by Chen and Cheng [4] was that of a 30-year-old man who presented with a large retroperitoneal seminoma. A subsequent ultrasound examination revealed an inhomogeneous echo pattern in the normal-sized right testis, which on orchiectomy showed extensive IGCNU, but neither invasive tumor nor scar was found despite exhaustive microscopic examination of paraffin blocks at multiple levels. The authors concluded that the retroperitoneal tumor represents a metastasis from the IGCNU of the testis. A question arises whether the retroperitoneal mass indeed represents a metastasis. If physical examination or ultrasound study of the testes is negative, is it reasonable to treat the retroperitoneal mass as a primary tumor? Assuming that it is a primary retroperitoneal GCT, what is the risk of developing a testicular GCT in such patients?

The frequency of subsequent testicular GCT in men who presented with an extragonadal GCT was reported recently. Hartmann et al. [5] reviewed the records of 635 patients presenting with an extragonadal GCT (341 mediastinal sites, 283 retroperitoneal sites, 1 cervical lymph node, and 10 unknown sites). Of 283 patients who were considered to have a primary retroperitoneal GCT, 12 (4.2%) developed a metachronous testicular tumor at a median interval of 42 months; and of 341 patients whose mediastinal GCTs were considered to be primary, 4 (1.1%) developed a metachronous testicular GCT at a median interval of 69 months. The risk of developing metachronous testicular GCT was statistically significantly higher in patients with an extragonadal GCT than in an age group-specific control population [standardized incidence ratio (SIR) of 62], at both mediastinal (SIR = 31) and retroperitoneal (SIR = 100) tumors. A retroperitoneal GCT was associated with a cumulative risk of 14.2%, and a primary mediastinal location was associated with a risk of 6.3% (nonsignificant difference, $P = 0.18$).

Also significantly associated with a high risk of metachronous testicular cancer were those with nonseminomatous GCT (in contrast to seminoma, SIR = 75). Among the 16 patients who developed a metachronous testicular cancer, most were initially diagnosed with nonseminomatous GCT ($n = 15$). By contrast, most of the testicular GCTs were diagnosed with seminoma ($n = 11$). In this study, it is unknown how vigorously the possibility of extragonadal GCT being a metastasis of a testicular GCT was sought during the initial phase. Because the report is based on data derived from multiple cancer centers, it is assumed that the possibility of metastasis was ruled out with reasonable assurance. It is interesting that metachronous testicular GCT occurred at two time periods, the first at approximately 2.5–4.0 years and the second at approximately 6.0–7.5 years after the initial manifestation of extragonadal GCT. Thus, one wonders if at least some of the cases of metachronous testicular GCT occurring after a short interval actually represent dormant testicular GCTs that were responsible for the retroperitoneal metastasis.

The presence of IGCNU has been observed in patients with an extragonadal GCT, more commonly with retroperitoneal GCT than with mediastinal GCT [6, 7]. The simultaneous presence of IGCNU and an extragonadal GCT suggests that the latter represents a metastasis of the testicular primary, although the two may be independent events unless invasive growth is demonstrated in the testis.

Spontaneous regression of the testicular GCT and replacement with a scar is a rare but well recognized phenomenon (Fig. 4-5-1). This probability appears to parallel the tendency of an individual tumor type to undergo necrosis. Among the several types of GCT, choriocarcinoma is most likely to undergo necrosis, followed in frequency by embryonal carcinoma and mixed GCTs. Regression is uncommon with testicular seminoma and probably does not occur in teratomas [8]. Balzer and Ulbright [9] analyzed 42 cases of testicular GCTs showing varying degrees of regression, ranging from more than 50% scarring to complete scarring. Thirty patients presented with symptoms of metastasis: seven with a testicular mass, two with elevated human chorionic gonadotropin, and one with testicular pain. Gross examination of orchiectomy specimens in 37 cases identified white to tan scars 0.6–2.4 cm in size in 33 patients. The lesion was circumscribed in 16 and ill-defined or stellate in

9; a scar was not apparent in 4. Microscopically, 90% of cases showed a single nodular scar, and the rest had a multinodular pattern. In all cases, tubular atrophy was evidenced by shrunken seminiferous tubules with a hyalinized basement membrane (Fig. 4-5-1) or with Sertoli cells only. Coarse intratubular, irregularly shaped dystrophic calcifications were identified in six cases. IGCNU was detected around the scar in 22 specimens. In some cases, Leydig cells in clusters were prominent. Microlith-type calcifications were seen both within and outside the scar. The single most useful feature diagnostic of regressed GCT (apart from residual invasive tumor) was the presence of IGCNU. However, IGCNU was evident in only 48% of their cases. In the absence of IGCNU,

aside from known metastasis, coarse intratubular calcifications, numerous small vessels, and clusters of Leydig cells were said to be helpful features to support the diagnosis of a regressed testicular GCT. Nevertheless, the differential diagnosis should include testicular infarct; diffuse atrophy does not occur in such testes and more often infarcted areas are multifocal and associated with vascular lesions (thrombi, vasculitis).

Another pathologic condition one should keep in mind is the testicular tumor with an exclusively intertubular growth pattern. This unusual presentation has attracted the attention of both urologists and pathologists because of the lack of overt clinical signs of a primary testicular mass [10]. Grossly, no mass

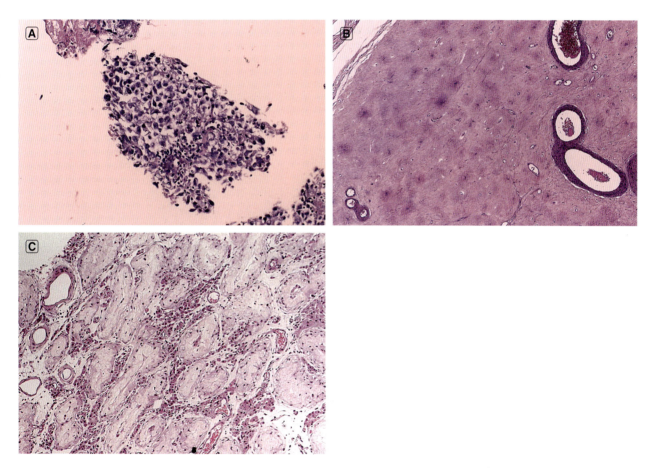

Fig. 4-5-1. A 54-year-old man presented with abdominal pain. Computed tomography (CT) scans demonstrated a midline retroperitoneal mass. Both testes are atrophic. Ultrasonographic examination demonstrated a discrete mass in the right testis. **A** A biopsy of the retroperitoneal mass was interpreted as consistent with a germ cell tumor. **B** Right orchiectomy specimen revealed a circumscribed white scar. **C** completely atrophic seminiferous tubules surrounded by clusters of Leydig cells were seen outside the scar. IGCNU was not identified. He responded to cisplatin-based chemotherapy. The residual mass that was resected revealed a nonseminomatous germ cell tumor

was presented, but an irregularly "firm area" was described in three cases and areas of discolorations in three. Microscopically, individual tumor cells were dispersed in the interstitium with lymphocytes and histiocytes. Clinically, three patients presented with infertility, two with cryptorchidism, two with metastasis, and one with testicular pain and atrophy (the presentation was unknown in the remaining four). None of the patients presented with a testicular mass. Ultrasonographic data were available in four: hypoechoic foci, a mass, calcifications and normal, in one each.

After appropriate management (resection of the retroperitoneal mass and/or chemotherapy), the patient should be followed. In a small percentage of patients, a metachronous testicular tumor may develop. If the interval between the two episodes is short (2–3 years), a testicular tumor that had remained dormant may be responsible for the retroperitoneal spread. If the interval between the initial retroperitoneal tumor and the subsequent testicular tumor is ≥4 years, the possibility that the patient has had two independent GCTs increases.

In summary, if one presents with a mediastinal GCT which is clearly isolated to the anterior mediastinum with no evidence of retroperitoneal lymph node involvement, it most likely is a primary GCT. If a patient presents with a retroperitoneal GCT, it can be either primary or metastatic. The final decision rests on the subsequent clinical course and pathology examination of the suspicious testicular lesion, if found.

References

1. Johnson DE, Appelt G, Samuels ML, Luna M (1976) Metastases from testicular carcinoma: study of 78 autopsy cases. Urology 8:234–239.
2. Bredael JJ, Vugrin D, Whitmore WF Jr (1982) Autopsy findings in 154 patients with germ cell tumors of the testis. Cancer 50:548–551.
3. Boehle A, Studer UE, Sonntag RW, Scheidegger JR (1985) Primary or secondary germ cell tumors? J Urol 135:939–943.
4. Chen KTK, Cheng AC (1989) Retroperitoneal seminoma and intratubular germ cell neoplasia. Hum Pathol 20:493–495.
5. Hartmann JT, Fossa SD, Nichols CR, Droz J-P, Horwich A, Gerl A, Beyer J, Pont J, Fizazi K, Hecker H, Kanz L, Einhorn L, Bokemeyer C (2001) Incidence of metachronous testicular cancer in patients with extragonadal germ cell tumors. J Natl Cancer Inst 93:1733–1781.
6. Heilemariam S, Engeler DS, Bannwart F, Amin MB (1997) Primary mediastinum germ cell tumor with intratubular germ cell neoplasia of the testis: further support for germ cell origin of these tumors—a case report. Cancer 79:1031–1036.
7. Daugaard G, Rorth M, von der Masse H, Skakkebaek N (1992) Management of extragonadal germ-cell tumors and the significance of bilateral testicular biopsies. Ann Oncol 3:283–289.
8. Tynski Z, MacLennan GT (2005) "Burnt-out" testicular germ cell tumors. J Urol 174:2013.
9. Balzer BL, Ulbright TM (2006) Spontaneous regression of testicular germ cell tumors: an analysis of 42 cases. Am J Surg Pathol 30:858–865.
10. Henley JD, Young RH, Wade CL, Ulbright TM (2004) Seminomas with exclusive intertubular growth: a report of 12 clinically and grossly inconspicuous tumors. Am J Surg Pathol 28:1163–1168.

Question 6

How does the late recurrence of testicular germ cell tumors occur? What are the prognostic factors to predict the late recurrence?

Answer

Germ cell tumors (GCTs) have become a model in contemporary medicine for a curable cancer with a combination of modalities such as surgery and chemotherapy. Nevertheless, 7%–16% of the patients still relapse, and most recurrences are seen within the first year. Late recurrence (recurrence after two disease-free years) is rare, seen in about 4% of patients. The risk is related to the initial stage of GCT, high levels of serum markers, presence of embryonal carcinoma in the orchiectomy specimen, and teratoma remaining in the retroperitoneal lymph nodes after chemotherapy. Teratoma is the most common type found in tissue removed at late recurrence, followed by atypical yolk sac tumors. Other types may be found at a lesser frequency. Late relapse is rarely, if ever, cured by chemotherapy alone. Thus, primary management is surgical. In about one-fourth of cases, non-GCT malignancies, including various types of sarcoma and adenocarcinoma, are found. Recurrence with teratoma alone has the best outcome, with approximately 80% of patients with no evidence of disease at follow-up.

Comments

Today, testicular germ cell tumor (GCT) is a curable disease with surgery and chemotherapy. An early-stage testicular GCT has a 95%–100% cure rate with orchiectomy followed by retroperitoneal lymph node dissection or surveillance with subsequent chemotherapy in case of relapse. Patients who remain disease-free for more than 2 years are considered to have a 99% cure rate [1]. Nevertheless, about 7%–16% of the patients relapse, and most of the recurrences are seen within the first year [2, 3].

Late recurrence (recurrence after two disease-free years) is rare. It may occur in patients with seminoma or nonseminomatous GCTs [4, 5]. The frequency has been reported at 0.6% [6, 7], 1.5% [8], 4.1% [4], 4.3% [3], and 8.0% [9]. The reported frequency varies depending on whether patients with high-stage (stage III) disease are included. In clinical stage I patients, the late relapse should be less than 1% [6].

Prognostic Factors to Predict High Risk of Late Recurrence

The clinical and pathologic features that may be associated with late recurrence are outlined in the following sections.

Initial Stage of GCT and Serum Markers

Among patients initially at clinical stage I (pathologic stages I, IIA, and IIB), none of the following variables—stage at initial presentation, primary tumor cell type including presence or absence of teratomatous elements, elevated markers [α-fetoprotein (AFP) and human chorionic gonadotropic (HGC)]—showed a statistically significant difference [10]. Reports encompassing all stages of GCTs indicate that initial stages are important for predicting a high risk of late relapse [3–5]. Data by Dieckmann et al. [5] from Germany point to more frequent relapse among patients initially with higher than stage I disease. According to Gerl et al. [3], the risk of late relapse was closely related to the levels of the GCT risk set by the Medical Research Council (MRC) of

England.[1] The risk was significantly lower in patients with good risk ($P < 0.01$).

The presenting positive serum markers were significant predictors of late relapse by Mead et al. [11] and Shahidi et al. (multivariate analysis by the latter group study: $P < 0.035$) [4].

Histologic Type of Initial Testicular GCT and Histologic Type of GCT Remaining After Initial Chemotherapy

One of the adverse factors set by the MRC is the presence of embryonal carcinoma in the resected testicular tumor [11]. Several reports stress that the presence of mature teratoma in specimens removed after chemotherapy is a risk of late recurrence [4, 5, 12, 13]. In particular, the presence of differentiated teratoma was a highly significant predictor of late recurrence ($P = 0.000$) [4]. Whether the postchemotherapy mature teratoma per se is capable of inducing either a more aggressive type of GCT or a non-germ-cell tumor is unknown. One risk is that such teratomas may coexist with non-germ-cell tumor elements [13, 14].

Initial Incomplete Dissection of Retroperitoneal Lymph Nodes

The Indiana University group emphasized that thorough clearance of lymphatic tissue in the appropriate templates of dissection remains critically important in the surgical management of GCT and that inadequate initial dissection of the retroperitoneal nodes is a significant causative factor for late recurrence [6, 7]. In their experience, the overall incidence of late relapse in patients undergoing primary retroperitoneal lymph node dissection from 1965 to 1989 was 0.6% (3/464) (Note that the period covered includes the pre-cisplatin era). All three patients had pathologic stage II disease at the initial retroperitoneal

node dissection. The site of relapse was in the chest [7]. Independently, Baniel et al. [6] at Indiana University analyzed referral cases with late relapse: 58% of patients with relapse in the retroperitoneum had received adjuvant chemotherapy after retroperitoneal lymph node dissection. Because the combination treatment should have aborted any future recurrence, the late relapse was attributed to inadequate dissection of the relevant lymphatic tissue. Data from many groups indicate that the retroperitoneal lymph nodes are the most frequent site of late recurrence [3, 5, 6, 10, 14], supporting Baniel group's contention. In the editorial comment on the Baniel article [6], Swanson of the MD Anderson Cancer Center commented, "The fact that many of the late relapses were in-field strongly suggests that inadequate retroperitoneal lymph node dissections may be responsible and that adjuvant chemotherapy following retroperitoneal dissection cannot prevent these relapses. This disease should be managed only by surgeons and oncologists with active ongoing experience" [15].

Gene Expression Profile of Early and Late Relapse

Tumors that relapse may have contained tumor tissue that was refractory to chemotherapy or may have transformed with time into a more resistant tumor. Attempts have been made to identify a group of genes in nonseminomatous GCTs in retroperitoneal metastases. A set of genes that can distinguish between early and late relapse have been identified. At this time their contribution to the late recurrence remains unknown [16]. Based on the gene expression study, we recently identified a novel GCT marker, glypican 3, which is present in components of yolk sac tumor, choriocarcinoma, and immature teratoma but not in benign testis, seminoma, or most embryonal carcinomas [17]. It appears to be a more sensitive marker for yolk sac tumor than α-fetoprotein (AFP). However, clinical utility of glypican 3 for detecting testicular GCTs or late recurrence needs to be further studied.

Pathologic Features of Tumors Resected at Late Recurrence

The most comprehensive study reported to date is, again, from the Indiana University group [14]. Specimens from 91 patients were analyzed. Altogether, 90% of the patients (for whom information was avail-

---

[1] The MRC (Medical Research Council) Study Group established the following as independently adverse features: (1) presence of liver, bone, or brain metastasis; (2) raised marker levels (AFP > 1000 kU/l or β subunit of HGC > 1000 IU/l); (3) presence of mediastinal lymph nodes >5 cm in diameter; (4) presence of ≥20 lung metastases; (5) increasing age; and (6) presence of embryonal carcinoma or fibrous tissue in the testicular tumor. The good-prognosis group has none of these features. A total of 66% of patients had none of these features. The poor-prognosis group is defined as patients who had at least one of these features [11].

able) received chemotherapy shortly after their initial diagnosis of testicular GCT. Most of the others were known to have stage I disease. Teratoma was the most common type, observed in 60% of patients. In 20 patients (22%), teratoma was the only type. Excluding teratomas that coexisted with other types of GCT, yolk sac tumor was the second most common type (47%). The yolk sac tumors had atypical histology in that the predominant types were glandular and clear cell, parietal, and pleomorphic types, often raising the differential diagnosis problems with non-germ-cell neoplasms. Other types of GCTs observed at a lesser frequency were embryonal carcinoma and, rarely, seminoma and choriocarcinoma. A striking feature is the occurrence of non-germ-cell tumors in 23% of the patients. They consisted of sarcomas (rhabdomyosarcoma, osteosarcoma, leiomyosarcoma, chondrosarcoma, undifferentiated sarcoma) and carcinoma (mostly adenocarcinoma). It is important to note that these cases are events of the status post chemotherapy. How much the histologic changes are caused by therapy and how much are caused by resistance to therapy is unknown.

Prognosis Associated with Late Recurrence

Data from Michael et al. [14] indicate that recurrence with teratoma alone had the best outcome, with 79% having no evidence of disease at last follow-up. Late recurrence with other types (yolk sac tumor, other GCTs, non-germ-cell tumors) had a much worse prognosis; less than 37% of patients were alive with no evidence of disease. The poorer response of patients of GCTs with yolk sac tumor components to cisplatin-containing chemotherapy than those without yolk sac tumor have been demonstrated in stage III patients [18]. These facts reflect the high resistance of further chemotherapy. Gerl et al. [3], however, reported that a small group of chemotherapy-pretreated patients may respond to additional chemotherapy.

How to Treat the Late Relapse

Patients who present with negative tumor markers should always undergo surgical treatment as the first mode of treatment. This especially applies to patients with reactivation of a mature teratoma. Moreover, a secondary non-GCT is an important diagnostic consideration that can be identified only by histologic examination of the resected tissue. If surgical margins are clear and tumor markers normalize postoperatively, patients probably would not benefit from adjunctive chemotherapy [3]. Late relapse is rarely, if ever, cured by chemotherapy alone. A unique trait of patients with late relapse is the almost uniformly refractory nature to chemotherapy. In Baniels' series [6], chemotherapy alone for late recurrence left only two patients continuously disease-free, and these two patients had not received cisplatin-based chemotherapy previously, indicating that late recurrence is associated with chemotherapy resistance. The primary management is surgical [6]. Gerl et al. [3], on the other hand, preferred chemotherapy after surgical resection and for patients with unresectable tumor. If tumor markers do not normalize after four cycles of chemotherapy, resection of localized disease should be reconsidered.

References

1. Einhorn LH (1990) Treatment of testicular cancer: a new and improved model. J Clin Oncol 8:1777–1781.
2. Einhorn LH (1981) Testicular cancer as a model for a curable neoplasm: the Richard and Hinda Rosenthal Foundation Award lecture. Cancer Res 41:3275–3280.
3. Gerl A, Clemm C, Schmeller N, Hentrich M, Lamerz R, Wilmanns W (1997) Late relapse of germ cell tumors after cisplatin-based chemotherapy. Ann Oncol 8:41–47.
4. Shahidi M, Norman AR, Dearnaley DP, Nicholls J, Horwich A, Huddart RA (2002) Late recurrence in 1236 men with testicular germ cell tumors. Cancer 95:520–530.
5. Dieckmann K-P, Albers P, Classen J, de Wit M, Pichlmeier U, Rick O, Mullerleile U, Kuczyk M (2005) Late relapse of testicular germ cell neoplasms: a descriptive analysis of 122 cases. J Urol 173:824–829.
6. Baniel J, Foster RS, Einhorn LH, Donohue JP (1995) Late relapse of clinical stage 1 testicular cancer. J Urol 154:1370–1372.
7. Donohue JP, Thornhill JA, Foster RS, Rowland RG, Bihrle R (1993) Primary retroperitoneal lymph node dissection in clinical stage A nonseminomatous germ cell testis cancer: review of the Indiana University experience 1965–1989. Br J Urol 71:326–335.
8. Borge N, Fossa SD, Ous S, Stenwig AE, Lien HH (1988) Late recurrence of testicular cancer. J Clin Oncol 6:1248–1253.
9. Read G, Stenning SP, Cullen MH, Parkinson MC, Horwich A, Kaye SB, Cook PA (1992) Medical Research Council prospective study of surveillance for stage I testicular teratoma. J Clin Oncol 10:1762–1768.
10. Baniel J, Foster RS, Gonin R, Messemer JE, Donohue JP, Einhorn LH (1995) Late relapse of testicular cancer. J Clin Oncol 13:1170–1176.

11. Mead GM, Stenning SP, Parkinson MC, Horwich A, Fossa SD, Wilkinson PM, Kaye SB, Newlands ES, Cook PA for the Medical Research Council Testicular Tumour Working Party (1992) The second Medical Research Council study of prognostic factors in non-seminomatous germ cell tumors: Medical Research Council Testicular Tumour Working Party. J Clin Oncol 10:85–94.

12. Tait D, Peckham MJ, Hendry WF, Goldstraw P (1984) Post-chemotherapy surgery in advanced nonsemino-matous germ-cell testicular tumours: the significance of histology with particular reference to differentiated (mature) teratoma. Br J Cancer 50:601–609.

13. Loehrer PJ, Mandelbaum I, Hui S, Clark S, Einhorn LH, Williams SD, Donohue JP (1986) Resection of thoracic and abdominal teratoma in patients after cisplatin-based chemotherapy for germ cell tumor: late results. J Thorac Cardiovasc Surg 92:676–683.

14. Michael H, Lucia J, Foster RS, Ulbright TM (2000) The pathology of late recurrence of testicular germ cell tumors. Am J Surg Pathol 24:257–273.

15. Swanson DA (1995) Editorial: low stage testis cancer is still potentially lethal. J Urol 154:1376–1377.

16. Sugimura J, Foster RS, Cummings OW, Kort EJ, Taka-hashi M, Lavery TT, Furge KA, Einhorn LH, Teh BT (2004) Gene expression profiling of early- and late-relapse nonseminomatous germ cell tumor and primitive neuroectodermal tumor of the testis. Clin Cancer Res 10:2368–2378.

17. Zynger DL, Dimov ND, Luan C, Toh BT, Yang XJ (2006) Glypican 3: a novel marker in testicular germ cell tumors. Am J Surg Pathol 30:1570–1575.

18. Logothesis CJ, Samuels ML, Trindade A, Grant C, Gomez L, Ayala A (1984) The prognostic significance of endodermal sinus tumor histology among patients treated for stage III nonseminomatous germ cell tumors of the testes. Cancer 53:122–128.

Part 5. Adrenals

Question 1

What are the pathologic criteria for distinguishing benign from malignant adrenal cortical neoplasms? What diseases should be considered for the differential diagnosis? Are there significant differences in clinical behavior between adult and pediatric adrenal cortical neoplasms?

Answer

One of the important criteria for malignancy is tumor size. Tumors weighing >100 g make up more than 90% of adrenal cortical carcinomas and only 6% of cortical adenomas. The presence of hemorrhage and/or necrosis may also be indicative of malignancy. The microscopic criteria set by the Weiss group has been commonly used. Those tumors fulfilling more than three of nine features should be regarded malignant. Among the carcinomas, those with >20 mitotic figures per 50 high power fields behave more aggressively than those with <20 mitoses.

The differential diagnosis of adrenal cortical carcinoma should include metastatic carcinomas (particularly lung carcinoma), renal cell carcinoma, hepatocellular carcinoma, and melanoma. Other tumors that may also be considered are pheochromocytoma and ganglioneuroma.

Adrenal cortical neoplasms are rare in children. Almost all pediatric patients with these tumors show evidence of hyperfunction; virilism is the predominant manifestation. The microscopic criteria set by Weiss may not apply for the pediatric tumors.

Comments

An adrenal mass is often discovered incidentally during abdominal computed tomography (CT) performed for other diagnosis. This poses an increasingly common clinical problem. The prevalence of these lesions ranges from 0.6% to 1.3% [1]. Autopsy studies have revealed incidental adrenal cortical adenomas in 1.9%–8.7% of cases [2, 3]. As scanning techniques continue to improve, adrenal masses will be discovered with increasing frequency [1]. Most of the incidentally discovered adrenal masses are clinically nonfunctional adrenal cortical adenomas [4]. In view of the high prevalence of adrenal masses coupled with the low prevalence of the hormonally active lesions, Ross and Aron [1] recommended that diagnostic efforts by biochemical screening should be directed only to those disorders of relatively high prevalence and only when clinical presentation warrants. Thus, if the patient is hypertensive, screening tests are performed for pheochromocytoma (determination of vanillylmandelic acid, metanephrine, or catecholamines) or an aldosterone-producing tumor (serum potassium concentration). Likewise, screening for an excess of glucocorticoids or androgens should be limited to patients with clinical features that suggest Cushing's syndrome or virilism. More recently, Young [5] proposed a set of clinical algorithms for diagnosing subclinical Cushing's syndrome, pheochromocytoma, primary aldosteronism, and adrenal metastasis from other sites.

The major concern for the surgical pathologist as well as the urologist is to determine if an adrenocortical tumor is benign (adenoma) or malignant (carcinoma) before and after surgery. If malignant, we must determine if it is of high grade or low grade. Although many patients with an adrenal carcinoma die of the disease within a few years, others live much longer before evidence of recurrence or metastasis appears [6].

Clinical Presentation

A bimodal peak in incidence has been reported for the development of adrenal cortical carcinoma—during the first and fifth decade of life [7]. Metastases are the initial manifestation of the disease in 15% [8] to 38% [9] of patients. The common sites are lungs, liver, peritoneum, lymph nodes, and bones [9]. Clinical evidence of cortical hyperfunction is observed in 26%–76% of patients [10]. Cushing's syndrome alone is the most common or mixed with virilization. The incidence of primary hyperaldosteronism as an isolated finding ranges from 1% to 6% [11]. The most common initial complaints are abdominal or flank pain; a palpable abdominal mass was detected in 30% of patients in one report [9]. Only 30% of patients had tumors confined to the adrenal gland on CT/ ultrasonography studies [9]. On the CT scan, an adrenocortical tumor usually is a well-defined mass with a smooth contour and is homogeneous [10]. The presence of virilization or feminization either alone or in combination with Cushing's syndrome may indicate malignancy, particularly in a large tumor weighing >100 g [8].

Gross Examination

Adrenal cortical carcinoma generally presents as a bulky mass. In one study, 70% of adrenal cortical carcinoma patients had invasion of the kidney, lymph nodes, liver, diaphragm, and/or pancreas at the initial operation [8]. Weight is an important consideration; tumors weighing >100 g comprise 93% of adrenal cortical carcinomas but only 6% of adrenocortical adenomas [12]. It is clear, however, that rarely some tumors weighing <40 g do metastasize [13, 14] (Figs. 5-1-1A, 5-1-2A, 5-1-3). Adrenal cortical adenomas generally weigh <50 g, and many weigh 10–40 g [15]. In the cut surface, the presence of hemorrhage and necrosis with or without cystic degeneration is suggestive of malignancy [10, 12]. The cut surface of the adrenal cortical adenoma is homogeneously yellow (Fig. 5-1-4) or orange-yellow (Fig. 5-1-5). Occasionally, areas of degeneration with fibrosis and cystic changes are seen, but confluent or geographic necrosis is uncommon [10].

Microscopic Examination

The features shared by malignant and benign tumors are large cells (larger than normal cortical cells) arranged in a trabecular, alveolar, or columnar pattern separated by sinusoids lined by an endothelial layer. The cells are compact with eosinophilic cytoplasm or, more commonly, microvesicular with lipids (Figs. 5-1-1B, 5-1-2B,C). Both types of cell may have hyaline globules and nuclear pseudoinclusions, features that are common in any neuroendocrine tumors. Nuclear pleomorphism or hyperchromasia in an adrenal tumor is not sufficient for a diagnosis of malignancy.

Among various microscopic criteria suggested by many investigators, the one proposed by Weiss et al. have been most widely used [6, 16]. Aside from two

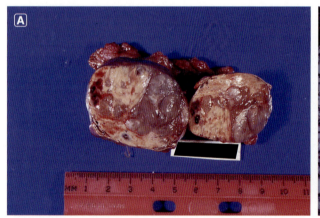
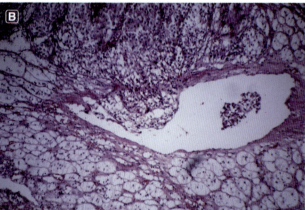

FIG. 5-1-1. Adrenocortical carcinoma with lung metastasis. The woman presented with mixed Cushing's syndrome and virilization. The tumor weighs 73 g. **A** The cut surface reveals dark-brown and yellow areas. **B** Microscopically, clear tumor cells are arranged in an alveolar pattern with invasion of venous space

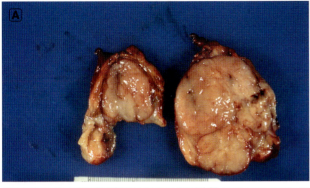

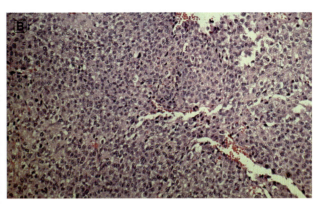

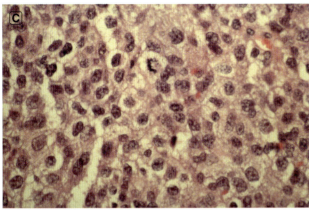

FIG. 5-1-2. **A** Adrenocortical carcinoma weighing 190 g. Note the atrophic cortex around the tumor mass. **B, C** Pale eosinophilic cells are arranged in sheets. One mitosis is demonstrated in **C**

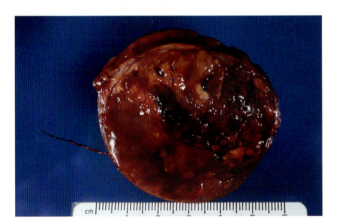

FIG. 5-1-3. Adrenocortical carcinoma with Cushing's syndrome, weighing 110 g. There are zonal areas of hemorrhage and a small focus of necrosis (*center, top*)

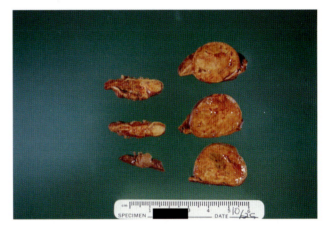

FIG. 5-1-4. Adrenocortical adenoma from a patient with Cushing's syndrome. The cut surface is homogeneous and yellow

gross features (weight and size), nine histologic features were studied.

- High-nuclear grade (grades 3 and 4 by the Fuhrman nuclear grading system used for evaluation of renal cell carcinoma) [17]
- Mitotic rate >20 per 50 high power fields (HPFs)
- Presence of atypical mitotic figures

- Clear cells occupying less than 25%
- Diffuse architecture
- Presence of microscopic necrosis
- Invasion of venous structure
- Invasion of sinusoidal architecture
- Invasion of capsule

Mitoses were evaluated by counting 10 random HPFs with the greatest number of mitoses. The authors

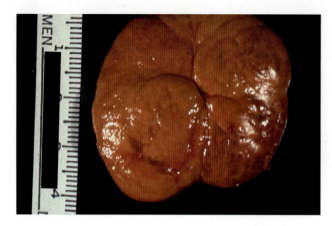

FIG. 5-1-5. Adrenocortical adenoma weighing 28 g. The cut surface bulges slightly and is uniformly orange-yellow

concluded that tumors fulfilling more than three of the nine features described above should be considered carcinoma. Furthermore, only one variable, mitotic rate of >20 mitoses/50 HPF, had a strong statistical association with patient outcome. Their 21 patients with carcinoma with >20 mitoses/50 HPF had a mean survival of 14 months, whereas the 21 patients with carcinoma with ≤20 mitoses/HPF had a mean survival of 58 months (p < 0.02).

Other parameters that have been tested for the differential diagnosis of carcinoma from adenoma are the cell proliferation index using Ki-67 or MiB-1 [18], determination of nucleolar organizer regions (AgNORs) [19], DNA ploidy analysis [20], and immunohistochemical staining for vimentin and cytokeratins. Other than the proliferation index, none of these techniques proved to be of any value. A high mean proliferative fraction (expressed as the number of MiB-1-positive nuclei/1000 cells) was 14.9 for adenoma, 31.5 for hyperplasia, and 208.1 for carcinomas [18]. None of benign lesions was positive to p53 immunostaining, whereas 9 of 20 adrenal cortical carcinomas were positive to p53 immunostaining (judged positive if >1% of nuclei were stained). The authors concluded that MiB-1 staining of more than 80 MiB-1-positive nuclei/1000 cells and positive p53 strongly suggested malignant behavior.

Differential Diagnosis of Adrenal Cortical Carcinoma from Other Malignant Tumors

To be considered for the differential diagnosis of adrenal cortical carcinoma are lung cancer, which is the most common type of metastatic carcinoma to the adrenal. Other malignant tumors to be considered are hepatocellular carcinoma, malignant melanoma, and renal cell carcinoma because these tumors share a microscopic appearance with adrenal cortical carcinoma: trabecular or alveolar arrangement of clear and eosinophilic cells bordered by vascular sinusoids. To date, there are no immunohistochemical markers specific for adrenocortical carcinoma. A number of markers have been tested, but only a few are useful, including cytokeratins, epithelial membrane antigen (EMA), and adrenal 4 binding protein (Ad4BP). Adrenocortical carcinomas are typically negative for cytokeratins [21–23] and EMA [22, 23], whereas renal cell carcinomas are positive for both markers [22–24]. Cytokeratin (AE1) is expressed by most hepatocellular carcinomas [22]. *Ad4BP* is a transcription factor that regulates the expression of enzymes involved in steroidogenesis. A comprehensive study on its expression was made by Sasano's group [25]. *Ad4BP* was expressed only by adrenal cortical carcinoma (8/8 cases) but not by any of the renal cell carcinomas (20 cases), hepatocellular carcinomas (10), malignant melanomas (8), or various other types (5 large cell carcinomas of lung, 3 pheochromocytomas, 6 ovarian and 3 uterine clear cell carcinomas). Although *Ad4BP* appears the best marker to distinguish adrenal cortical carcinoma from other malignant tumors, it may have limited value in distinguishing adenoma from carcinoma in the adrenal gland.

If hepatocellular carcinoma is clinically suspected, immunohistochemical staining for hepatocyte antigen should be used because of its extremely high sensitivity [26]. To rule in malignant melanoma, markers such as HMB45, S100, and melanin A may be used.

Pediatric Adrenal Cortical Neoplasms

There is a distinct difference between adult and childhood adrenal tumors. Adrenal cortical tumors are far less common in the pediatric than the adult population. It is three to five times as common in girls as in boys [27, 28], in contrast to the female/male ratio of 1.5:1.0 in adults [10]. Adult adrenocortical carcinomas are functional in 26%–76% of cases, and Cushing's syndrome with or without virilism is the most common manifestation [10]. In contrast, 90%–100% of pediatric cases show evidence of hyperfunction, with virilism being the predominant manifestation [27, 28]. Some of them also are associated with Cushing's syndrome. The microscopic criteria set by Weiss [16] tend to overdiagnose many cases that follow a benign course. Tumor size ($>200\,cm^3$) [27] and weight ($>500\,g$) [29] predict an unfavorable outcome.

References

1. Ross NS, Aron DC (1990) Hormonal evaluation of the patient with an incidentally discovered adrenal mass. N Engl J Med 323:1401–1405.

2. Abecasses M, McLoughlin MJ, Langer B, Kudlow JE (1985) Serendipitous adrenal masses: prevalence, significance, and management. Am J Surg 149:783–788.

3. Hedeland H, Ostberg G, Hokfelt B (1968) On the prevalence of adrenocortical adenoma in an autopsy material in relation to hypertension and diabetes. Acta Med Scand 184:211–214.

4. Mansmann G, Lau J, Balk E, Rothberg M, Miyachi Y, Bornstein SR (2004) The clinically inapparent adrenal mass: update in diagnosis and management. Endocr Rev 25:309–340.

5. Young WF Jr (2007) The incidentally discovered adrenal mass. N Engl J Med 356:601–610.

6. Weiss LM, Medeiros LJ, Vickery AL (1989) Pathologic features of prognostic significance in adrenocortical carcinoma. Am J Surg Pathol 13:202–206.

7. Wooten MD, King DK (1993) Adrenal cortical carcinoma: epidemiology and treatment with mitotane and a review of the literature. Cancer 72:3145–3155.

8. Cohn K, Gottesman L, Brennan M (1986) Adrenocortical carcinoma. Surgery 100:1170–1177.

9. Venkatesh S, Hickey RC, Sellin RV, Fernandez JF, Samaan NA (1989) Adrenal cortical carcinoma. Cancer 64:765–769.

10. Lack EE (1997) Tumors of the adrenal gland and extra-adrenal paraganglia. In: Atlas of tumor pathology 19. Armed Forces Institute of Pathology, Washington, DC.

11. Lack EE, Travis D (1995) Diagnostic problems in surgical pathology of the adrenal glands. Mod Pathol 8: 312–332.

12. Sasano H (2006) Histopathology and immunohistochemistry of adrenal cortical adenoma and carcinoma. Presented at the United States and Canadian Academy of Pathology Annual Meeting, February 2006, Atlanta.

13. LeFevre M, Gerard-Marchant R, Gubler JP, Chaussain JL, Lemerle J (1983) Adrenal cortical carcinoma in children: 42 patients treated from 1958 to 1980 at Villejuif. In: Humphrey GB, Grindey GB, Dehner LP, Acton RT, Pycher TJ (eds) Adrenal and endocrine tumors in children. Martinus Nijhoff, Boston, pp 265–276.

14. Gandour MJ, Grizzle WE (1986) A small adrenocortical carcinoma with aggressive behavior: an evaluation of criteria for malignancy. Arch Pathol Lab Med 110:1076–1079.

15. Neville AM, O'Hare MJ (1985) Histopathology of the human adrenal cortex. Clin Endocrinol Metab 14:791–820.

16. Weiss LM (1984) Comparative histologic study of 43 metastasizing and nonmetastasizing adrenal cortical tumors. Am J Surg Pathol 8:163–170.

17. Fuhrman SA, Lasky LC, Limas C (1982) Prognostic significance of morphologic parameters in renal cell carcinoma. Am J Surg Pathol 6:655–663.

18. Vargas MP, Vargas HI, Kleiner DE, Merino MJ (1997) Adrenocortical neoplasms: role of prognostic markers MiB-1, p 53, and RB. Am J Surg Pathol 21:556–562.

19. Sasano H, Saito Y, Sato I, Sasano N, Nagura H (1990) Nuclear organizer regions in human adrenocortical disorders. Mod Pathol 3:591–595.

20. Suzuki T, Sasano H, Nisikawa T, Rhame J, Wilkinson DS, Nagura H (1992) Discerning malignancy in human adrenocortical neoplasms; utility of DNA flow cytometry and immunohistochemistry. Mod Pathol 5:224–231.

21. Cote RJ, Cordon-Cardo C, Reuter VE, Rosen PP (1990) Immunopathology of adrenal and renal cortical tumors: coordinated change in antigen expression is associated with neoplastic conversion in the adrenal cortex. Am J Pathol 136:1077–1084.

22. Gaffey MJJ, Traweek ST, Mills SE, Travis WD, Lack EE, Medeiros LJ, Weiss LM (1992) Cyto-keratin expression in adrenocortical neoplasia: an immunohistochemical and biochemical study with implications for the differential diagnosis of adrenocortical, hepatocellular, and renal cell carcinoma. Hum Pathol 23:144–153.

23. Wick MR, Cherwitz DL, McGlennan RC, Dehner LP (1986) Adrenocortical cacrcinoma: an immunohistochemical comparison with renal cell carcinoma. Am J Pathol 122:343–352.

24. Medeiros LJ, Michie SA, Johnson DE, Warnke RA, Weiss LM (1988) An immunoperoxidase study of renal cell carcinomas: correlation with nuclear grade, cell type, and histologic pattern. Hum Pathol 19:980–987.

25. Sasano H, Shizawa S, Suzuki T, Takayama K, Fukuya T, Morohashi K, Nagura H (1995) Transcription factor adrenal 4 binding protein as a marker of adrenocortical malignancy. Hum Pathol 26:1154–1156.

26. Chu PG, Ishizawa S, Wu E, Weiss LM (2002) Hepatocyte antigen as a marker of hepatocellular carcinoma: an immunohistochemical comparison to carcinoembryonic antigen, CD10, and alpha-fetoprotein. Am J Surg Pathol 26:978–988.

27. Ribeiro RC, Neto RS, Schell MJ, Lacerda L, Sambaio GA, Cat I (1990) Adrenocortical carcinoma in children: a study of 40 cases. J Clin Oncol 8:67–74.

28. Mendonca BB, Lucon AM, Menezes CAV, Saldanha LB, Latronico AC, Zerbini C, Madureira G, Domenice S, Albergaria MAP, Camargo MHA, Halpern A, Liberman B, Arnhold IJP, Bloise W, Andriolo A, Nicolau W, Silva FAQ, Wroclaski E, Arap S, Wajchenberg BL (1995) Clinical, hormonal and pathological findings in a comparative study of adrenocortical neoplasms in childhood and adulthood. J Urol 154: 2004–2009.

29. Cagle PT, Hough AJ, Pysher TJ, Page DL, Johnson EH, Kirkland RT, Holcombe JH, Hawkins EP (1986) Comparison of adrenal cortical tumors in children and adults. Cancer 57:2235–2237.

Question 2

When a patient presents with a clinical picture of adrenal cortical hyperfunction, what would be the anatomic changes in the adrenal cortex?

Answer

Three major functional disorders of the adrenal glands are hypercortisolism, hyperaldosteronism, and virilization/feminization. Each type of these disorders may be due to cortical hyperplasia, cortical adenoma, or carcinoma. Cushing's syndrome (hypercortisolism), the most common, can be caused by many pathologic processes. It may be due to bilateral cortical hyperplasia (70%) stimulated by adrenocorticotropic hormone (ACTH) released from a pituitary micro- or macroadenoma (Cushing's disease). Secretion of ectopic ACTH is a less common cause of Cushing's syndrome (approximately 10%) and comes from nonpituitary tumors such as small-cell carcinomas of the lung, bronchial carcinoid tumors, and others. Adrenal cortical adenoma and carcinoma account for most ACTH-independent sources of hypercortisolism (approximately10%–20%). Primary cortical hyperplasia being responsible for Cushing's syndrome is uncommon. The adrenal causes of hyperaldosteronism are primarily aldosterone-producing cortical adenomas and, rarely, carcinoma and primary cortical hyperplasia. Adrenal cortical neoplasms with virilism or feminization can be potentially malignant. Most cortical neoplasms in children are hyperfunctional with virilism and some are also associated with Cushing's syndrome.

Comments

The three major pathologic changes that take place in the adrenal cortex are hyperplasia, either diffuse or nodular, adenoma, and carcinoma. These lesions may or may not be functional depending on whether the amount of hormones produced is sufficient to produce symptoms. Sasano's group [1, 2] stated that incidentally discovered adrenocortical lesions show immunoreactivity of all the enzymes involved in corticosteroidogenesis, indicating that they can synthesize cortisol and possibly biologically active corticosteroids but in amounts that may not be sufficient to cause symptoms [1]. Adrenal cortical carcinomas, however, are less efficient in steroidogenesis [3]. Hyperfunction of the adrenal cortex can be classified into three groups: hypercortisolism (Cushing's syndrome), hyperaldosteronism, and virilization and feminization.

Hypercortisolism (Cushing's Syndrome)

Excluding the Cushing's syndrome due to exogenous glucocorticoids, Orth [4] classified 630 cases of Cushing's syndrome into the following groups depending on the underlying mechanisms. The most common group is corticotropin-dependent Cushing's syndrome. It includes (1) Cushing's disease due to pituitary adenomas (68%); (2) ectopic corticotropin syndrome due to corticotropin release from nonpituitary tumors, most commonly small cell carcinomas of the lung but also carcinoid tumors of the lung and endocrine tumor of the pancreas (12%); and (3) ectopic corticotropin-releasing hormone syndrome (clinically indistinguishable from ectopic corticotropin syndrome) (<1%). A second group consists of corticotropin-independent Cushing's syndrome. It includes (1) adrenocortical adenoma (10%); and (2) adrenocortical carcinoma (8%), micronodular hyperplasia (1%), and macronodular hyperplasia (<1%).

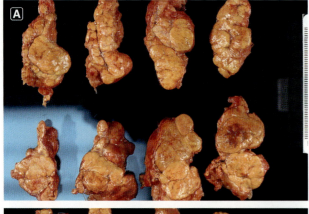

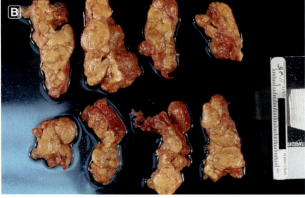

FIG. 5-2-1. **A, B** Bilateral macronodular cortical hyperplasia (MMAD). This 47-year-old woman presented with Cushing's syndrome

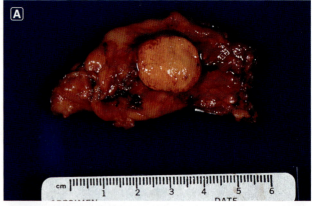

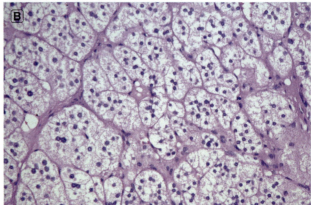

FIG. 5-2-2. **A** Cortical adenoma from a patient with hyperaldosteronism. It is a discrete yellow tumor. **B** Microscopically, it is composed of clear cells in an alveolar pattern surrounded by delicate vascular sinusoids

The third group is pseudo-Cushing's syndrome, which includes major depressive disorder (1%) and alcoholism (<1%).

Primary cortical hyperplasia is uncommon. Two types of primary bilateral adrenocortical hyperplasia have been described in association with Cushing's syndrome. The first is massive macronodular adrenocortical disease (MMAD) (Fig. 5-2-1), which affects older adults [5]. The nodules are usually >3mm in diameter. A second type, primary pigmented nodular adrenal disease (PPNAD), also known as micronodular adrenal disease [5, 6], is often associated with Carney complex 1.[1] It occurs in children and young adults <30 years of age. Macronodular hyperplasia with Cushing's syndrome may occur in patients with multiple endocrine neoplasia type 1 (MEN 1) [10].

Hyperaldosteronism (Conn's Syndrome)

The anatomic lesions capable of producing primary hyperaldosteronism are adrenocortical adenoma (Fig. 5-2-2), including "black" adenoma [11, 12], diffuse and/or micronodular adrenocortical hyperplasia, and rarely MEN 1 [13]. In a report from the Mayo Clinic, adenoma accounted for 54% of cases of hyperaldosteronism and bilateral cortical hyperplasia for 45% [14].

Virilization or Feminization

The adrenal causes of virilization or feminization are congenital adrenal hyperplasia, adrenal cortical adenoma, and carcinoma. Adrenal cortical neoplasms with virilization or feminization are uncommon in

---

[1] Carney complex 1 is a disease complex of dominant inheritance and consists of gastric leimyosarcoma, pulmonary chondroma, extraadrenal paraganglioma, cardiac myxoma, cutaneous myxoma, myxomatous fibroadenoma of the breast, Cushing's syndrome, cutaneous lentigenes, blue nevus, and large cell calcifying Sertoli cell tumor of the testis [7–9].

adults. They are potentially malignant [15]. Most cortical neoplasms in the pediatric population manifest as virilism.

In summary, there are many causes for adrenal cortical hyperfunction. In most cases, it is impossible to determine if the lesion is hormonally active and, if active, the type of hormone it may be producing based on morphologic features alone.

References

1. Sasano H, Suzuki T, Sano T, Kameya T, Sasano N, Nagura H (1991) Adrenocortical oncocytoma: a true nonfunctioning adrenocortical tumor. Am J Surg Pathol 15:949–956.
2. Suzuki T, Sasano H, Sawai T, Tsunoda K, Nisikawa T, Abe K, Yoshinaga K, Nagura H (1992) Small adrenocortical tumors without apparent clinical endocrine abnormalities: immunolocalization of steroidogenic enzymes. Pathol Res Pract 188:883–889.
3. D'Agata R, Malozowski S, Barkan A, Cassorla F, Loriaux D (1987) Steroid biosynthesis in human adrenal tumors. Horm Metab Res 19:386–388.
4. Orth DN (1995) Cushing syndrome. N Engl J Med 332:791–803.
5. Stratakis CA, Kirschner LS (1998) Clinical and genetic analysis of primary bilateral adrenal disease (micro- and macro-nodular disease) leading to Cushing syndrome. Horm Metab Res 30:456–463.
6. Travis WD, Tsokos M, Doppman JL, Nieman L, Chrousos GP, Cutler GB Jr, Loriaux DL, Norton JA (1989) Primary pigmented nodular adrenocortical disease: a light and electron microscopic study of eight cases. Am J Surg Pathol 13:921–930.
7. Carney JA, Sheps SG, Go VLW, Gordon H (1977) The triad of gastric leiomyosarcoma, functioning extra-adrenal paraganglioma and pulmonary chondroma. N Engl J Med 296:1517–1518.
8. Carney JA, Hruska LS, Baeuchamp GD, Gordon H (1986) Dominant inheritance of the complex of myxomas, spotty pigmentation, and endocrine overactivity. Mayo Clin Proc 61:165–172.
9. Manthos CL, Sutherland RS, Sims JE, Perloff JJ (1993) Carney's complex in a patient with hormone-producing Sertoli cell tumor of the testicles. J Urol 150:1511–1512.
10. Miyagawa K, Ishibashi M, Kasuga M, Kanazawa Y, Yamaji T, Takaku F (1998) Multiple endocrine neoplasia type I with Cushing's disease, primary hyperparathyroidism, and insulin-glucagonoma. Cancer 61:1232–1236.
11. Caplan RH, Virata RL (1974) Functional black adenoma of the adrenal cortex: a rare cause of primary aldosteronism. Am J Clin Pathol 62:97–103.
12. Cohen RJ, Brits R, Phillips JI, Botha JR (1991) Primary aldoseteronism due to a functional black (pigmented) adenoma of the adrenal cortex. Arch Pathol Lab Med 115:813–815.
13. Ballard HS, Frame B, Hartsock RJ (1964) Familial multiple endocrine adenoma—peptic ulcer complex. Medicine 43:481–516.
14. Young WF Jr, Hogan MJ, Klee GG, Grant CS, van Heerden JA (1990) Primary aldosteronism: diagnosis and treatment. Mayo Clin Proc 65:96–110.
15. Lack EE (1997) Tumors of the adrenal gland and extra-adrenal paraganglia. In: Atlas of Tumor Pathology 19. Armed Forces Institute of Pathology, Washington, DC.

Question 3

What is the difference between pheochromocytoma and paraganglioma? What are the familial syndromes that have pheochromocytoma as a component? What are the pathologic features of pheochromocytoma indicating malignancy?

Answer

The terms pheochromocytoma and paraganglioma are often used interchangeably because morphologically and functionally these entities are the same. Strictly speaking, however, paragangliomas that arise in the adrenal medulla are defined as pheochromocytomas, and those outside the adrenal gland are called paragangliomas. Most of pheochromocytomas and paragangliomas are functional, synthesizing and secreting catecholamines (epinephrine and norepinephrine).

Although most pheochromocytomas occur sporadically, they may develop in association with several familial syndromes including multiple endocrine neoplasia (MEN) types 2a and 2b and von Hippel-Lindau, von Recklinghausen, and Sturge-Weber diseases.

Only 10% of (adrenal) pheochromocytomas are malignant. The frequency of malignant (extraadrenal) paragangliomas is higher, ranging from 14% to 80%. The diagnosis of malignant pheochromocytoma is based on evidence of extensive local invasion or, more reliably, by the evidence of metastasis. Features suggestive of malignant behavior are greater tumor size, extensive necrosis, and extraadrenal location. The presence of nuclear atypia in pheochromocytoma or paraganglioma does not indicate malignant behavior.

Comments

The sympathoadrenal neuroendocrine system is an integrated complex composed of the paraganglia and the adrenal medulla in association with the sympathetic nervous system. Paraganglia are a collection of specialized neural crest cells, termed chromaffin cells, occurring outside the adrenal medulla, most commonly lying close to or within the capsules of the ganglia of the sympathetic trunk and of the collateral abdominal ganglia [1]. These cells, called pheochromocytes because of their brown-black color after exposure to potassium chromate (Zenker's fixative), synthesize and secrete catecholamines in response to signals from preganglionic nerve fibers in the sympathetic nervous system [2]. The adrenal medulla is the major source of catecholamines (epinephrine and norepinephrine). Epinephrine (adrenaline) is secreted into the vascular system. The extraadrenal portion of the paraganglion system is divided into four groups based on its anatomic distribution, innervation, and microscopic structure: (1) branchiomeric; (2) intravagal; (3) aorticosympathetic; and (4) visceral-autonomic [3]. Neoplasms arising from the branchiomeric and intravagal paraganglia are usually negative for chromaffin and are rarely functional [4, 5].

The most important diseases of the adrenal medulla are neoplasms. They include neoplasms of chromaffin cells (pheochromocytomas) and neuronal neoplasms (including neuroblastoma and more mature ganglioneuroma). The aorticosympathetic paraganglia are found along the aorta between the renal arteries and around the iliac bifurcation. The organs of Zuckerkandl are paraganglia that are also present in this area. The visceral-autonomic paraganglia make up a poorly defined group that occurs in association with blood vessels or visceral organs such as the bladder [4]. Tumors arising from the aorticosympathetic and visceral autonomic paraganglia are most often positive for chromaffin and functional [4, 6].

The nomenclature of neoplasms arising from the paraganglion system was confusing before the work of Glenner and Grimley [3]. Enzinger and Weiss [5] stated that "the most rational approach is that paragangliomas be named according to their anatomic sites and further modified depending on whether functional activity is documented clinically. Thus, the common nonfunctional carotid body tumor would be designated 'carotid body paraganglioma, nonfunctional.'" Following this definition, a bladder paraganglioma is called a paraganglioma, functional. Other researchers, however, emphasized the functional status. Thus, a functioning paraganglioma in the bladder is designated an extraadrenal pheochromocytoma, and a nonfunctioning tumor is called a paraganglioma. Although designation of tumors by functional status sounds reasonable, it must be realized that not all adrenal pheochromocytomas are functioning and that the functional status of extraadrenal paragangliomas is not always clear. Nevertheless, the designation extraadrenal pheochromocytoma has been used in the literature [1, 4]. From pathologists' point of view, without knowledge of their functionality, we prefer to use the term pheochromocytoma for adrenal tumors and paraganglioma for extraadrenal tumors.

Adrenal Pheochromocytoma and Its Salient Features

Pheochromocytoma arises from chromaffin cells of the adrenal medulla. The normal adrenal medulla and paraganglia consist of two types of cell: (1) chief cells that are arranged in clusters and contain neurosecretory granules that store catecholamines; and (2) sustentacular cells that surround a group of chief cells. The chief cells are immunohistochemically reactive to antibodies to neuroendocrine markers such as neuron-specific enolase (NSE) [7] and chromogranin A [1, 8], whereas sustentacular cells are readily identified immunohistochemically by antibodies to S-100 protein [6, 8, 9]. Pheochromocytomas/paragangliomas comprise also chief cells and sustentacular cells. The cell ratio varies among tumors, the significance of which is discussed shortly.

Clinically malignant pheochromocytomas are uncommon. A diagnosis of malignant pheochromocytoma is based on evidence of extensive local invasion or, more reliably, evidence of metastasis. The reported incidence of malignant pheochromocytomas ranges from 2.4% to 14.0% [10–14]. If local inva-

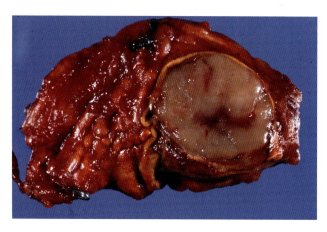

FIG. 5-3-1. Pheochromocytoma. It is a clearly demarcated mass with a typical gray to light-tan cut surface

sion is not demonstrated, what features could suggest malignant clinical course? The typical gross appearance of pheochromocytomas is shown in Figs. 5-3-1, 5-3-2, 5-3-3, and 5-3-4. Benign tumors (based on the clinical course) measure usually <5 cm in diameter and exhibit a gray to tan, slightly bulging cut surface often discolored dark brown owing to hemorrhage.

Despite a number of studies, there are no reliable pathologic criteria by which malignancy can be predicted. Based on a study of 60 adrenal pheochromocytomas, Medeiros et al. [14] found that malignant tumors tended to demonstrate greater weight (mean weight 759 g vs. 156 g for benign tumors) and extensive necrosis (100% vs. 51%), and all malignant tumors were composed of small cells. The Linnoila group [15] had 98 cases of pheochromocytoma with adequate follow-up information (64 clinically benign and 34 malignant, 75 adrenal and 21 extraadrenal[2]). Sixteen parameters were selected for study, including nonhistologic (age, sex, race, location, size, solid vs. cystic, and unicentric vs. coarsely nodular/multinodular), and histologic factors (architecture, necrosis, mitotic rate, nuclear hyperchromasia/pleomorphism, invasion, extensive local invasion and/or vascular invasion, cytoplasmic hyaline globules, cytologic features resembling ganglion cells, and proteinaceous material resembling colloid). The data were subjected to logistic regression analysis. Features found more frequently in malignant tumors were male predominance ($P = 0.002$, two-sided P value),

---

[2] The location of the remaining two cases was not stated.

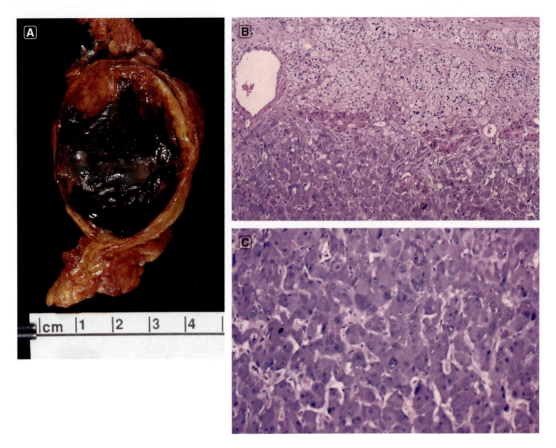

FIG. 5-3-2. **A** Pheochromocytoma. An extensive area of hemorrhage is evident in the cut surface. The normal adrenal tissue is in the lower portion of the photograph. **B, C** The tumor borders sharply without a capsule on the zona reticularis (a narrow band of eosinophilic cells). Basophilic cells with oncocytic features are arranged in a thin anastomosing trabecular pattern. The nuclear size and shape exhibit some pleomorphism

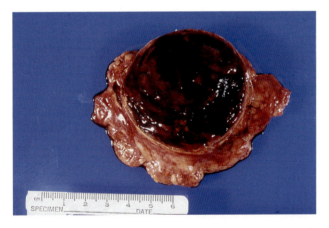

FIG. 5-3-3. Pheochromocytoma. The cut surface reveals mottled to confluent areas of hemorrhage. Note a thin rim of the cortex. The tumor is clinically benign

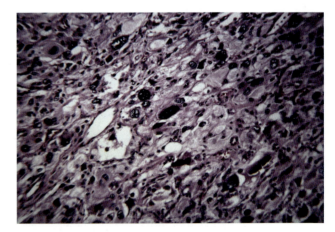

FIG. 5-3-4. Pheochromocytoma exhibiting striking cellular pleomorphism. It is clinically benign

extraadrenal location ($P < 0.0001$), greater tumor weight (mean 383 g vs. 73 g for nonmalignant tumors), confluent tumor necrosis, and the presence of vascular invasion and/or extensive local invasion. Intracytoplasmic hyaline globules were seen in 59% and 32% of benign and malignant tumors, respectively ($P = 0.001$). Of the 16 parameters, 4 (extraadrenal location, coarse nodularity of the primary tumor, confluent tumor necrosis, absence of hyaline globules) were most predictive of malignancy.

Adrenal Pheochromocytomas in Association with Familial Syndromes

Although most adrenal pheochromocytomas occur sporadically, about 10% of them arise in association with one of several familial syndromes, including (1) MEN 2a (medullary thyroid carcinomas and C-cell hyperplasia, adrenal pheochromocytomas and adrenal medullary hyperplasia, and parathyroid hyperplasia); (2) MEN 2b (medullary thyroid carcinomas and C-cell hyperplasia, pheochromocytomas and adrenal medullary hyperplasia, mucosal neuromas, angiomatosis, and Marfanoid features); (3) von Hippel-Lindau disease (renal, hepatic, pancreatic, and epididymal cysts; renal cell carcinomas; pheochromocytomas; angiomatosis; and cerebellar hemangioblastomas); (4) von Recklinghausen syndrome (neurofibromatosis, café au lait skin spots, schwannomas, meningiomas, gliomas, and pheochromocytomas; (5) Sturge-Weber (cavernous hemangiomas of the 5th cranial nerve distribution, and pheochromocytomas) [2].

About 95% of sporadic pheochromocytomas are solitary, and 5% are bilateral. In the familial setting, more than 50% of tumors are bilateral [1].

Composite Pheochromocytoma

Composite pheochromocytoma is a rare variant of pheochromocytoma that has additional components, such as neuroblastoma, ganglioneuroblastoma, or ganglioneuroma (Fig. 5-3-5), This phenomenon was observed in 3% of the sympathoadrenal paragangliomas, and all four cases arose in the adrenal glands as a unilateral solitary mass [15].

Primitive neuroectodermal cells are postulated to give rise to two types of cell: pheochromoblasts and neuroblasts [1]. The former, as they mature, become medullary cells in the adrenal gland, and the latter are the source of ganglion cells and schwann cells. It is not surprising, then, if neoplasms of bidirectional differentiation and maturation at varying stages develop. In the Linnoila series, one of the four cases was clinically malignant.

Extraadrenal Paragangliomas

Five to ten percent of sporadic paragangliomas/pheochromocytomas are extraadrenal [16], and most of them are located intraabdominally. The largest group is superior paraaortic in location and includes those located adjacent to the adrenal glands. The second group consists of those located along the inferior paraaortic region. Most tumors at this location arise from the remnant of the organs of

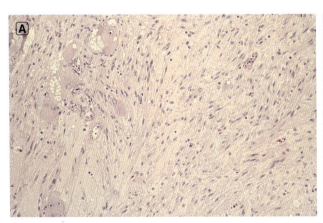 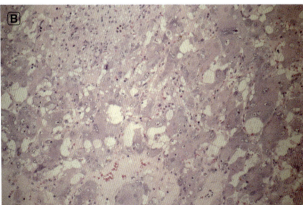

Fig. 5-3-5. Composite pheochromocytoma and ganglioneuroma of the adrenal gland. **A** In the ganglioneuromatous portion, clearly identifiable ganglion cells are within the schwannian cell stroma. **B** In this field, basophilic pheochromocytoma cells resemble neuronal or ganglion cells and are arranged in an anastomosing pattern. A small nest of schwannian cells is present

Zuckerkandel. The third group is those occurring in the urinary bladder [17]. Symptoms and signs indicative of excess catecholamine secretion have been reported in 25%–86% [16, 18, 19].

In comparison to (adrenal) pheochromocytomas, more aggressive behavior of (extraadrenal) paragangliomas has been well documented. The reported frequency of malignant tumors ranges from 14% to 50% [10, 12, 13, 16, 18–20] compared to 10% malignant (adrenal) pheochromocytomas. In Linnoila's series cited above [15], 17 of the 21 (80%) extraadrenal paragangliomas were clinically malignant. Some investigators have reported that the absence of sustentacular cells in adrenal pheochromocytomas [9] and extraadrenal paragangliomas [6] indicates a malignant clinical outcome.

References

1. Lack EE (1997) Tumors of the adrenal gland and extraadrenal paraganglia. In: Atlas of tumor pathology 19. Armed Forces Institute of Pathology, Washington, DC.
2. Kumar V, Abbas AH, Fausto N (2005) Robbin's pathologic basis of disease. Elsevier Saunders, Philadelphia, pp 1218–1219.
3. Glenner GG, Grimley PM (1974) Tumors of the extra-adrenal paraganglion system (including chemoreceptors). In: Atlas of tumor pathology. fascicle 9. Armed Forces Institute of Pathology, Washington DC, p 1.
4. Whalen RK, Althausen AF, Daniels GH (1992) Extraadrenal pheochromocytoma. J Urol 147:1–10.
5. Enzinger FM, Weiss SW (1995) Soft tissue tumors. Mosby, St. Louis, pp 965–990.
6. Kliewer KE, Cochran AJ (1989) A review of the histology, ultrastructure, immunohistology, and molecular biology of extra adrenal paragangliomas. Arch Pathol Lab Med 113:1209–1218.
7. Lloyd RV, Shapiro B, Sisson JC, Kalff V, Thompson NW, Beierwaltes WA (1984) An immunohistochemical study of pheochromocytomas. Arch Pathol Lab Med 108:541–544.
8. Lloyd RV, Blaivas M, Wilson BS (1985) Distribution of chromogranin and S100 protein in normal and abnormal adrenal medullary tissues. Arch Pathol Lab Med 109:33–35.
9. Unger P, Hoffman K, Pertsemlidis D, Thung S, Wolfe D, Kaneko M (1991) S100 protein-positive sustentacular cells in malignant and locally aggressive adrenal pheochromocytomas. Arch Pathol Lab Med 115:484–487.
10. Melicow MM (1977) One hundred cases of pheochromocytoma (107 tumors) at the Columbia-Presbyterian Medical Center, 1926-1976: a clinicopathological analysis. Cancer 40:1987–2004.
11. Modlin IM, Farndon JR, Shepherd A, Johnston ID, Kennedy TL, Montgomery DA, Welbourn RB (1979) Pheochromocytomas in 72 patients: clinical and diagnostic features, treatment and long term results. Br J Surg 66:456–465.
12. ReMine WH, Chong GC, van Heerden JA, Sheps SG, Harrison EG Jr (1974) Current management of pheochromocytoma. Ann Surg 179:740–747.
13. van Heerden JA, Sheps SG, Hamberger B, Sheedy PF II, Poston JG, ReMine WH (1982) Pheochromocytoma: current status and changing trends. Surgery 91:367–373.
14. Medeiros LJ, Wolf BC, Balogh K, Federman M (1985) Adrenal pheochromocytoma: a clinicopathologic review of 60 cases. Hum Pathol 16:580–589.
15. Linnoila RI, Keiser HR, Stenberg SM, Lack EE (1990) Histology of benign versus malignant sympathoadrenal paragangliomas: clinicopathologic study of 120 cases including unusual histologic features. Hum Pathol 21:1168–1180.
16. Lack EE, Cubilla AL, Woodruff JM, Lieberman PH (1980) Extra-adrenal paragangliomas of the retroperitoneum: a clinicopathologic study of 12 tumors. Am J Surg Pathol 4:109–120.
17. Fries JG, Chamberlin JA (1968) Extra-adrenal pheochromocytoma: literature review and report of a cervical pheochromocytoma. Surgery 63:268–279.
18. Hayes WS, Davidson AJ, Grimley PM, Hartman DS (1990) Extraadrenal retroperitoneal paraganglioma: clinical, pathologic and CT findings. AJR Am J Roentgenol 155:1247–1250.
19. Sclafani LM, Woodruff JM, Brennan MF (1990) Extra-adrenal retroperitoneal paragangliomas: natural history and response to treatment. Surgery 108:1124–1130.
20. Scott HW Jr, Halter A (1985) Oncologic aspect of pheochromocytoma: the importance of follow-up. Surgery 96:1061–1066.

Subject Index